Three
eek loan

Please return on or before the last date below

Metallothionein in Biology and Medicine

Metallothionein
in
Biology and Medicine

Edited by

Curtis D. Klaassen, Ph.D.

Department of Pharmacology, Toxicology, and Therapeutics
University of Kansas Medical Center
Kansas City, Kansas

and

Kazuo T. Suzuki, Ph.D.

National Institute for Environmental Studies
Onogawa, Tsukuba, Japan

CRC Press
Boca Raton   Ann Arbor   Boston   London

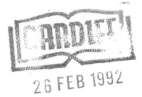
Library of Congress Cataloging-in-Publication Data

Metallothionein in biology and medicine / editors, Curtis D. Klaassen
and Kazuo T. Suzuki.
    p.   cm.
    Includes bibliographical references and index.
    ISBN 0-8493-8832-5
    1. Metallothionein—Physiological effect. 2. Metallothionein—
Analysis. 3. Metallothionein—Therapeutic use. I. Klaassen,
Curtis D. II. Suzuki, Kazuo T.
    [DNLM: 1. Metallothionein.   QU 55 M5895]
QP552.M47M48   1991
591.19'245—dc20
DNLM/DLC
for Library of Congress   91-18711
                                                CIP

Developed by Telford Press

PREFACE

Metallothionein was first isolated as a specific cadmium-binding protein and has been considered by heavy metal toxicologists, to play an important role in protecting the living body from hazardous heavy metals such as cadmium and mercury. Metallothionein has been more recently utilized as a model for protein and coordination chemistry as well as a useful tool for the study of regulation mechanisms of gene expression. The promotor region of the metallothionein gene has often been used in gene technology as an easily controllable promoter of transgenic mice. In addition, metallothionein has also been shown to protect the body from the harmful action of chemicals other than heavy metals, as well as from endogenously generated hazardous substances, such as active oxygen. The side effects of some anticancer drugs and radiation damage, probably due to free radicals formed, have been shown to be prevented by inducing metallothionein synthesis in the target organs. On December 10–14, 1989, a meeting was held in Honolulu, Hawaii, on "Metallothionein in Biology and Medicine". This book brings to the reader the proceeding of that meeting.

CONTRIBUTORS

Masakazu Adachi
Japan Immunoresearch
Laboratories, Co., Ltd.
Gunma, Japan

M. Akkerman
University of Maryland
Program in Toxicology
Baltimore, Maryland

Glen K. Andrews, Ph.D.
Biochemistry and Molecular
Biology
University of Kansas Medical
Center
Kansas City, Kansas

Yasunobu Aoki, Ph.D.
National Institute for
Environmental Studies
Ibaraki, Japan

Toshihiko Ariyoshi
School of Pharmaceutical Sciences
Nagasaki University
Nagasaki, Japan

Koji Arizono, Ph.D.
School of Pharmaceutical Sciences
Nagasaki University
Nagasaki, Japan

Rüdiger Bartsch
Gesellschaft für Strahlen-und
Umweltforschung mbH
München
Neuherberg, Germany

Mrinal R. Bhave, Ph.D.
Frederick Cancer Research and
Development Center
National Cancer Institute
Frederick, Maryland

Ian Bremner, D.Sc.
Deputy Director
The Rowett Research Institute
Aberdeen, Scotland

George M. Cherian, Ph.D.
The University of Western Ontario
Department of Pathology
London, Ontario, Canada

Mark Chernaik, Ph.D.
Biochemistry Department
Johns Hopkins University
School of Hygiene and Public
Health
Baltimore, Maryland

Mary Cismowski, Ph.D.
Biochemistry Department
Johns Hopkins University
School of Hygiene and Public
Health
Baltimore, Maryland

Chris Cody, Ph.D.
Biochemistry Department
Johns Hopkins University
School of Hygiene and Public
Health
Baltimore, Maryland

Valeria Culotta, Ph.D.
Laboratory of Chemistry
National Cancer Institute
National Institutes of Health
Bethesda, Maryland

Rodney R. Dietert
Cornell University
Ithaca, New York

Michael Dunn, Ph.D.
Food Science and Human
Nutrition
University of Hawaii
Honolulu, Hawaii

Lawrence P. Fernando, Ph.D.
Biochemistry and Molecular
  Biology
University of Kansas Medical
  Center
Kansas City, Kansas

Ernest Foulkes, Ph.D.
College of Medicine
University of Cincinnati
Cincinnati, Ohio

Bruce A. Fowler, Ph.D.
The University of Maryland
Baltimore, Maryland

Peter Fürst, Ph.D.
Laboratory of Chemistry
National Cancer Institute
National Institutes of Health
Bethesda, Maryland

R.E. Gandley
University of Maryland
Program in Toxicology
Baltimore, Maryland

Justine S. Garvey, Ph.D.
Visiting Research Associate
Department of Biology
California Institute of Technology
Pasadena, California

Abdul Ghaffar
National Institute for
  Environmental Studies
Ibaraki, Japan

Rebecca Hackett, Ph.D.
Laboratory of Chemistry
National Cancer Institute
National Institutes of Health
Bethesda, Maryland

Dean Hamer, Ph.D.
Cell Regulation Section
National Cancer Institute
Bethesda, Maryland

Hiroki Hashiba
Institute of Medical Science
University of Tokyo
Tokyo, Japan

Tsao Hsu, Ph.D.
Laboratory of Chemistry
National Cancer Institute
National Institutes of Health
Bethesda, Maryland

Stella Hu
Laboratory of Chemistry
National Cancer Institute
National Institutes of Health
Bethesda, Maryland

P.C. Huang, Ph.D.
Biochemistry Department
Johns Hopkins University
School of Hygiene and Public
  Health
Baltimore, Maryland

Takehiro Igawa
Otsuka Pharamceutical Co., Ltd.
Tokushima, Japan

Takumi Imai
Faculty of Pharmaceutical
  Sciences
Osaka University
Osaka, Japan

Nobumasa Imura, Ph.D.
School of Pharmaceutical Sciences
Kitasato University
Tokyo, Japan

Mesayosmi Inagawa, Ph.D.
School of Medicine
University of Tokyo
Tokyo, Japan

Carla Inouye, B.S.
Department of Pharmacology
University of California, San
Diego
La Jolla, California

Jeremias H.R. Kägi, M.D.
Biochemisches Institut der
Universität Zürich
Zürich, Switzerland

Ravi Kambadur, Ph.D.
Laboratory of Chemistry
National Cancer Institute
National Institutes of Health
Bethesda, Maryland

Mika Karasawa, Ph.D.
Institute of Medical Science
University of Tokyo
Tokyo, Japan

Michael Karin, Ph.D.
Department of Pharmacology
College of Medicine
University of California
La Jolla, California

Sanae Kawahara
National Institute for
Environmental Studies
Ibaraki, Japan

Umeko Kawaharada
College of Medical Care and
Technology
Gunma University
Maehashi, Gunma, Japan

William C. Kershaw, Ph.D.
Department of Pharmacology
University of Kansas Medical
Center
Kansas City, Kansas

Masami Kimura, Ph.D.
Central Institute for Experimental
Animals
Kawasaki, Japan

Curtis D. Klaassen, Ph.D.
Department of Pharmacology
University of Kansas Medical
Center
Kansas City, Kansas

Dominik Klein
Gesellschaft für Strahlen-und
Umweltforschung mbH
München
Neuherberg, Germany

Etsuko Kobayashi
National Institute for
Environmental Studies
Ibaraki, Japan

Shizuko Kobayashi, Ph.D.
Kyoritsu College of Pharmacy
Tokyo, Japan

Toshiaki Koizumi, Ph.D.
Frederick Cancer Research and
Development Center
National Cancer Institute
Frederick, Maryland

Yutaka Kojima
Department of Environmental
Medicine
Graduate School of Environmental
Science
Hokkaido University
Kita-ku, Sapporo, Japan

Toshio Kuroki
Institute of Medical Science
University of Tokyo
Tokyo, Japan

Lois D. Lehman-McKeeman, Ph.D.
Department of Pharmacology
University of Kansas Medical Center
Kansas City, Kansas

L.Y. Lin, Ph.D.
Department of Biochemistry
The Johns Hopkins University
School of Hygiene and Public Health
Baltimore, Maryland

M.M. Lipsky
Department of Pathology
University of Maryland
Medical School
Baltimore, Maryland

Tamio Maitani, Ph.D.
National Institute of Hygienic Sciences
Tokyo, Japan

R.K. Mehra, Ph.D.
Division of Hematology-Oncology
University of Utah Medical Center
Salt Lake City, Utah

Charles C. McCormick, Ph.D.
Department of Poultry and Avian Sciences
The Division of Nutritional Sciences
Cornell University
Ithaca, New York

Tsutomu Mimura
Faculty of Pharmaceutical Sciences
Osaka University
Osaka, Japan

Minehiro Moriyama
Daiichi College of Pharmaceutical Sciences
Fukuoka, Japan

Akira Naganuma, Ph.D.
School of Pharmaceutical Sciences
Kitasato University
Tokyo, Japan

Katsuyuki Nakajima, Ph.D.
Japan Immunoresearch Laboratories, Co., Ltd.
Gunma, Japan

Tadashi Niioka
Department of Environmental Medicine
Graduate School of Environmental Science
Hokkaido University
Kita-ku, Sapporo, Japan

Hisao Nishimura
Aichi Medical University
Aichi, Japan

Noriko Nishimura
Aichi Medical University
Aichi, Japan

Nancy A. Noble
Department of Medicine
University of Utah
School of Medicine
Salt Lake City, Utah

Satomi Onosaka
Faculty of Nutrition
Kobe-Gakuin University
Ikawadani-cho, Nishi-ku, Kobe
Hyogo, Japan

Noriko Otaki
National Institute of Industrial Health
Kanagawa, Japan

Alan Perantoni, Ph.D.
Frederick Cancer Research and Development Center
National Cancer Institute
Frederick, Maryland

Michael H. Rayner, Ph.D.
National Institute for
Environmental Studies
Ibaraki, Japan

In-Koo Rhee, Ph.D.
Department of Biochemistry
The Johns Hopkins University
School of Hygiene and Public
Health
Baltimore, Maryland

Aileen Robertson
Department of Nutrition and
Dietetics
Raigmore Hospital
Inverness, Scotland

Yukio Saito
National Institute of Hygienic
Sciences
Tokyo, Japan

Masao Sato, Ph.D.
Division of Environmental
Pollution Research
Research Laboratory
Fukushima Medical College
Fukushima, Japan

Masahiko Satoh
School of Pharmaceutical Sciences
Kitasato University
Tokyo, Japan

Zahir A. Shaikh, Ph.D.
Department of Pharmacology and
Toxicology
University of Rhode Island
Kingston, Rhode Island

Petra Skroch, Ph.D.
Department of Pharmacology
University of California, San
Diego
La Jolla, California

M. Smith
Department of Pathology
University of Maryland
Medical School
Baltimore, Maryland

C. Sugawara, Ph.D.
Department of Public Health
Sapporo Medical College
Chuo-ku, Sapporo, Japan

Naoki Sugawara, Ph.D.
Department of Public Health
Sapporo Medical College
Chuo-ku, Sapporo, Japan

Karl H. Summer, Ph.D.
Gesellschaft für Strahlen-und
Umweltforschung mbH
München
Neuherberg, Germany

Hiroyuki Sunaga
National Institute for
Environmental Studies
Ibaraki, Japan

Junko S. Suzuki
Kyoritsu College of Pharmacy
Tokyo, Japan

Kazuo T. Suzuki
National Institute for
Environmental Studies
Ibaraki, Japan

Keiji Suzuki
College of Medical Care and
Technology
Gunma University
Maehashi, Gunma, Japan

Akiko Tanahe
School of Pharmaceutical Sciences
Nagasaki University
Nagasaki, Japan

Keiichi Tanaka
Faculty of Nutrition
Kobe-Gakuin University
Ikawadani-cho, Nishi-ku, Kobe
Hyogo, Japan

Takeshi Tani
Otsuka Pharamceutical Co., Ltd.
Tokushima, Japan

Chiharu Tohyama, Ph.D.
National Institute for
  Environmental Studies
Ibaraki, Japan

Kazutake Tsujikawa, Ph.D.
Faculty of Pharmaceutical
  Sciences
Osaka University
Osaka, Japan

Milan Vašák
Biochemisches Institut der
  Universität Zürich
Zürich, Switzerland

Michael P. Waalkes, Ph.D.
Frederick Cancer Research and
  Development Center
National Cancer Institute
Frederick, Maryland

Zakaria Z. Wahba, Ph.D.
Frederick Cancer Research and
  Development Center
National Cancer Institute
Frederick, Maryland

Michael Webb, D.Sc.
10 Lagham Park
South Godstone
Surrey, England

D.R. Winge, Ph.D.
Division of Hematology-Oncology
University of Utah Medical Center
Salt Lake City, Utah

Anne M. Wood
Deputy Director
The Rowett Research Institute
Aberdeen, Scotland

Kunitoshi Yoshihira
National Institute of Hygienic
  Sciences
Tokyo, Japan

TABLE OF CONTENTS

Cd-Hem Method and Its Application

Satomi Onosaka and Keiichi Tanaka
Faculty of Nutrition
Kobe-Gakuin University
Ikawadani-cho, Nishi-ku, Kobe
Hyogo, Japan

SUMMARY

The concentration of metallothionein (MT) in tissues was determined by the Cd-hem method and biological roles of MT were examined. The MT concentration in mouse liver increased after a preinjection of a number of compounds: organic solvents, fatty acids, hepatotoxins and oriental medicines. The preventive effect of MT against acute Cd toxicity was observed if the MT concentration in the liver was raised to over 100 μg/g by a preinjection of the compounds. A simultaneous injection of nitrosodimethylamine (NDMA) inhibited MT induction and Zn uptake but did not affect Cd uptake by the liver. The concentration of MT was high in human liver, but was decreased in patients with hepatic diseases, especially cancer. These results indicate that increasing the MT concentration is a useful tool in clarifying the biological roles of MT.

INTRODUCTION

Metallothionein (MT) is a low molecular metal-binding protein (Kägi and Vallee, 1960, 1961). Metals such as Zn, Cu, Cd and Hg are bound to cysteine residues of thionein to form MT. The biosynthesis of MT is induced by many compounds, particularly metals (Piscator, 1964; Webb, 1972; Piotrowski et al., 1974) and hormones (Etzel et al., 1979). Besides these, the concentration of MT is also increased by physiological stresses (Oh et al., 1978) and physical stimuli (Shiraishi et al., 1986).

Biological roles of MT include decreasing effects of acute heavy metal toxicity (Suzuki and Yoshikawa, 1974) and involvement in metabolism of Zn and Cu (Richard and Cousins, 1975). MT is also reported to protect against X-irradiation (Matsubara, 1985) and depress a side-effect of an anti-cancer drug (Naganuma et al., 1987).

In this study, the Cd-hem method for MT determination is presented. The MT concentration in tissues determined by the Cd-hem method is shown after various kinds of treatments. The biological roles of MT are clarified by application of the Cd-hem method. The MT concentration in human tissues are presented.

Cd-hem METHOD

Affinity of MT for Cd is extremely high, and Cd-MT is heat stable (Kägi and Vallee, 1960, 1961). To develop the Cd-hem method, these properties were utilized. An outline of the Cd-hem method is shown in Figure 1. Tissue supernatant was added with a Cd solution to saturate all the metal-binding sites of MT by substituting MT-bound Zn with Cd. Thereafter, hemolysate was added to bind excess Cd and was subsequently removed by heat treatment. After repeating the heat-treatment process three times, most of the Cd still present in supernatant was bound to MT. In previous studies, the molar ratio of MT to MT-bound metal was assumed to be 1:6 (Onosaka and Cherian, 1981). The MT concentration in the tissues is calculated here assuming the 1:7 ratio (Diete et al., 1986; Furey et al., 1986). Metal concentrations in the tissues were determined after ashing when necessary.

Several methods were reported for MT determination. Each method has its own advantages. For example, HPLC-AAS has the ability to analyze metal composition of MT (Suzuki, 1980). Radioimmunoassay can be used for urine or blood (Chang et al., 1980; Tohyama and Shaikh, 1981). Because of the lower affinity of MT for Cd than for Hg or Cu, Hg- or Cu-MT can not be determined by the Cd-hem method. But, this method is useful to determine the MT concentration in tissues after MT induction, because most of metal-binding sites of induced MT are occupied by Zn (Winge et al., 1975).

In the following experiments, male mice, ddY strain, 32 to 39 g, were used. The mice were usually injected s.c. with compounds, and the MT concentration was determined 24 h after the last injection.

METHOD

```
Tissue
   | 0.25 M sucrose(x5 vol.)
   | homogenize
Homogenate
```

```
12000 rpm, 20min.
Supernatant(0.5ml)                        Homogenate(0.5 ml)

   30 mM Tris—HCl      1.9 ml            HNO₃—HClO₄
   Cd(10 ppm)          1.0 ml

   hemolysate  0.2 ml ⎤
   100°C, 1 min.       ⎬ 3 times
   3000 rpm, 5 min.   ⎦                  3000 rpm, 5 min.

Supernatant                              Supernatant
        ──► AAS(Cd)                             ──► AAS(Zn,Cd,Cu)
            ⇓                                        ⇓
       Metallothionein                          Metals
```

Figure 1. An outline of the Cd-hem method.

EFFECTS OF STRESSES ON MT CONCENTRATION

Effects of stresses were examined because mice were injected with compounds at sub-lethal doses in many cases (Table I).

Several effects of starvation on MT levels were observed. In the first place, the MT concentration in the liver was increased (Bremner et al., 1973). Secondly, its concentration remained below 100 µg/g. Thirdly, the MT concentration also increased in the pancreas. And fourth, the increase of MT by starvation had no effect on acute Cd toxicity (Figure 2).

The MT concentration in the liver also increased by cutting the abdomen (Brady, 1981) but no increase was observed in the pancreas.

TABLE I.
Effect of Stresses on Metallothionein Concentration in Mouse Tissues

Stress	Metallothionein (mg/kg tissue)		
	Liver	Kidney	Pancreas
None	12 ± 4	10 ± 3	219 ± 97
Starvation	88 ± 27^a	15 ± 3	518 ± 82^a
Sham operation	116 ± 35^a		186 ± 9

$^a p < 0.01$.

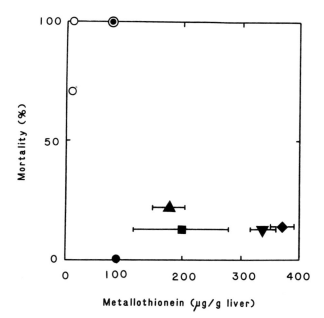

Figure 2. Relationship between metallothionein concentration in the mouse liver and the mortality. Mice (10 to 12) were injected with either olive oil (10 ml/kg, i.p.), phytine (500 mg/kg, i.p.), heptane (5 ml/kg, s.c.), thiopronine (1000 mg/kg, s.c.) or shosaikoto (1000 mg/kg, s.c.), or starved for 24 h. The MT concentration in the liver of three mice of each group was determined 24 h after the injections or starvation. The other mice were injected with Cd (10 mg/kg, s.c.) 24 h after the injections or starvation, and the mortality of each group was determined 3 d after the Cd injection. Mice of the control groups were injected s.c. with Cd alone. The concentration of MT indicates mean ± s.d. of three mice. (○) control; (●) olive oil; (▼) phytine; (◆) heptane; (■) thiopronine; (▲) shosaikoto; (◎) starvation.

TABLE II.
Effect of Hepatotoxins on Metallothionein Concentration in Mouse Liver

Hepatotoxin	Metallothionein (mg/kg liver)
None	17 ± 5
o-Acetaminophenol	88 ± 28[a]
Acetaminophen	160 ± 18[b]
Bromobenzene	130 ± 47[a]
Carbon tetrachloride	298 ± 31[b]
Galactosamine	15 ± 2
6-Mercaptopurine	414 ± 77[b]
Naphthylisocyanate	194 ± 116
Naphthylisothiocyanate	113 ± 56[a]

[a] $p < 0.05$.
[b] $p < 0.01$.

EFFECTS OF COMPOUNDS ON MT CONCENTRATION

There are a number of reports on MT induction. However, the tissue's response is specific to the injected compound (Onosaka and Cherian, 1981, 1982). Therefore, effects of compounds on the MT concentration were examined in the liver, kidney and pancreas separately.

Besides metals (Piscator, 1964; Webb, 1972; Piotrowski et al., 1974), organic solvents increased the MT concentration in the liver (Waalkes et al., 1984). It should be noted that the time course of the MT concentration after heptane injection was different from that after Zn injection. The MT concentration reached 464 µg/g 48 h after the injection, thereafter decreasing by a constant amount: 100 µg/g/d (Onosaka et al., 1988c). Hepatotoxins (Kotsonis and Klaassen, 1979), and related compounds also increased the MT concentration in the liver (Table II). Among 15 compounds causing fatty liver, 8 compounds, boric acid, cerium, chloroform, colchicine, orotic acid, safrol, tannic acid and toluenediamine, resulted in an elevated MT concentration. Particularly, colchicine was as potent as Cd which is recognized as the most potent inducer of MT (Onosaka et al., 1989). These results indicate that the MT concentration in the liver increases in such a case of hepatic disorder.

It is believed that MT is induced easily in the liver and kidney. As mentioned above, there are a number of treatments for increasing MT in the liver. However, no treatment other than metal injection was found to induce MT in the kidney (Table III). The injection of Bi, Cd or Zn resulted in high concentrations of MT in the kidney.

The MT concentration in the pancreas of normal mice was about 200 µg/g (Table I). The high level was maintained after growth (Onosaka et al., 1988a). This indicates that MT-bound Zn is the main chemical form of Zn in the pancreas of normal mice.

The MT concentration in the pancreas is highest after Zn administration (Oh et al., 1979). The induction of MT in the pancreas is sensitive to Zn-deficiency (Onosaka and Cherian, 1982). These findings suggest important roles of MT in the pancreas. The MT concentration was increased by an injection of alloxane, streptozotocin or benzene (Onosaka et al., 1988a,c). But, the increase might not be due to a direct effect of these compounds since the MT levels were as high as those after starvation (Table I). However, injection of hexane resulted in a decrease of the MT concentration in pancreas (Onosaka et al., 1988d).

The characteristics of these compounds were applied to clarify the biological roles of MT in following experiments.

PREVENTIVE EFFECT OF MT AGAINST ACUTE Cd TOXICITY

As biological roles of MT, catalysis, storage, immune phenomena or detoxication were proposed in the first paper of MT (Kägi and Vallee, 1960). Several compounds were injected to conclude the preventive effect of MT against acute Cd toxicity (Table IV).

Preinjection of Zn decreased the mortality of mice for acute Cd toxicity. An increase in the dose of Cd diminished the effect, but mice could tolerate 30 mg Cd/kg after increasing the dose of Zn, i.e., elevating the pre-existing amount of MT. However, it is unclear which tissue is responsible for Cd tolerance because MT is induced in the pancreas, liver, kidney and small intestine by Zn (Onosaka and Cherian, 1982).

It is uncertain why mice died after Cd injection. If the MT concentration is increased only in the liver, and mice tolerate a lethal dose of Cd, this indicates that MT in the liver plays an important role in preventing acute

TABLE III.
Effect of Compounds on Metallothionein
Concentration in Mouse Kidney

Compound	Metallothionein (mg/kg kidney)
None	11 ± 6
$Bi(NO_3)_2$	218 ± 64^b
K_2CrO_4	77 ± 29^a
$NiCl_2$	93 ± 18^b
$UO_2(CH_3COO)_2$	110 ± 12^b
$ZnSO_4$	227 ± 15^b

$^a p < 0.05$; $^b p < 0.01$.

TABLE IV.
Effect of Metallothionein Against
Acute Cadmium Toxicity

Injected metal (mg/kg)		
Zn	Cd	Mortality (%)
0	10	8/8 (100)
10	10	0/7 (0)[a]
10	15	6/7 (86)
50 × 4	30	1/8 (13)[a]

[a]$p < 0.01$.

Cd toxicity (Figure 2). Most of the mice died within three days after the injection of Cd at the dose of 10 mg/kg. Five compounds including an oriental medicine, a drug for hepatic diseases and organic solvent were preinjected. Mortality of the mice was decreased significantly by the pre-injection of these compounds ($p < 0.05$). A common property of these compounds was only that an increase of MT was observed in the liver. The required MT level in the liver was estimated to be 100 μg/g.

The MT concentration in the liver reached about 100 μg/g after starvation. But, the mortality of the mice was not decreased. This discrepancy is presently under investigation.

A protective effect of MT in the kidney was tested (Onosaka et al., 1986). Mice did not die after an injection of Cd or cysteine alone, but all mice died after a simultaneous injection of the both compounds. The mortality of the mice decreased after a preinjection of Bi, Ni or Zn. No significant relationship was observed in the liver, but a negative correlation was found between the MT concentration in the kidney and the mortality. This indicates that MT in the kidney also prevents Cd toxicity.

INVOLVEMENT OF MT IN Zn UPTAKE

It was reported that both mRNA and MT synthesis appeared to be necessary for hepatic Zn uptake (Richards and Cousins, 1975). If an inhibition of MT induction does not affect uptake of an injected metal, it is clear that MT is not involved in the uptake of the metal. Nitrosodimethylamine (NDMA) was used to inhibit the MT induction (Figure 3).

The concentrations of MT and Zn in the liver increased after Zn injection. The induction was inhibited by NDMA, and the concentrations of MT and Zn decreased in the liver as the dose of NDMA increased. No increase of the Zn concentration was observed in the case of complete inhibition of the MT induction since the Zn concentration in the liver was as same as that in normal mice: 20 μg.

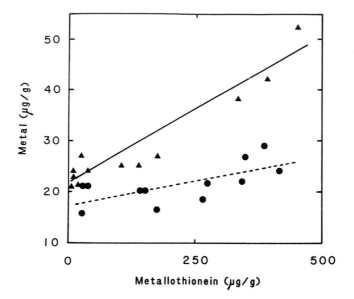

Figure 3. Effect of nitrosodimethylamine on metal uptake by liver. Mice were injected simultaneously with NDMA (0, 0.05, 0.2 or 1.0 ml/kg, s.c.) and Cd (3 mg/kg, s.c.), or with NDMA (0-1.0 ml/kg) and Zn (50 mg/kg, s.c.). The concentrations of MT and the injected metal in the liver were determined 10 h after the injections. The solid line shows the relationship between concentrations of MT and Zn in the mouse liver. The dotted line shows the relationship between concentrations of MT and Cd in the liver. (●) Cd injected; (▲) Zn injected.

The concentrations of MT and Cd increased after Cd injection. The induction of MT by Cd was inhibited dose-dependently by NDMA. However, the Cd concentration in the liver did not decrease to the same extent. It was 17 μg/g even if the induction was inhibited completely.

These results indicate that MT may be involved in Zn uptake. In contrast to Zn, MT is not related to the uptake of Cd by the liver.

MT CONCENTRATION IN HUMAN TISSUES

Little is known about MT concentrations in human tissues. The MT concentration in human liver obtained from patients was determined (Figure 4).

A positive correlation was found between the Zn and MT concentrations. If the Zn level in the liver of a normal person is assumed to be 50 μg/g, the MT concentration is about 450 μg/g based on regression line analysis. Therefore, MT is a normal component in the human liver, and MT-bound Zn is a major chemical form of Zn.

It is known that Zn concentration in the human liver decreases in the case of hepatic diseases: cirrhosis, hepatitis and cancer. It is clear that the decrease is related to the variation of MT concentration since the concentrations of Zn and MT were closely correlated (Onosaka et al., 1985). It should be emphasized that the MT concentration in the malignant tissue was lower than that in the non-malignant tissue.

Human pancreases were obtained from 20 patients. The mean of MT concentration determined by the Sephadex® G-75 method was 194 (0 to 834) μg/g (Onosaka et al., 1988b). It has already been reported that the MT concentration in the human kidney is high and correlates to the Cd level in the kidney (Cherian, 1986).

These results suggest that the MT concentration varies with the animal species under study. It is clear that the MT concentration is high in the human liver, kidney and pancreas.

ACKNOWLEDGMENTS

We are very grateful to our co-workers, particularly Drs. K. Kobashi, S. Tashiro, and S. Nishiyama.

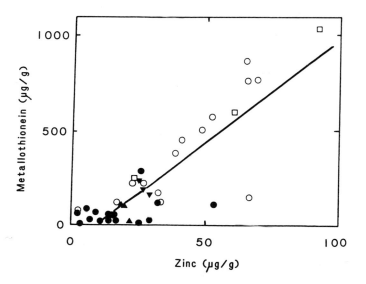

Figure 4. Concentrations of zinc and metallothionein in human liver. (○) non-malignant; (●) malignant; (□) diabetes; (▼) cirrhosis; (▲) hepatitis.

REFERENCES

Brady FO (1981): Synthesis of rat hepatic zinc thionein in response to the stress of sham operation. *Life Sci.* 28: 1647.

Bremner I, Davies NT, and Mills CF (1973): The effect of zinc deficiency and food restriction on hepatic zinc proteins in the rat. *Biochem. Soc. Transact.* 1: 982.

Chang CC, Vander Mallie RJ, and Garvey JS (1980): A radio-immunoassay for human metallothionein. *Toxicol. Appl. Pharmacol.* 55: 94.

Cherian MG (1986): Metallothionein levels in liver and kidney of Canadians—a potential indicator of environmental exposure to cadmium. *Arch. Environ. Health.* 44: 319.

Dieter HH, Muller L, Abel J, and Summer K-H (1986): Determination of Cd-thionein in biological materials: comparative standard recovery by five current methods using protein nitrogen for standard calibration. *Toxicol. Appl. Pharmacol.* 85: 380.

Etzel KR, Shapiro SG, and Cousins RJ (1979): Regulation of liver metallothionein and plasma zinc by the glucocorticoid dexamethasone. *Biochem. Biophys. Res. Commun.* 89: 1120.

Furey WF, Robbins AH, Clancy LL, Winge DR, Wang BC, and Stout CD (1986): Crystal structure of Cd,Zn metallothionein. *Science* 231: 704.

Kägi JHR and Vallee BL (1960): Metallothionein: a cadmium- and zinc-containing protein from equine renal cortex. *J. Biol. Chem.* 235: 3460.

Kägi JHR and Vallee BL (1961): Metallothionein: a cadmium- and zinc-containing protein from equine renal cortex II. Physicochemical properties. *J. Biol. Chem.* 236: 2435.

Kotsonis FN and Klaassen CD (1979): Increase in hepatic metallothionein in rats treated with alkylating agents. *Toxicol. Appl. Pharmacol.* 51: 19.

Matsubara J (1985): Alternation of radiosensitivity in metallothionein induced mice and a possible role of Zn-Cu-thionein in GSH-peroxidase system. *2nd Int. Meet. on Metallothionein.* Zürich.

Naganuma A, Satoh M, and Imura N (1987): Prevention of lethal and renal toxicity of cis-diamminedichloropalatinum(II) by induction of metallothionein synthesis without compromising its antitumor activity in mice. *Cancer Res.* 47: 983.

Oh SH, Deagen JT, Whanger PD, and Weswig PH (1978): Biological function of metallothionein. V. Its induction in rats by various stresses. *Am. J. Physiol.* 234: E282.

Oh SH, Nakaue H, Deagen JT, Whanger PD, and Abscott GH (1979): Accumulation and depletion of zinc in chick tissue metallothioneins. *J. Nutr.* 109: 1720.

Onosaka S and Cherian MG (1981): The induced synthesis of metallothionein in various tissues of rat in response to metal. I. Effect of repeated injection of cadmium salts. *Toxicology* 22: 91.

Onosaka S and Cherian MG (1982): The induced synthesis of metallothionein in various tissues of rats in response to metal. II. Influence of zinc status and specific effect on pancreatic metallothionein. *Toxicology* 23: 11.

Onosaka S, Min KS, Fukuhara C, Tanaka K, Tashiro S, Furuta M, and Yasutomi T (1985): Concentration of metallothionein in human tissues. *Eisei Kagaku.* 31: 352.

Onosaka S, Min KS, Fukuhara C, and Tanaka K (1986): Role of renal metallothionein in acute cadmium toxicity in mice. *Eisei Kagaku.* 32: 109.

Onosaka S, Min KS, Fujita Y, Tanaka K, Shin I, and Okada Y (1988a): High concentration of pancreatic metallothionein in normal mice. *Toxicology* 50: 27.

Onosaka S, Min KS, Fujita Y, Tanaka K, Hara K, Enzan H, Nakamura K, and Nishiyama S (1988b): Concentration of metallothionein in human pancreas. *Eisei Kagaku.* 34: 92.

Onosaka S, Ochi Y, Min KS, Fujita Y, and Tanaka K (1988c): Influences of compounds on metallothionein concentration in mouse tissues. I. Increase of hepatic metallothionein concentration by organic solvents and fatty acids. *Eisei Kagaku.* 34: 440.

Onosaka S, Ochi Y, Min KS, Fujita Y, and Tanaka K (1988d): Influences of compounds on metallothionein concentration in mouse tissues. II. Decrease of pancreatic metallothionein concentration by *n*-hexane. *Eisei Kagaku.* 34: 446.

Onosaka S, Ochi Y, Min KS, Fujita Y, and Tanaka K (1989): Influences of compounds on metallothionein concentration in mouse tissues. III. Effects of hepatotoxins. *Eisei Kagaku.* 35: 162.

Piotrowski JK, Trojanowska B, Wisniewska-Knypl JM, and Bolanowska W (1974): Mercury binding in the kidney and liver of rats repeatedly exposed to mercuric chloride: induction of metallothionein by mercury and cadmium. *Toxicol. Appl. Pharmacol.* 27: 11.

Piscator M (1964): On cadmium in normal human kidneys together with a report on the isolation of metallothionein from livers of cadmium-exposed rabbits. *Nord. Hyg. Tidskr.* 45: 76.

Richards MP and Cousins RJ (1975): Mammalian zinc homeostasis: requirement for RNA and metallothionein synthesis. *Biochem. Biophys. Res. Commun.* 64: 1215.

Shiraishi N, Yamamoto H, Takeda Y, Kondoh S, Hayashi H, Hahimoto K, and Aono K (1986): Increased metallothionein content in rat liver and kidney following X-irradiation. *Toxicol. Appl. Pharmacol.* 85: 128.

Suzuki KT (1980): Direct connection of high-speed liquid chromatograph (equipped with gel permeation column) to atomic absorption spectrophotometer for metalloprotein analysis: metallothionein. *Anal. Biochem.* 102: 31.

Suzuki Y and Yoshikawa H (1974): Role of metallothionein in the liver in protection against cadmium toxicity. *Ind. Health.* 12: 141.

Tohyama C and Shaikh ZA (1981): Metallothionein in plasma and urine of cadmium-exposed rats determined by a single-antibody radioimmunoassay. *Fund. Appl. Toxicology* 1: 1.

Waalkes MP, Hjelle JJ, and Klaassen CD (1984): Transient induction of hepatic metallothionein following oral ethanol administration. *Toxicol. Appl. Pharmacol.,* 74: 230.

Webb M (1972): Binding of cadmium ions by rat liver and kidney. *Biochem. Pharmacol.* 21: 2751.

Winge DR, Rremakumar R, and Rajagopalan KV (1975): Metal-induced formation of metallothionein in rat liver. *Arch. Biochem. Biophys.* 170: 242.

Chapter 2

A Cd-Saturation Assay for Cu-Containing Metallothionein

Karl H. Summer, Rüdiger Bartsch,
and Dominik Klein
Institute for Toxicology
GSF Research Center
Neuherberg, Germany

ABSTRACT

A rapid and sensitive Cd-saturation method to determine Cu-containing metallothionein (MT) is described. The main features of this assay are: high molecular weight Cd-binding compounds are denatured with acetonitrile (50% final concentration), Cu bound to MT is removed with ammonium tetra-thiomolybdate, excessive tetrathiomolybdate and its Cu-complexes are removed with the anion exchanger DEAE-Sephacel®, apothionein is saturated with Cd and excessive Cd is bound to the cation exchanger Chelex-100®. The thiomolybdate assay is capable of reliably detecting 14 ng MT and thus is particularly suited to measure MT in small tissue samples (e.g., biopsies), in extrahepatic tissues and in cultured cells. Moreover, the combination of the thiomolybdate assay with the recently developed Cd-Chelex® assay (Bartsch et al., 1990) also makes it possible to measure the relative Cu-load of MT, provided the amount of non-Cu-thionein exceeds 100 ng, the detection limit of the Cd-Chelex® assay.

INTRODUCTION

Investigating the role of metallothionein (MT) in Cu-metabolism requires an accurate, sensitive and yet simple method to quantify Cu-containing MT. Since such a method is not available, Cu-thionein is mainly determined by gel filtration chromatography and subsequent metal analysis of the MT fractions. This rather insensitive and time consuming technique, however, is not suitable for determination of basal levels of Cu-thionein in tissues from control animals or MT contents of small probes such as biopsies.

The metal-independent immunological methods (Vander Mallie and Garvey, 1979; Thomas et al., 1986), although being sensitive, cannot distinguish Cu-containing MT from MT that contains metals other than Cu. The determination of MT by an Ag-saturation method also has been reported (Scheuhammer and Cherian, 1986). Due to the higher affinity of the protein to Ag as compared to Cu, this method seems promising to quantify also Cu-containing MT. However, the stoichiometry of Ag-thionein is not sufficiently established yet.

With the known molar ratio of Cd to MT of 7, a Cd-saturation assay, as a simple and accurate method to measure Zn,Cd-thioneins (Waalkes et al., 1985; Dieter et al., 1986), without chromatographical steps, would be superior to analyze Cu-containing MT, provided Cu can be removed from the protein prior to Cd-saturation.

The present study describes a fast and simple assay for Cu-thionein using ammonium tetrathiomolybdate to sequester Cu from Cu-containing MT (Bremner and Mehra, 1983; Allen and Gawthorne, 1987) and subsequent saturation of the apothionein with radiolabeled Cd.

MATERIALS AND METHODS

Chemicals

^{109}Cd (37 MBq/μg Cd) in 0.1 M HCl was obtained from Amersham Buchler, Braunschweig, Germany; ammonium tetrathiomolybdate was supplied by Ventron-Alfa, Karlsruhe, Germany; Cd_5,Zn_2-thionein from rabbit liver, CM-Sephadex® (40 to 200 μm), DEAE-Sephacel® (40 to 150 μm) and bovine serum albumin (BSA), RIA grade, were purchased from Sigma Chemie, Deisenhofen, Germany; cadmium chloride, standard solution for AAS, was obtained from Aldrich, Steinheim, Germany; Chelex-100® (100 to 200 mesh) was supplied by Bio-Rad, Munich, Germany; $Cu(CH_3CN)_4ClO_4$ was synthesized according to Hemmerich and Sigwart (1963), recrystallized twice from acetonitrile, dried in a desiccator over silica gel and stored under argon at 4°C; all other chemicals used were of the highest purity available.

Before use, ion-exchange resins were washed with 10 volumes of 10 mM Tris-HCl, 1 M NaCl, pH 7.4, and equilibrated with 10 volumes of 10 mM Tris-HCl, 85 mM NaCl, pH 7.4. All solutions used in the assays were degassed by sonification and saturated with nitrogen at 4°C.

Animals

Male Wistar rats (inbred strain, Neuherberg, Germany) weighing 180 to 200 g were fed a standard laboratory diet (Altromin, Lage, Germany) *ad libitum* and had free access to tap water. For MT induction, rats were injected i.p. daily on two consecutive days with 10 mg Zn^{2+} or 3 mg Cu^{2+} per kg b.w. in 0.9% NaCl. Animals were killed 18 h after the last treatment.

Human Liver

Post-mortem specimens were obtained from a 41-year-old male after suicidal death and from 5 children aged 2.5 to 14 months with the sudden infant death syndrome. The reports on the histological examinations revealed no indication of liver diseases. Liver biopsies (Menghini technique) from patients with primary biliary cirrhosis and Wilson's disease were supplied by the Krankenhaus der Barmherzigen Brüder, Munich, and were kept at −80°C until measurements.

Cells

Human foreskin fibroblasts from two children aged 4 and 10 years were provided by the Dermatologische Klinik, LMU, Munich. Cells were grown in Dulbecco's modified Eagle's Medium (DMEM) (NordVacc, Sweden) containing 10% fetal bovine serum (Gibco, Paisley, Scotland) and cultivated in a humidified environment of 7% CO_2 at 37°C. Confluent monolayer cultures grown on Falcon petri dishes (10 cm diameter) were incubated 48 h with 10 ml complete medium containing 0.3 to 760 μM Cu. For homogenization, medium was decanted and after washing the dishes with 4 × 5 ml ice-cold PBS, the cells were harvested with a rubber policeman in 0.5 ml of 10 mM Tris-HCl, 85 mM NaCl, pH 7.4 per dish. Cells were lysed by freezing and thawing five times.

Preparation of Cytosols

Samples of post-mortem livers were homogenized with four volumes of 10 mM Tris-HCl, pH 7.4 at 0°C with a Potter Elvehjem homogenizer. Biopsies (3 to 8 mg wet weight) were homogenized by ultrasonification in 0.4 ml 10 mM Tris-HCl for 3 s. Tissue and cell homogenates were centrifuged at $100,000 \times g$ (60 min, 0°C), and the supernatant fractions (S100) were used for MT and metal determinations. Cytosolic protein was measured with the Biuret method or according to Lowry et al. (1951).

Thiomolybdate Assay

In a 1.5 ml vial filled with argon, 0.05 or 0.1 ml sample was mixed with the same volume of acetonitrile. After 3 min, 0.5 ml of buffer A (10 mM Tris-HCl, 85 mM NaCl, pH 7.4) and 0.1 ml of CM-Sephadex® (66% v/v suspension in buffer A) were added. The mixture was shaken for 3 min under argon and incubated with 0.05 ml BSA solution (30 mg/ml buffer A, daily freshly prepared). After 2 min, 0.02 ml of a daily freshly prepared ammonium tetrathiomolybdate solution (1.3 mg/ml buffer A) was added, and after 2 min, the mixture was shaken with 0.1 ml DEAE-Sephacel® (66% v/v suspension in buffer A) for 3 min under argon. After centrifugation ($8,000 \times g$, 5 min), 0.6 ml of the supernatant fraction was incubated with 0.01 ml ^{109}Cd-labeled CdCl$_2$ solution (0.66 mM Cd in buffer A, 0.5 mCi/mg Cd) for 5 min, 0.1 ml of Chelex-100® (66% v/v suspension in buffer A) was added and the mixture was shaken for 15 min. After centrifugation ($8,000 \times g$, 5 min), 0.5 ml of the supernatant fraction was mixed with 0.5 ml acetonitrile and after 3 min, the precipitate was removed by centrifugation ($8,000 \times g$, 5 min) and 0.9 ml of the supernatant fraction analyzed for Cd with the gamma counter (Autogamma 5000, Canberra-Packard, Frankfurt, Germany).

Determination of the Cu-Load of MT

Samples were analyzed with both the thiomolybdate assay and the Cd-Chelex® assay (Bartsch et al., 1990) which is capable to determine Zn(Cd)-thioneins only. The relative Cu-load of MT was then calculated from the different results of both assays.

In Vitro Preparation and Characterization of Cu-Containing MT

Dilutions of the S100 from liver homogenates or of the stock solution of purified Zn-thionein (11), quantified with the Cd-Chelex® assay, were incubated under argon with the same volume of a solution of Cu(CH$_3$CN)$_4$ClO$_4$ in acetonitrile for 3 min. The added moles of Cu per mol MT were 6 to 50 for the purified Zn-thionein, 10 to 62 for MT in the hepatic S100 of the Zn-treated rat and 7 to 100 for MT in the hepatic cytosol of the 41-year-old individual. The resulting Cu-containing MT (0.1 to 3 μg) were analyzed with the Cd-Chelex® and the thiomolybdate assay omitting the first addition of acetonitrile.

Cu-saturated MT, obtained by incubating purified Zn-thionein with $Cu(CH_3CN)_4ClO_4$ in a molar ratio of added Cu/MT of 16, was further characterized after dialysis against 10 mM Tris-HCl, pH 7.4. Gel filtration chromatography (Spherogel® TSK 2000 SW, 7.5 × 300 mm, 10 μm, mobile phase 50 mM Tris-HCl, 150 mM NaCl, pH 7.0, saturated with nitrogen; flowrate 0.5 ml/min; fraction size 0.5 ml; detection of absorbance at 254 nm; calibrated with Cd_5,Zn_2-thionein) revealed a single band with the relative elution volume $V_e/V_0 = 1.8$ to 2.3, typical for MT. All of the Cu was found in the MT-fractions. Moreover, 100% exchange of Zn against Cu was confirmed as no Zn could be detected in the MT fractions. EPR-spectra of the Cu-thionein showed only EPR-inactive diamagnetic Cu(I). Oxidation with hydrogen peroxide resulted in a resonance peak, whereas the corresponding amount of hydrogen peroxide alone caused no signal (data not shown).

RESULTS

One major requirement for the reliable determination of Cu-containing MT with this Cd-saturation method is the quantitative sequestration of Cu by ammonium tetrathiomolybdate. Moreover, both the Cu-thiomolybdate complexes and excessive thiomolybdate have to be removed without affecting MT. This was achieved with DEAE-Sephacel® and by performing the test in 10 mM Tris-HCl, 85 mM NaCl, pH 7.4. MT with varying Cu content, obtained by exchanging MT-bound Zn against Cu *in vitro* and MT contents of the S100 of liver homogenates from Zn- or Cu-treated rats and of human liver were determined with the Cd-Chelex® assay in presence and absence of DEAE-Sephacel®. Independent of the samples, DEAE-Sephacel® did not influence the determination of MT with various Cu-loads of 0 to 100%.

After shaking thiomolybdate solutions [100 nmoles with or without Cu(I) or Cu(II)] with DEAE-Sephacel®, neither tetrathiomolybdate nor Cu could be detected photometrically or by AAS, respectively (results not shown).

The quantitative removal of Cu from MT was investigated with gel filtration chromatography: Before and after addition of thiomolybdate and DEAE-Sephacel®, hepatic S100 fractions from a Cu-treated rat (Figure 1A) and Cu-thionein obtained from purified Zn-thionein by adding Cu(I) (Figure 1B) were chromatographed and analyzed for Cu. The treatment with thiomolybdate and DEAE-Sephacel® resulted in a total removal of MT-bound Cu.

The specificity of the thiomolybdate assay for MT in biological probes was examined with gel filtration chromatography and metal analysis. The thiomolybdate assay was performed with hepatic S100 from a Cu-treated

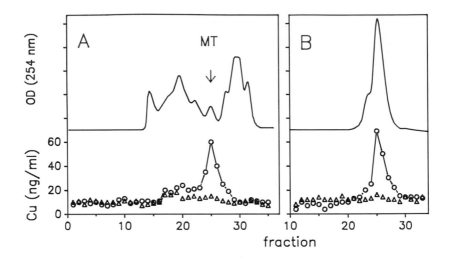

Figure 1. Efficiency of $(NH_4)_2MoS_4$ to remove Cu from Cu-containing MT. Cu-distribution of chromatographically separated hepatic cytosol from a Cu-treated rat (A) and of Cu-thionein obtained from purified Zn-thionein (mol Cu added/mol MT = 15) (B) before (O–O) and after (△–△) addition of $(NH_4)_2MoS_4$ and DEAE-Sephacel®.

rat and the final supernatant fraction was chromatographically separated. Whereas Cu was virtually absent, Cd was exclusively found in the MT fractions (Figure 2), additionally demonstrating the effectiveness of acetonitrile to denature cytosolic high molecular weight proteins.

Furthermore, up to 0.1 mM, the Cd-binding thiols glutathione and cysteine, which are not denatured by acetonitrile, did not impair the test results (data not shown).

The quality of the thiomolybdate assay was investigated with *in vitro* prepared Cu-thionein. Various dilutions of hepatic S100 from a Zn-treated rat, human liver cytosol and a stock solution of purified Zn-thionein, were incubated with Cu(I) to yield different molar ratios of Cu/MT. The samples were analyzed for MT with both the Cd-Chelex® and the thiomolybdate assay. Whereas with the Cd-Chelex® assay MT recovery declined with increasing molar ratios of Cu/MT, recovery of MT with the thiomolybdate assay was $100 \pm 10\%$ and thus was independent of the sample type, MT-amount (0.1 to 3.0 μg) and the Cu-content of MT (Figure 3).

From the difference of the results obtained with the Cd-Chelex® and the thiomolybdate assay, the relative Cu-load of MT was calculated.

Linearity and sensitivity of the thiomolybdate assay were determined with various dilutions of the hepatic S100 from a Cu-treated rat. MT could be reliably determined within the range of 0.014 to 3.2 μg (Figure 4). The upper limit of the assay can be extended further by using more thiomolybdate and Cd.

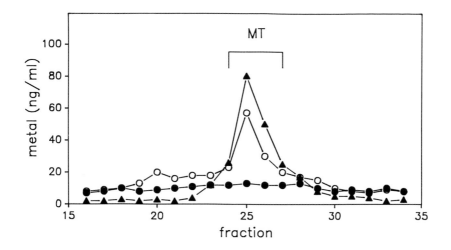

Figure 2. Metal distribution of gel chromatographically separated hepatic cytosol from a Cu-treated rat before and after the thiomolybdate assay. Cu in the native cytosol (O–O); Cu (●–●) and Cd (▲–▲) of the same sample after the assay.

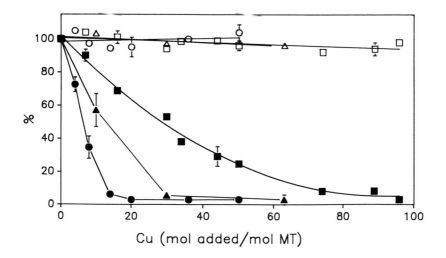

Figure 3. Recovery of Cu-containing MT with the thiomolybdate (open symbols) and the Cd-Chelex® assay (filled symbols). Cu-containing MT were prepared from Zn(Cd)-thioneins (0.1 to 3 μg) by adding $Cu(CH_3CN)_4ClO_4$. Purified Zn-thionein from rat liver (O,●); hepatic cytosol from a Zn-treated rat (△,▲) and human liver cytosol (□,■); mean ± S.D. (n = 3 to 6).

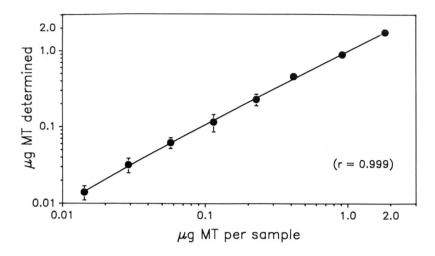

Figure 4. Linearity and sensitivity of the thiomolybdate assay for Cu-containing MT. Dilutions of hepatic cytosol from a Cu-treated rat (60 μg MT/ml) were analyzed with the thiomolybdate assay (mean ± S.D., n = 3).

The presented method was then applied for quantification of MT in Cu-treated cultured human fibroblasts, and in human liver biopsies of patients with Wilson's disease and primary biliary cirrhosis. Additionally, the relative Zn-, or Cu-load of MT were determined.

Incubation of the fibroblasts with $CuCl_2$ up to 130 μM did not rise the MT-content, although the cytosolic Cu-levels were increased about 4-fold at 130 μM Cu compared to cells grown in basal medium. The initial decrease in the Zn-load of MT reflects the incorporation of Cu into MT. Incubation of the cells with more than 200 μM Cu led to a dose-dependent MT accumulation and a further decrease of the Zn-load of MT down to 10% at 760 μM Cu (Figure 5).

Biopsies of patients with Wilson's disease showed high MT-contents of 30.2 ± 11.7 μg/mg cytosolic protein. Patients with primary biliary cirrhosis, revealed hepatic MT-levels of 3.6 to 10.5 μg/mg cytosolic protein (Table 1). In both diseases, the hepatic MT content correlated with the levels of cytosolic Cu (r = 0.988, n = 11, data not shown).

DISCUSSION

With the thiomolybdate assay, a fast and sensitive method to determine Cu-containing MT in biological tissues was developed. The new features of this Cd-saturation assay include the precipitation of high molecular weight Cd-binding proteins by acetonitrile, the removal of MT-bound Cu by am-

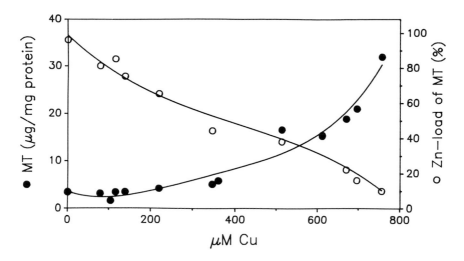

Figure 5. MT and Zn-load of MT in cultured human skin fibroblasts. Cells were incubated with $CuCl_2$ and MT was analyzed in the cytosolic fractions with the thiomolybdate and the Cd-Chelex® assay. The Zn-load of MT was calculated from the results of both assays.

TABLE I.
MT and Cu-Load of MT in Wilson's Disease (WD)
and Primary Biliary Cirrhosis (PBC)

Liver specimens	Cu (ng/mg protein)[a]	MT (µg/mg protein)[a]	Cu-load of MT (%)
Control[b]	135 ± 62 (6)	3.8 ± 2.3 (6)	14 ± 13 (6)
WD[c]	3271 ± 1642 (3)	30.2 ± 11.7 (3)	57 ± 12 (3)
PBC[c]	428 ± 420 (8)	6.5 ± 2.9 (8)	36 ± 21 (8)

[a]Cytosolic protein.
[b]Post-mortem livers from individuals without indication of liver diseases.
[c]Biopsies, mean ± S.D., number of individuals in parenthesis.

monium tetrathiomolybdate, the removal of excessive thiomolybdate and its Cu-complexes by DEAE-Sephacel® and the binding of excessive Cd by Chelex-100®. This approach avoids both, heating of the samples which is not practicable with the heat-labile Cu-thionein and the possible enclosure of MT into heat-denatured hemoglobin as well as the removal of Cd from Cd-thionein by excessive hemoglobin (Eaton and Toal, 1982), inherent problems of conventional Cd-heme assays.

The disappearance of the typical absorption spectrum (results not shown), the gel filtration and metal analysis data indicate that ammonium tetrathiomolybdate was effective in quantitatively sequestrating Cu from Cu-containing MT, confirming data from others (Bremner and Mehra, 1983; Kay et al., 1987). Oxidation of the intermediately formed apothionein was avoided by using nitrogen saturated solutions and by carrying out the test procedures in an atmosphere of argon until Cd-saturation. Furthermore, oxidation of the apothionein might also be prevented by tetrathiomolybdate with its highly negative redox potential (Kelleher and Mason, 1986).

Although Cd-saturation assays in general measure the Cd-binding capacity rather than the protein itself, chromatographic analysis and metal determinations with AAS demonstrate the specificity of the thiomolybdate assay for MT (Figure 2).

Quality of the assay in recovering Cu-thioneins was assessed by using *in vitro* prepared Cu-thioneins from different biological sources as standard. These samples showed the same characteristics as physiological Cu-containing MT with respect to metal-binding, chromatographic behavior and oxidation state of MT-bound Cu.

With its performance to reliably measure 14 ng MT, the thiomolybdate assay, although less sensitive than immunological tests (Tohyama et al., 1981; Thomas et al., 1986) is more sensitive than conventional Cd-saturation assays and thus is particularly suited to determine MT in small tissue samples (e.g., liver biopsies of a few milligrams wet weight) and in extrahepatic tissues or cell cultures with low MT concentrations.

Being capable of quantifying Cu-containing MT, and, in combination with the Cd-Chelex® assay, also to determine the Cu-load of MT, the thiomolybdate assay is considered to be superior to present available assays for Cu-thioneins.

The presented results on increased MT-levels in Cu-treated cultured human fibroblasts and on the involvement of MT in liver diseases associated with Cu-accumulation (Figure 5 and Table 1), provide further evidence that the thiomolybdate assay is a useful and sufficiently sensitive tool for quantitative studies on the contribution of Cu-containing MT in the metabolism and toxicity of Cu.

ACKNOWLEDGMENT

The authors wish to thank Drs. G.A. Drasch and J. Eisenburg for supplying the samples of human liver and J. Lichtmannegger for valuable contributions and expert technical assistance.

REFERENCES

Allen JD and Gawthorne JM (1987): Effect of molybdenum treatments on the distribution of Cu and metallothionein in tissue extracts from rats and sheep. *J. Inorg. Biochem.* 31: 161.

Bartsch R, Klein D, and Summer KH (1990): The Cd-Chelex® assay: a new sensitive method to determine metallothionein containing zinc and cadmium. *Arch. Toxicol.* 64:177.

Bremner I and Mehra RK (1983): Metallothionein: some aspects of its structure and function with special regard to its involvement in copper and zinc metabolism. *Chemica Scripta* 21: 117.

Dieter HH, Müller L, Abel J, and Summer KH (1986): Determination of Cd-thionein in biological materials: comparative standard recovery by five current methods using protein nitrogen for standard calibration. *Toxicol. Appl. Pharmacol.* 85: 380.

Eaton DL and Toal BF (1982): Evaluation of the Cd/hemoglobin affinity assay for the rapid determination of metallothionein in biological tissues. *Toxicol. Appl. Pharmacol.* 66: 134.

Hemmerich P and Sigwart C (1963): $Cu(CH_3CN)_2^+$, ein Mittel zum Studium homogener Reaktionen des einwertigen Kupfers in wässriger Lösung. *Experientia* 19: 488.

Kay J, Cryer A, Brown MW, Norey CG, Bremner I, Overnell J, Parten B, and Dunn BM (1987): N-terminal sequence of metallothionein from rainbow trout. *Biochem. Soc. Trans.* 15: 453.

Kelleher CA and Mason J (1986): Reversible inhibition of ovine ceruloplasmin by thiomolybdates. *Int. J. Biochem.* 18: 629.

Lowry OH, Rosebrough NJ, Farr AL, and Randall RJ (1951): Protein measurement with the folin phenol reagent. *J. Biol. Chem.* 193: 265.

Scheuhammer AM and Cherian MG (1986): Quantification of metallothioneins by a silver-saturation method. *Toxicol. Appl. Pharmacol.* 82: 417.

Thomas DG, Linton HJ, and Garvey JS (1986): Fluorometric ELISA for the detection and quantitation of metallothionein. *J. Immunol. Methods* 89: 239.

Tohyama C, Shaikh ZA, Ellis KJ, and Cohn SH (1981): Metallothionein excretion in urine upon cadmium exposure: its relationship with liver and kidney cadmium. *Toxicology* 22: 181.

Vander Mallie RJ and Garvey JS (1979): Radioimmunoassay of metallothioneins. *J. Biol. Chem.* 254: 8416.

Waalkes MP, Garvey JS, and Klaassen CD (1985): Comparison of methods of metallothionein quantification: cadmium radioassay, mercury radioassay, and radioimmunoassay. *Toxicol. Appl. Pharmacol.* 79: 524.

Chapter

3

The Development and Utilization of Immunological Probes for Detection/Quantitation of Metallothionein

*Justine S. Garvey**
Department of Biology
Syracuse University
Syracuse, New York

INTRODUCTION

Immunological assays are characterized by specificity and sensitivity. Protocols may be designed to quantitate either of the two principal reagents, antigen and antibody. In the context of this paper, the metal-binding protein metallothionein (MT) is antigen and antibody is a reagent obtained by prior immunization with MT. Both MT and antibody vs. MT are appropriately detected and/or quantitated in an optimized binding reaction in which the antibody serves as a probe. The limitations on specificity/sensitivity of an antibody probe are attributable to the affinity of the antibody combining site for the antigenic determinant, analogous to a key-lock combination. There are two emphases in this paper, one aimed at providing a brief background

*Present position: Visiting Research Associate, Division of Biology, California Institute of Technology, Pasadena, CA.

of the development of immunological reagents and methods for detection and quantitation of MT, and the second reviewing selected studies in which the developed reagents and methods were utilized. Both emphases are on the author's contributions; however, in the section on *Development of Reagents and Assays,* a background of contributions by others is cited while in the section on *Utilization of the RIA and ELISA* the concern is with contributions, selected and not inclusive, of the author to various areas of MT research.

DEVELOPMENT OF REAGENTS AND ASSAYS

Polyclonal Antibody and Radioimmunoassay (RIA)

Antibodies for investigative purposes are produced by either polyclonal (conventional) immunization or by monoclonal (i.e., hybridoma) procedures. Although much still remains unknown about these procedures, they have the unique property of providing a reagent, antibody, that specifically binds to a small region, usually 5 to 7 amino acids (either continuous or discontinuous in sequence), of a protein antigen. In 1976, a project was initiated in my laboratory that was aimed at production in rabbits of an antibody with specificity for MT. An isoform of rat liver MT was visualized as pure by Coomassie blue staining of the sample after electrophoresis in a nondenatured polyacrylamide gel. MT that was treated with glutaraldehyde was the immunogen that provided a high affinity antibody reagent which had complete cross-reactivity in immunological assays with mammalian MTs, the apoprotein and metal-chelated with Zn, Cu, Cd or Hg (Vander Mallie and Garvey, 1978, 1979). The assay that was then developed for quantitation of MT (Garvey et al., 1982) is a double-antibody competitive fluid phase radioimmunoassay (RIA). The basic format has remained unchanged since the first publication (*vide supra*); however, parameters of the assay have been continuously optimized, this need often arising because of sample variations. The protocols for development of logit-log regressions (standard curves) and the statistical processing of data derive primarily from the analyses of Rodbard and colleagues (Rodbard et al., 1968, 1970, 1976; Rodbard, 1971, 1974). A prototypic response curve (Garvey, 1989) is shown in Figure 1. Typically, a logit-log rendition of the data permits quantitation of mammalian MTs with circa 5% accuracy over the region 100–20,000 pg MT; extensions of the principal regression permit quantification with decreased accuracy to ca. 100,000 pg and to ca. 10 pg MT.

There have been several reports by others of immunization with MT and characterization of a polyclonal antibody in an RIA (Brady and Kafka, 1979; Tohyama and Shaikh, 1981; Mehra and Bremner, 1983; Nolan and

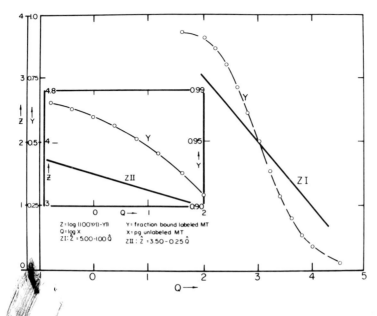

Figure 1. Typical standard curve for MT: Radioimmunoassay. The sigmoid response (Y vs. Q) is linearized when converted to logit-log form (Z vs. Q). Accuracy of quantitation of unknowns is customarily ± 5% over the central region. The characteristic correlation coefficient (in excess of 0.99 over the central region) of the regression decreases to 0.80–0.85 for the extension (insert) developed over the concentration range 100 to 1 pg competing MT. A similar correlation coefficient characterizes extensions beyond 20,000 pg competing MT. (Adapted from Garvey, 1989.)

Shaikh, 1986). In these reports both the protocols for immunization and the format of the RIA varied as likewise the reported sensitivity for MT detection. One of these RIAs is claimed to be specific for one isoform only of rat MT (Mehra and Bremner, *vide supra*). Waalkes et al. (1985) and Dieter et al. (1987) have performed comparisons of the accuracy of the RIA and other assays in common use for measuring MT in samples. Both experiments confirm that the RIA is more work-intensive than the non-immunological assays but it is usually found to be more accurate and its sensitivity provides the only capability for detecting and quantitating MT in physiological fluids of very low MT content.

Enzyme-Linked Immunosorbent Assay (ELISA)

The incentive for development of an ELISA (Thomas et al., 1986) was to provide an alternate capability to the RIA, especially in the screening of monoclonal antibodies (MAbs) where use of a radioisotope appeared more of a hindrance than an advantage. Bound antigen and antibody are measured in both the RIA and ELISA; the basic principle of the two reactions is the same. The primary difference to be exploited in the two assays is the label that provides the signal from which quantitation is derived. When enzyme detection can provide the sensitivity of a radiolabel, then the choice of assay used may clearly favor the ELISA. The initial assessment of the ELISA was made in terms of its performance relative to the RIA. Accordingly, the same pair of antibodies were used as in the RIA, i.e., polyclonal antibody (rabbit) produced vs. rat liver MT as primary antibody and anti-rabbit IgG (goat) as secondary antibody. Both colorimetric and fluorometric substrates were used, chosen appropriately for evaluation with beta-galactosidase or alkaline phosphatase. In a competition between solid phase MT and fluid phase MT the detection of competitor MT was in approximately the range as found in the RIA (Figure 2). The fluorometric method was then selected for most applications of the ELISA, although the colorimetric method has seen much application in the screening of MAbs. It was demonstrated that cytosolic MT, because of its typically high concentrations in tissues such as liver and kidney, could be readily quantitated by ELISA; physiological

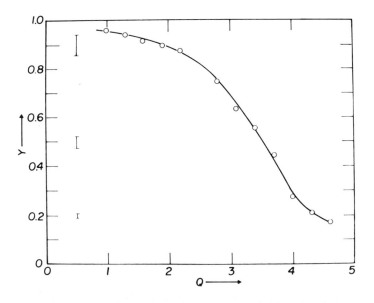

Figure 2. Typical standard curve for MT: ELISA. The sigmoid response (Y vs. Q) may be linearized as in the RIA when expressed in logit-log form (Z vs. Q); Y, Z and Q defined as in Figure 1. In logit-log form the accuracy is comparable to that of the RIA. Error bars indicate the range of typical standard errors at $Y = 0.9$, 0.5, and 0.2 when quantitating unknowns. (Adapted from Thomas et al., 1986.)

fluids such as serum and urine, because of interfering substances, necessitated prior sample preparation. In the case of the RIA such additional procedures have not been necessary. Grider et al. (1989) have developed a colorimetric ELISA for assay of MT in human liver samples obtained at autopsy. Applications in this regard gave results which compared favorably to those obtained by the Cd-heme method.

Production and Assessment of Monoclonal Antibodies

The objective of this phase of research was two-fold: to obtain reagents of other specificities than had been derived from polyclonal techniques, and to obtain reagents of useful specificities for MT detection/quantitation with the advantage provided by monoclonal over polyclonal antibody production, i.e., unlimited supply. As is made abundantly clear in previous and following sections, and particularly the section on *Analysis of Antigenic Determinants of MT,* the principal antigenic determinants recognized by the polyclonal antibody are on the beta domain (residues 1–30) of the mammalian MT molecule. Thus, one goal of MAb production was obtaining clones reactive with the alpha domain (residues 31–61) of the molecule. For use as immunogen in MAb production a human MT isoform was either conjugated to keyhole limpet hemocyanin (KLH) with a bifunctional agent or injected simply as an emulsion in adjuvant (RIBI, Hamilton, MT). The initial injection was made into multiple sites of LOU/MN rats. The secondary immunization was with the same immunogen as used for the initial injection but was made intrasplenic 3 to 4 d prior to splenectomy. The splenocytes obtained were fused with rat myeloma cells designated 1R983F that were provided by Prof. Hérve Bazin, Brussels. The salient points of cell culture, hybridoma selection, production of ascites, and purification of culture supernatants by an affinity matrix were adapted from publications of Prof. Bazin (reviewed in Bazin et al., 1986 and DeClerq et al., 1986). Two principal strategies of the fluorometric ELISA were intended to bias MAb selection of (a) high affinity by use of minimal antigen for binding, and of (b) IgG class by use of a secondary antibody-enzyme conjugate that had anti-rat IgG binding specificity. The antigen capture format of the ELISA (van Heyningen, 1986), essentially as used in Thomas et al. (1986), but lacking competition from fluid phase antigen, permitted a ranking of several clones of MAbs as shown in Figure 3. A different ELISA format, known as "sandwich" because antigen is bound between two layers of antibody (Van Regenmortel, 1988), was used as a further demonstration of binding of the MAbs to the alpha fragment. To a coating of polyclonal antibody (anti-rat liver MT produced in rabbits) was added human MT. In the next incubation step solutions of previously unreacted MAb, and also the same MAb already reacted with the alpha fragment by an incubation step, were

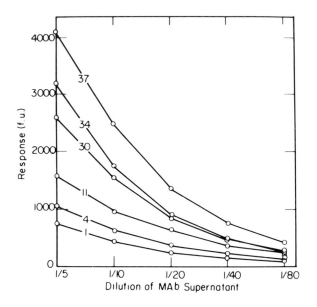

Figure 3. Relative binding affinity of MAbs to the alpha fragment of MT. A panel of rat-rat hybridomas selected in an ELISA for binding to human MT-2 (the immunogen) were cloned twice and expanded by *in vitro* culture. Supernatants from confluent cultures were tested for binding to the alpha fragment of rat apoMT-1, a gift from Dr. Dennis Winge, University of Utah Medical School. The ELISA procedure was essentially as described in Thomas et al., 1986. The response in fluorometric units (f.u.), corrected for the response lacking MAb (20 f.u.), is measured after a 45 min. ambient temperature incubation with substrate. Not shown are the response curves of MAb 32 (similar to MAb 34), MAb 2 (similar to MAb 11), MAbs 22 and 33 (intermediate to the responses of MAbs 11 and 4), MAbs 3 and 18 (similar to MAb 1). As noted in the text, further testing is in progress to define the binding region of the alpha fragment.

added in separate wells of the polyclonal antibody-human MT complex. The final binding reaction with an antibody (specific for rat IgG) conjugated to enzyme and followed by substrate cleavage permits detection of the MAb reaction with the alpha fragment; the competitive inhibition of that reaction gives strong indication that an antigenic determinant on the alpha fragment is recognized. This experiment is still in progress, not only for definitive characterization of the alpha fragment specificity but of MAbs with other specificity.

At least three groups of investigators have published findings with MT used as immunogen for MAb production (Masui et al., 1983; Talbot et al., 1986; Kikuchi et al., 1988). Unlike the rat-rat hybridomas described by the author, these reports concern mouse-mouse hybridomas. Unique cross-reactive patterns with MTs and different Ig classes characterize the first report; only the IgM class is described in the other two reports. The results of the third study concern one clone well-characterized in a competitive RIA with synthetic peptides of human MT-2. The authors conclude that the MAb recognizes as an antigenic determinant of MT the amino terminal peptide (residues 1–7) since inhibition is obtained with both the beta domain as a peptide (residues 1–29 in this case) and the mentioned amino terminal peptide. Also, competition was lacking with the carboxyl terminal peptide of residues 29 to 35 and the alpha domain.

Development of the Western Blot Assay

The Western blot is a three-step procedure: (1) resolution of a mixture of proteins (antigens) by gel electrophoresis followed by (2) direct replica transfer to a membrane, and (3) treatment of the membrane with antibody followed by sensitive visualization of the immunological reaction. Of these steps electrophoresis is the most demanding in technical expertise. However, because electrophoresis is a common tool for both physical and biological scientists, the sensitive detection and characterization provided by an immunological reaction is made more readily available to those scientists via the Western blot. Thus, the time commitment should be less than that necessary to master such sensitive immunological assays as the RIA and ELISA. Still, the unique properties of MT (e.g., 20 of the 61 residues in mammalian MTs are cysteine involved in the chelation of 7 divalent metals or 10 to 11 univalent metals) can lead to behavior that imposes challenges to the development of a satisfactory Western blot for the protein (Aoki et al., 1986; Aoki and Suzuki, 1987; Timms and Hagen, 1989; Maiti et al., 1988; Chatterjee and Maiti, 1987; Andersen and Daae, 1988).

Of the two recent developments in electrophoresis of MT that are solutions to anomalous migration of the protein in SDS-PAGE, i.e., either carboxymethylation of the cysteine residues of MT (Otsuka et al., 1988) or use of an optimal concentration of 2-ME in sample preparations (Hidalgo et al., 1988a), the latter was used with 2-ME at 50 mM concentration rather than the usual concentration of 5% in SDS-PAGE (Laemmli, 1970). Isoforms of human MT, prepared in the author's laboratory from autopsied human liver tissue, were Cd-MTs because of the treatment of the cytosol with Cd during the isolation of the MTs. A PAGE gel of the two human MT isoforms, together with synthetic alpha and beta fragments, is shown with silver staining (Figure 4A) and with immunodetection (Figure 4B). Thus the conditions for the Western blot, as optimized in the author's laboratory, have provided an improved procedure for reliable results with MT. Moreover, the Western blot provided further evidence to confirm the experimental demonstration that the polyclonal antibody recognizes continuous

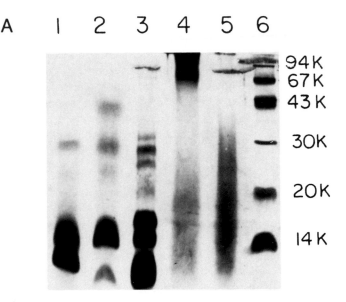

Figure 4. SDS-PAGE electrophoresis of human liver MT isoforms and domain fragments with detection by silver staining and by Western blotting (Lin and Garvey, unpublished results). **4A.** Samples, containing 50 m*M* 2-mercaptoethanol, were pre-heated 5–10 min. in boiling water prior to loading, 1–3 μg/lane, onto a 0.75 mm thick 15% SDS-gel. Separation is shown after 3 h at 150 V in a SE 300 unit (Hoefer Scientific Instruments, San Francisco) that was cooled in tap water. The silver stained samples are: human liver MT-2, preparation II (lane 1); human liver MT-1, preparation II (lane 2); low molecular weight SDS-17 standards (Sigma) (lane 3); synthetic beta fragment (residues 1–30) of human liver MT-2, provided by Dr. Dean Wilcox, Dept. of Chemistry, Dartmouth College (lane 4); synthetic alpha fragment (residues 31–61) of human liver MT-2, also provided by Dr. Dean Wilcox (lane 5); and low molecular weight standards, Pharmacia (lane 6). **4B.** A western blot is shown of a 15% SDS-gel for which electrophoresis was similar to that described in Figure 4A. The samples, shown after electrophoretic transfer [40 V for 3 h to an Immobilon type P membrane (Millipore)] are: the synthetic human MT-2 fragments provided by Dr. Wilcox, alpha (lane 1) and beta (lane 2); human liver MT-1 (lane 3); and human liver MT-2 (lane 4). Prior to the immunodetection procedure [incubation with anti-MT specific polyclonal antibody prepared by Vander Mallie and Garvey, 1978; followed by an incubation with the second antibody, purified goat anti-rabbit IgG conjugated to alkaline phosphatase; followed by detection with the substrate solution that contained 5-bromo-4-chloro-3-indoyl phosphate (BCIP, Sigma), the color enhancer nitroblue tetrazolium (NBT, Sigma) and MgCl$_2$] each of the membranes shown had a different overnight treatment at 4°C to determine the influence of a refolding treatment, i.e., (A) PBS, (B) 125 m*M* 2-ME, and (C) 4 *M* urea. As noted in the section on *Analysis of Antigenic Determinants of MT,* the negligible difference in reaction products found by the three treatments is not unexpected in view of past theoretical structural predictions (Garvey, 1984) and the experimental demonstrations that the polyclonal antibody recognized sequential determinants (Winge and Garvey, 1983).

A   **B**   **C**

1 2 3 4   1 2 3   4   1 2   3   4

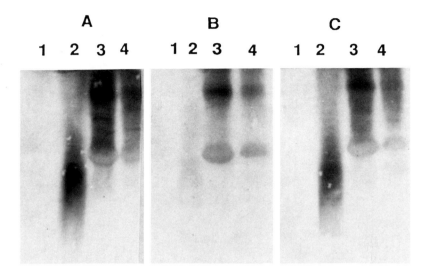

Figure 4. (continued.)

antigenic determinants on the beta domain (Winge and Garvey, 1983; see discussion in section below on *Analysis of Antigenic Determinants of MT*).

Immunocytochemical Localization of MT

There have been numerous studies of MT in tissues based on a reaction with specific antibody and subsequent microscopic detection of the antibody-antigen complex (Hart et al., 1989; Elmes et al., 1989; Clarkson et al., 1985; Banerjee et al., 1982; Nartey et al., 1987; Danielson et al., 1982). The techniques have varied, but like all immunological reactions, the critical reagent is the primary antibody; producing laboratories have commonly provided others with this reagent. The author has provided numerous investigators with the polyclonal antibody and/or MAbs specific in their reactivity with MT as described in previous sections. Thus far, all communications on results obtained by others using these reagents have been highly positive. An example of results obtained by the optimized procedure developed in Dr. Margaret Elmes' laboratory is shown in Figure 5.

UTILIZATION OF THE RIA AND ELISA

Analysis of Antigenic Determinants of MT

Prior to the publication of crystal structure data (Furey et al., 1986) the author developed a theoretical analysis of protein structure and antigenicity

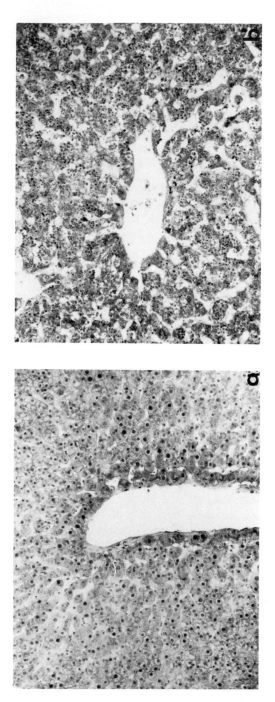

Figure 5. Immunocytochemical localization of MT in human liver. Metallothionein immunoreactivity is demonstrated using the polyclonal anti-MT antibody produced in the author's laboratory and a second antibody staining method (immunoperoxidase, haematoxylin counterstain) developed at the University of Wales College of Medicine (Clarkson et al., 1985). (a) Normal human liver. Cytoplasmic and nuclear immunostaining of MT is present in liver cells with a perivenular accentuation of the cytoplasmic staining. (b) Fetal human liver, gestation 22 wks. The cytoplasm of all liver cells is uniformly immunostained for MT. Primitive blood cell nuclei stained with hematoxylin are prominent. (c) Diagnostic liver biopsy from a case of untreated Wilson's disease. Strong immunostaining of clusters of surviving liver cells is prominent against a background of chronic inflammation. (d) Diagnostic liver biopsy from the same case of Wilson's disease after 1 year of penicillamine therapy. Regenerated liver cells showing near normal MT immunostaining are seen in focal areas of chronic inflammation. (Photomicrographs [original magnification ×125) and histology/pathology assessment courtesy of M.E. Elmes and B. Jasani.)

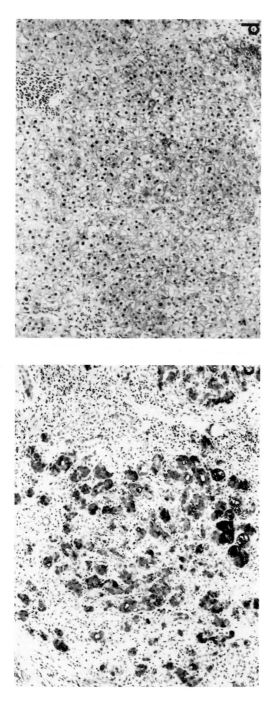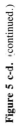

Figure 5 c-d. (continued.)

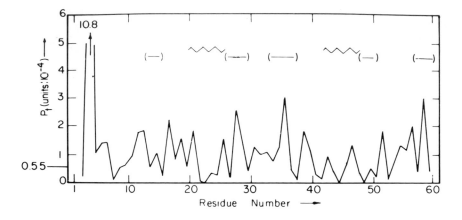

Figure 6. Secondary structure profile of human MT-2. Probabilities P_t for sequential tetra-peptides to form a reverse turn are plotted with values indicated at the center of each tetra-peptide; calculations are based on the protocols of Chou and Fasman (Chou and Fasman, 1977, 1978; Fasman, 1980). The average value for P_t from their analysis of 29 proteins is 0.55×10^{-4}. Also indicated are candidate beta chains (——) and helices (∿∿) predicted by the same protocols. Various boundary conditions and secondary conditions make the stable existence of the candidate chains and helices unlikely. (Adapted from Garvey, 1984.)

for application to the MT molecule (Garvey, 1984). The analysis was based on the protocols of Chou and Fasman (Chou and Fasman, 1977, 1978; Fasman, 1980) for predicting secondary structure from sequence information and of Hopp and Woods (1981) for predicting hydrophilic regions of high probability of acting as principal antigenic sites. All mammalian MTs were predicted to have no stable alpha or beta structure and to exist primarily as reverse turns and random coils (Figure 6). The regions of high probability to act as principal antigenic sites included the invariant amino terminal residues 1 to 7, the series of residues 20–25, and residues 42 to 46 and 52 to 58. Experiments confirmed the first two mentioned sites as the principal determinants of MT (Winge and Garvey, 1983); the alpha domain, residues 31 to 61, has consistently been shown to be of minimal antigenicity with respect to the polyclonal antibody, indicating the influence of neighboring hydrophobicity and tertiary conformation (Winge and Garvey, 1983; Winge et al., 1986). Confirmation of these findings with respect to the principal determinants of MT comes from a report by Japanese investigators (Kikuchi et al., 1988). They produced a MAb of IgM class and studied its binding to various synthetic human MT peptides. They found binding only by the invariant amino terminal heptapeptide and by the beta fragment (residues 1 to 29 in this case) and not by peptides of the alpha domain. All the sub-sequent findings by others regarding mammalian MT structure as determined by x-ray crystallography (Furey et al., 1986) and by spectroscopic analyses

(Otvos et al., 1987; Vašák, 1986) support the immunological findings and the central concepts expressed above. The study of MT crystal structure has shown that the two domains have limited contact and that the charged residues in positions 20, 22, and 25 (lysines in the case of human MT) may be in proximity to the amino terminus in solution (Furey et al., 1986). This possibility has been particularly prominent in the reports of the Scripps protein group (Getzoff et al., 1988) concerning antibodies as catalytic "enzyme" reagents and suggesting that antigenic determinants are associated with a moving boundary of the protein structure. Mobility of the residues of an antigenic determinant, such as might characterize reverse turns, has also been emphasized by others (Westhof et al., 1984) as well as by the Scripps group (Tainer et al., 1984). With respect to spectroscopic studies it has been demonstrated that the beta domain is characterized by very high kinetic properties of the bound metals, orders of magnitude higher than kinetic properties in the alpha domain (Otvos et al., 1987). This complements the studies associating mobility with antigenicity and supports the experimental finding of the immunodominance of the beta domain. Studies have also revealed that folding as a structural feature of the MT molecule is little affected by metal binding (Vašák, 1986). This has significance in that the polyclonal antibody probe binds equally well to the apoprotein or to MTs with varying degrees of metal chelation (Winge and Garvey, 1983; Laib et al., 1985) and with different metals chelated (Garvey, 1982).

MT as a Biomarker of Metal Toxicity

The complete immunological cross-reactivity of mammalian MTs when precipitated with the polyclonal antibody was an early and important finding. In the case of sequenced human MT provided by Dr. J.H.R. Kägi, this led to a standardization of the RIA and an immediate utilization of the assay for MT quantitation in urine (Chang et al., 1980; Roels et al., 1983; Falck et al., 1983; Nordberg et al., 1982) and in serum (Falck et al., 1983; Nordberg et al., 1982) of occupational groups exposed to cadmium. Various other assays designed to assess MT and metal status in chronic occupational cadmium exposure leading to impaired renal function were performed at the discretion of the laboratories providing the samples for subsequent analysis by RIA by the author. The focus on MT in urine and serum was encouraged by the potential value of MT as a non-invasive biological monitor of toxicities due to heavy metal exposure, particularly those associated with cadmium. A very significant relationship was found between log Cd and log MT in urine (Figure 7). As a corollary to these investigations involving MT in human physiological fluids a survey was made providing data on normal levels of MT in urine and serum (Garvey, 1984). The typical range for normal serums is from 0.01 ng/ml to 1 ng/ml; concentrations above 2 ng/

ml should be considered abnormal. The typical range for normal urines is from less than 1 ng/ml to 10 ng/ml; concentrations above 10 ng/ml should be considered abnormal. MT levels are orders of magnitude higher in liver and kidney cytosols.

The influence of extended exposure to cadmium in the environment is shown in an RIA of liver tissue taken at autopsy from a worker in a battery factory who had developed metastatic carcinoma originating in the lung. MT levels in the liver tissue were 20-fold higher than levels in normal liver tissue assayed at the same time (Garry et al., 1986). In co-investigations with Dr. Beth Hart, University of Vermont, determinations were made of MT content in cell isolates from lung tissues of rats exposed by Dr. Hart

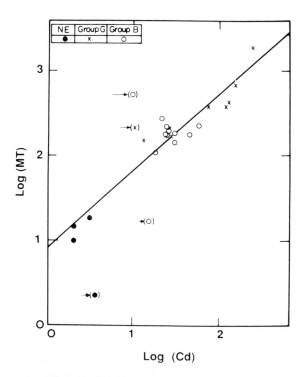

Figure 7. Relation between MT and Cd in urine of Cd-exposed workers. Analysis of RIA data relating MT and Cd concentrations in urine of Cd-exposed and non-exposed humans. MT and Cd concentrations are expressed in μg/g creatinine in urine. NE indicates nonexposed; exposed subjects are from two differing occupational environments, G and B. The regression (20 responses) has a correlation coefficient of 0.962; 4 variant respones (arrows) are not included. (Adapted from Garvey, 1982.)

to cadmium aerosols (Hart and Garvey, 1986). MT levels in alveolar macrophages rose dramatically with increased exposure and suggest that MT synthesis followed by Cd sequestration is responsible in part for the adaptive response of the lung to Cd exposure. A related study on the effect of exposure of rats to high oxygen levels gives support to the proposed role of MT as an intracellular defense mechanism during periods of oxidative stress (Hart et al., 1989).

Analyses have been performed on physiological fluids of patients treated with proprietary drugs, e.g., auranofin (a gold compound) and cis-platin (a platinum compound), in which the metal is the principal agent for successful treatment and also the presumed agent for subsequent toxicities. One study involved equine MTs with varying amounts of chelated gold to determine changes in binding to the polyclonal antibody (Laib et al., 1985); a slight increase in affinity was observed as gold content increased, indicating that the antibody is heteroclitic. Another study involved cell lines developed by Dr. Anne Glennas (Norway) to investigate the role of MT in response to the use of the gold compound, auranofin, in treatment of rheumatoid arthritis (Glennas et al., 1986). The MT content in epithelial cell lines made resistant to cadmium was significantly enhanced as was also the case with auranofin-treated cells. A study of platinum MTs was initiated by questions concerning the toxic reactions at times encountered when cis-diamminedichloroplatinum (cis-DDP or cis-platin) is used in treatment of tumors. It was determined that Pt-MT is formed via substitution of Pt for Zn or Cd in existing MTs rather than by directly inducing MT and that cellular mechanisms vary in the response to the cis or trans form of the compound (Zelazowski et al., 1984).

MT as a Biomarker of Genetic Disease and of Tumors

It is noted that several studies on this subject are still in progress. MT has been studied in certain genetic diseases to ascertain its possible role in the faulty metal metabolism associated with these pathologies. An example is Wilson's disease in which faulty copper metabolism is a universal characteristic as is the pathology of the liver; this is seen in Figure 5, illustrating the technique of immunocytochemical localization. MT levels in both serum and urine have been determined by RIA by the author, contributing to a study in which clinical data will be correlated with diagnosed and undiagnosed Wilson's disease in members of pedigreed families; the clinical site of this patient group is the University of Utah Medical School.

Patients with spina bifida (faulty zinc metabolism) have been found to have increased serum MT and Zn levels compared to their age and sex matched controls (Zimmerman et al., 1985). MT was found to be present at a greatly increased level compared to normal levels in a cell line established from a Menkes' disease patient (faulty Cu metabolism). There was no altered uptake and/or change in the transport kinetics of the metal as might be expected if MT functions in a protective role (a conclusion communicated by Dr. Murray Ettinger, University of Buffalo Medical School; the author provided the MT results). The presence of MT has been shown convincingly in the mouse Ehrlich cell ascites tumor, the results derived from an *in vivo* model for the study of the associated Zn deficiency and arrested cell metabolism (Kraker et al., 1988). And the finding of MT in tumors of lung tissue has led to an hypothesis that MT is a potential biomarker for tumors of the lung (unpublished data from an investigation with Dr. Beth Hart, University of Vermont Medical School).

It may be concluded from these studies that the association of MT with abnormal metabolism is a curious rather than a profound one. However, this conclusion is not likely to persist if the interrelationship of metals and MT levels in the normal metabolism of the cell, e.g., in the hepatocyte, is made a targeted goal of future study.

Assays of MT in Fetal/Maternal Tissues

It has long been known from studies of cadmium exposure in the environment that levels of MT and Cd in tissues and fluids are both sex-dependent and age-dependent, although correlations are not as obvious as in the MT and Cd relationship shown in Figure 7. And as shown in Figure 5, almost every cell of the fetal human liver not only demonstrated MT but at an enhanced concentration compared to that found more discreetly confined (perivenular) in the adult. In a recent investigation (Hart et al., 1990), levels of MT were studied by RIA in post-natal lung tissues of rats and shown to be increased about 4-fold over the adult levels; a dramatic decline in concentration to the normal adult level occurred within several days following birth. The author assayed MT by RIA in cytosols from tissues of lactating mice prepared in the laboratory of Dr. M. Bhattacharrya, Argonne National Laboratories. Liver, kidneys and duodenum showed a heightened MT level that was specific for the lactation period. A manuscript has been submitted (Solaiman et al., 1991) with the results (protein values). Dr. Bhattacharrya has communicated to the author that MT mRNA measured in the total liver RNA shows the same relative level as the protein values for similar days of lactation and weaning.

Role of MT in Psychogenic Stress and in Response to Hormones

A major series of experiments involving MT in response to stress in rats and the influence of various hormones on the response was performed in collaboration with scientists at the Universidad Autonoma, Barcelona,

Spain. Typically, cytosols and physiological fluids prepared in Spain were then assayed by RIA or ELISA by the author. The studies included the relation of MT synthesis and transport and metal levels in conditions of stress (restraint, food/water deprivation), as a function of sex, age, and pregnancy, and as influenced by glucocorticoids, glucagon, catecholamines, corticosterone, and endogenous opioids (Hidalgo et al., 1986a,b, 1987a,b, 1988a–e; Armario et al., 1987). The results confirm that simple restraint is a principal inducer of MT in liver, that adrenergic blockade has minimal effect on MT production during restraint, that endogenous opioids are involved in MT regulation *in vivo* and that MT is a multi-regulated protein. Glucocorticoids were found not essential to MT induction during stress. Chronic stress produced a significant increase in serum MT in prepuberal rats, an indication of an age-related response. Acute treatment with ACTH reduced MT response to stress, indicating an inhibitory effect of glucocorticoids on liver MT regulation. The glucocorticoid, corticosterone, specifically has an inhibitory role in this respect. The results challenge some popular views concerning glucocorticoid influence on MT induction and emphasize that the process of hormonal control of induction of MT in liver by stress is unclear at this writing.

MT as a Biomonitor of Environmental Pollution by Metals and Other Agents

The biological role of MT appears to involve the responsiveness of a species to not only metals but to stress factors, e.g., crowding and temperature. MT may then serve as a biomonitor of environmental changes affecting endogenous species. In a study of tissue cytosols from feral moose and reindeer in Sweden, it was found that MT levels increased with age, reflecting the longer exposure to cadmium in the environment (Wikner et al., 1988). Clearly, the polyclonal antibody can serve as a probe of other toxin-exposed feral mammalian species. In the case of non-mammalian species, little attention has thus far been afforded to development of antibody probes for detection of other candidate biomonitors, e.g., the MT-like molecules designated class II and class III (Kägi and Kojima, 1987b). That detection of these molecules requires development of specific probes has a significant source in the attention afforded in the period 1980 to 1988 to the analyses by the author's laboratory using the RIA and ELISA in studies oriented on whether the isolates of various metal-binding proteins were reactive with the polyclonal antibody and thus might be MTs or candidate MTs. Included were proteins from mammals and other vertebrates, invertebrates, micro-organisms and plants. A rather imposing amount of information has been cataloged to show that the antigenic determinants recognized by the polyclonal antibody are the invariant amino terminal residues of mammalian MTs and those of the region of residues 20–25 (Winge and Garvey, 1983; Winge et al., 1986). Non-mammalian MTs which do not exhibit these determinants have been uniformly minimally reactive or non-reactive in the RIA and ELISA. Species studied and reported upon include *Salmo gairdneri* (Kay et al., 1986), *Ostrea lutaria* and *Crassotrea glomerata* (Nordberg et al., 1986), *Euglena gracilis* (Gingrich et al., 1986), *Placopecten magellanicus* (Fowler et al., 1988) and chicken (McCormick et al., 1988). Species studied at the request of other investigators and found minimally or non-reactive and not yet reported upon include *Crassotrea virginica, Callianassa tyrhena, Scylla serrata, Pleuronectes platessa, Drosophila melanogaster, Mytilus edulis, Neurospora crassa*, and *Agrostis gigantea*. This body of negative data on non-mammalian species emphasizes the power of immunological detection with respect to specificity, whereas the body of positive data on mammalian species, especially in the quantitation of serum MT (Garvey and Chang, 1981; Garvey, 1984), emphasizes the sensitivity of the polyclonal antibody in its reaction with the unique structural features of mammalian MTs. This encourages the production of a panel of species-specific MTs to serve as environmental biomonitors, the prototypic MTs drawn from all three classes of metal-binding proteins designated by Kägi and Kojima (1987b). In addition to detection/quantitation the collected data should contribute to elucidation of aspects of evolutionary development and of the role of these molecules in cellular metabolism.

SUMMARY COMMENTS

The immunological methods described in this paper provide investigators of the properties, functions, and potential applications of metallothionein with a spectrum of research tools of demonstrated utility and importance. The principal assays thus far developed for quantitation of the protein (RIA, ELISA) have been successfully applied to accurate analysis of MT in cytosols and physiological fluids of mammalian species; these immunological methods have proven particularly useful in quantitation of MT in normal serum. Immunocytochemical studies are beginning to provide critical information concerning MT in cellular processes; continued analyses promise to clarify numerous basic uncertainties about MT metabolism and transport. The Western blot promises to become a useful method for relatively rapid assessment and characterization of MT, especially when used in conjunction with cross-disciplinary studies (biochemical, molecular-biological, physiological, and toxicological). The demonstrated utility of the polyclonal antibodies thus far developed should receive significant complementation from the increasing production of monoclonal antibodies. Practical applications of the immunological methods mentioned have included quantiation of MT in tissues and fluids of humans and other mammals, including feral species, exposed to metals of toxic potential (particularly cadmium, gold, and platinum), of humans suffering metal-associated diseases (Wilson's disease, Menkes' disease, tumors), and of animals exposed to stress and toxic environments. The methods have been used to establish that certain candidate MTs (metal-thiolate polypeptides) from various invertebrates, micro-organisms and plants were either not MTs or were of sequence distinctly variant from that of mammalian MTs. This latter capability suggests that the development of antibody probes specific for a particular species has utility not only for application in assessment of environmental toxins and stresses as these impact feral species but also for application in studies of evolutionary development. Such a program might be initiated with the production of antibody probes, each specific for a prototypic member of a closely related group (aquatic, avian, plant), the family of probes including individuals with specificity for all three classes (I, II, III) of metal-thiolate polypeptides.

ACKNOWLEDGMENTS

The word processing expertise of Joyce Cattelane and funding by NIEHS are gratefully acknowledged. David Campanille, M.D., is thanked for contributing to the preparation of human liver MT isoforms.

REFERENCES

Andersen RA and Daae HL (1988): Preparation of metallothionein from rat liver and studies of its properties with respect to use as a standard in gel permeation chromatography, polyacrylamide gel systems, autoradiography and western blotting. *Comp. Biochem. Physiol.* 90B: 59.

Aoki Y, Kunimoto M, Shibata Y, and Suzuki KT (1986): Detection of metallothionein in nitrocellulose membrane using Western blotting technique and its application to identification of cadmium-binding proteins. *Anal. Biochem.* 157: 117.

Aoki Y and Suzuki KT (1987): Characterization of cadmium-binding proteins detected in rat liver by the Western blotting technique. *J. Biochem. Toxicol.* 2: 67.

Armario A, Hidalgo J, Bas J, Restrepo C, Dingman A, and Garvey JS (1987): Age-dependent effects of acute and chronic intermittent stresses on serum metallothionein. *Physiol. Behav.* 39: 277.

Banerjee D, Onosaka S, and Cherian MG (1982): Immunohistochemical localization of metallothionein in cell nucleus and cytoplasm of rat liver and kidney. *Toxicol.* 24: 95.

Bazin H, Cormont F, and De Clerq L (1986): Purification of rat monoclonal antibodies. *Meth. Enzymol.* 121: 638.

Brady FO and Kafka RL (1983): Radioimmunoassay of rat liver metallothionein. *Anal. Biochem.* 98: 89.

Chang CC, Lauwerys R, Bernard A, Roels H, Buchet JP, and Garvey JS (1980): Metallothionein in cadmium-exposed workers. *Environ. Res.* 23: 422.

Chatterjee A and Maiti IB (1987): Purification and immunological characterization of catfish (*Heteropneustes fossilis*) metallothionein. *Mol. Cell. Biochem.* 78: 55.

Chou PY and Fasman GD (1977): β-turns in proteins. *J. Mol. Biol.* 116: 135.

Chou PY and Fasman GD (1978): Prediction of the secondary structure of proteins from their amino acid sequence. *Adv. Enzymol.* 47: 45.

Clarkson JP, Elmes ME, Jasani B, and Webb M (1985): Histological demonstration of immunoreactive zinc metallothionein in liver and ileum of rat and man. *Histochem. J.* 17: 343.

Danielson KG, Ohi S, and Huang PC (1982): Immunochemical detection of metallothionein in specific epithelial cells of rat organs. *Proc. Nat. Acad. Sci. U.S.A.* 79: 2301.

De Clerq L, Cormont F, and Bazin H (1986): Generation of rat-rat hybridomas with the use of the LOU 1R983F nonsecreting fusion cell line. *Meth. Enzymol.* 121: 234.

Dieter HH, Muller L, Abel J, and Summer KH (1987): Metallothionein-determination in biological materials: interlaboratory comparison of 5 current methods. *Op. Cit.* (Kägi and Kojima, 1987a), p. 351.

Elmes ME, Clarkson JP, Mahy NJ, and Jasani B (1989): Metallothionein and copper in liver disease with copper retention—a histopathological study. *J. Pathol.* 158: 131.

Falck FY, Fine LJ, Smith RG, Garvey JS, Schork AM, England BG, McClatchey KD, and Linton HJ (1983): Metallothionein and occupational exposure to cadmium. *Brit. J. Ind. Med.* 40: 305.

Fasman GD (1980): Prediction of protein conformation from the primary structure. *Ann. N.Y. Acad. Sci.* 348: 147.

Fowler BA, Gould E, Garvey JS, and Bakewell WE (1988): Comparative studies on the 45,000 Dalton cadmium-binding protein (45K CdBP) from the Scallop, *Placopecten Magellanicus*: immunological properties and copper competition studies. In, Roesijadi B and Spies RB, Eds., *Marine Environmental Research, Vol. 24,* Elsevier Applied Science, Essex, England, p. 141.

Furey WF, Robbins AH, Clancy LI, Winge DR, Wang BC, and Stout CD (1986): Crystal structure of Cd, Zn metallothionein. *Science* 231: 704.

Garry VF, Pohlman BL, Wick MR, Garvey JS, and Zeisler R (1986): Chronic cadmium intoxication: tissue response in an occupationally exposed patient. *Am. J. Indust. Med.* 10: 153.

Garvey JS and Chang CC (1981): Detection of circulating metallothionein in rats injected with zinc or cadmium. *Science* 241: 805.

Garvey JS (1982): The application of a radioimmunoassay for sensitive detection of metallothionein (thionein) in physiologic fluids of humans and rats. In, Porter GA Ed., *Nephrotoxic Mechanisms of Drugs and Environmental Toxins,* Plenum, New York, p. 437.

Garvey JS, Vander Mallie RJ, and Chang CC (1982): Radioimmunoassay of metallothioneins. *Meth. Enzymol.* 84: 121.

Garvey JS (1984): Metallothionein: structure/antigenicity and detection/quantitation in normal physiological fluids. *Environ. Health Perspect.* 54: 117.

Garvey JS (1989): Metallothionein: a potential biomonitor of exposure to environmental toxins. In, Shugart LR and McCarthy JF, Eds., *Biological Markers of Environmental Contaminants* (ACS Symposium Proceedings, Los Angeles, 25-30 Sept. 1988). Lewis, p. 267.

Getzoff ED, Tainer JA, Lerner RA, and Geysen HM (1988): The chemistry and mechanism of antibody binding to protein antigens. *Adv. Immunol.* 43: 1.

Gingrich DJ, Weber DN, Shaw CF, Garvey JS, and Petering DH (1986): Characterization of a highly negative and labile binding protein induced in *Euglena gracilis* by cadmium. *Environ. Health Perspect.* 65: 77.

Glennas A, Hunziker PE, Garvey JS, Kägi JHR, and Rugstad HE (1986): Metallothionein in cultured human epithelial cells and synovial rheumatoid fibroblasts after *in vitro* treatment with auranofin. *Biochem. Pharmacol.* 35: 2033.

Grider A, Kao K-J, Klein PA, and Cousins RJ (1989): Enzyme-linked immunosorbent assay for human metallothionein: correlation of induction with infection. *J. Lab. Clin. Med.* 113: 221.

Hart BA and Garvey JS (1986): Detection of metallothionein in bronchoalveolar cells and lavage fluid following repeated cadmium inhalation. *Environ. Res.* 40: 391.

Hart BA, Voss GW, and Garvey JS (1989): Induction of pulmonary metallothionein following oxygen exposure. *Environ. Res.* 50: 269.

Hart BA, Voss GW, and Garvey JS (1990): Native metallothionein in rat lung during postnatal development. *Biol. Neonate* 59: 236.

Hidalgo J, Armario A, Flos R, Dingman A, and Garvey JS (1986a): The influence of restraint stress in rats on metallothionein production and corticosterone and glucagon secretion. *Life Sci.* 39: 611.

Hidalgo J, Armario A, Flos R, and Garvey JS (1986b): Restraint stress-induced changes in rat liver and serum metallothionein and in zinc metabolism. *Experientia* 42: 1006.

Hidalgo J, Garvey JS, and Armario A (1987a): The role of catecholamines and glucagon on serum and liver metallothionein in response to restraint stress. *Rev. Esp. Fisiol.* 43: 433.

Hidalgo J, Giralt M, Garvey JS, and Armario A (1987b): Sex and restraint stress differences in rat metallothionein and Zn levels. *Rev. Esp. Fisiol.* 43: 427.

Hidalgo J, Bernues J, Thomas DG, and Garvey JS (1988a): Effect of 2-mercaptoethanol on the electrophoretic behavior of rat and dogfish metallothionein and chromatographic evidence of a naturally occurring metallothionein polymerization. *Comp. Biochem. Physiol.* 89C: 191.

Hidalgo J, Campmany L, Borras M, Garvey JS, and Armario A (1988b): Metallothionein response to stress in rats: role in free radical scavenging. *Am. J. Physiol.* 255: E518.

Hidalgo J, Giralt M, Garvey JS, and Armario A (1988c): Are catecholamines positive regulators of metallothionein synthesis during stress in the rat? *Horm. Metabol. Res.* 20: 530.

Hidalgo J, Giralt M, Garvey JS, and Armario A (1988d): Physiological role of glucocorticoids in basal and stress conditions. *Am. J. Physiol.* 254: E71.

Hidalgo J, Giralt M, Garvey JS, and Armario A (1988e): Differences between pregnant and nulliparous rats in basal and stress levels of metallothionein. *Biol. Neonate* 53: 148.

Hopp TP and Woods KR (1981): Prediction of protein antigenic determinants from amino acid sequences. *Proc. Nat. Acad. Sci. U.S.A.* 78: 3824.

Kägi JHR and Kojima Y, Eds. (1987a): *Metallothionein II (Experientia Suppl.* 52), Birkhäuser-Verlag, Basel, pp. 755.

Kägi JHR and Kojima Y (1987b): Chemistry and biochemistry of metallothionein. In *Op. Cit.* (Kägi and Kojima, 1987a), p. 25.

Kay J, Thomas DG, Brown MW, Cryer A, Shurben D, Solbe JF del G, and Garvey JS (1986): Cadmium accumulation and protein binding patterns in tissues of the rainbow trout, *Salmo gairdneri*. *Environ. Health Perspect.* 65: 133.

Kikuchi Y, Wada N, Irie M, Ikebuchi H, Sawada J-I, Terao T, Nakayama S, Iguchi S, and Okada Y (1988): A murine monoclonal anti-metallothionein autoantibody recognizes a chemically synthesized amino-terminal heptapeptide common to various animal metallothioneins. *Mol. Immunol.* 25: 1033.

Kraker AJ, Krakower G, Shaw III CF, Petering DH, and Garvey JS (1988): Zinc metabolism in Ehrlich cells: Properties of a metallothionein-like zinc-binding protein. *Cancer Res.* 48: 3381.

Laemmli UK (1970): Cleavage of structural proteins during the assembly of the head of bacteriophage T4. *Nature* 227: 681.

Laib JE, Shaw III CF, Petering DH, Eidsness MK, Elder RC, and Garvey JS (1985): Formation and characterization of aurothioneins: Au, Zn, Cd-Thionein, Au, Cd-Thionein, and (Thiomalato-Au)$_x$-thionein. *Biochem.* 24: 1977.

Maiti IB, Hunt AG, and Wagner GJ (1988): Seed-transmissible expression of mammalian metallothionein in transgenic tobacco. *Biochem. Biophys. Res. Commun.* 150: 640.

Masui T, Utakoji T, and Kimura M (1983): Monoclonal antibodies to metallothionein from Cd^{2+}-resistant Chinese hamster lung fibroblasts. *Experientia* 39: 182.

McCormick CC, Fullmer CS, and Garvey JS (1988): Amino acid sequence and comparative antigenicity of chicken metallothionein. *Proc. Nat. Acad. Sci. U.S.A.* 85: 309.

Mehra RK and Bremner I (1983): Development of a radioimmunoassay for rat liver metallothionein-I and its application to the analysis of rat plasma and kidneys. *Biochem. J.* 213: 459.

Nartey N, Cherian MG, and Banerjee D (1987): Immunohistochemical localization of metallothionein in human thyroid tumors. *Am. J. Pathol.* 129: 177.

Nolan CV and Shaikh ZA (1986): Determination of metallothionein in tissues by radioimmunoassay and by cadmium saturation method, *Anal. Biochem.* 154: 213.

Nordberg GF, Garvey JS, and Chang CC (1982): Metallothionein in plasma and urine of cadmium workers. *Environ. Res.* 28: 179.

Nordberg M, Nuottaniemi I, Cherian MG, Nordberg GF, Kjellstrom T, and Garvey JS (1986): Characterization studies on the cadmium-binding proteins from two species of New Zealand oysters. *Environ. Health Perspect.* 65: 57.

Otsuka F, Koizumi S, Kimura M, and Ahsawa M (1988): Silver staining for carboxymethylated metallothioneins in polyacrylamide gels. *Anal. Biochem.* 168: 184.

Otvos JD, Engeseth HR, Nettesheim DG, and Hilt CR (1987): Interprotein metal exchange reactions of metallothionein. In *Op. Cit.,* Kägi and Kojima, 1987a, p. 171.

Rodbard D, Rayford PL, Cooper JA, and Ross GT (1968): Statistical quality control of radioimmunoassays, *J. Clin. Endocrinol.* 28: 1412.

Rodbard D and Lewald JE (1970): Computer analysis of radioligand assay and radioimmunoassay data. *Acta Endocrinol.* (Copenhagen) 64 (Suppl. 147), 79.

Rodbard D (1971): Statistical aspects of radioimmunoassay. In, Odell WD and Daughaday WH, Eds., *Competitive Protein Binding Assays.* Lippincott, Philadelphia, p. 204.

Rodbard D (1974): Statistical quality control and routine data processing for radioimmunoassays and immunoradiometric assays. *Clin. Chem.* 20: 1255.

Rodbard D, Lenox RH, Wray HL, and Ramseth D (1976): Statistical characterization of the random errors in the radioimmunoassay dose-response variable. *Clin. Chem.* 22: 350.

Roels H, Lauwerys R, Buchet JP, Bernard A, Garvey JS, and Linton HJ (1983): Significance of urinary metallothionein in workers exposed to cadmium. *Int. Arch. Occup. Environ. Health* 52: 159.

Solaiman D, Bhattacharrya MH, Miyazaki W, and Garvey JS (1991): Lactation-specific increases in metallothionein contents of mouse liver, kidneys, and duodenum. *Eur. J. Biochem. Tox., submitted.*

Tainer JA, Getzoff ED, Alexander H, Houghten RA, Olson AJ, Lerner RE, and Hendrickson WA (1984): The reactivity of anti-peptide antibodies is a function of the atomic mobility of sites in a protein. *Nature* 312: 127.

Talbot BG, Bilodeau G, and Thirian J-P (1986): Monoclonal antibodies against metallothioneins and metalloproteins. *Mol. Immunol.* 23: 1133.

Thomas DG, Linton HJ, and Garvey JS (1986): Fluorometric ELISA for the detection and quantitation of metallothionein. *J. Immunol. Meth.* 89: 239.

Timms BG and Hagen JA (1989): Immunohistochemical localization of metallothionein in the rat prostate gland during postnatal development. *The Prostate* 14: 367.

Tohyama C and Shaikh ZA (1981): Metallothionein in plasma and urine of cadmium-exposed rats determined by a single-antibody radioimmunoassay. *Fund. Appl. Toxicol.* 1: 1.

Vander Mallie RJ and Garvey JS (1978): Production and study of antibody produced against rat cadmium thionein. *Immunochem.* 15: 857.

Vander Mallie RJ and Garvey JS (1979): Radioimmunoassay of metallothioneins. *J. Biol. Chem.* 254: 8416.

van Heyningen V (1986): A simple method for ranking the affinities of monoclonal antibodies. *Meth. Enzymol.* 121: 472.

Van Regenmortel MHV (1988): Solid phase immunoassays. In, Regenmortel MHV, Briand JP, Muller S, and Plaue S, Eds., *Synthetic Polypeptides as Antigens,* Elsevier, New York, p. 145.

Vašák M (1986): The spatial structure of metallothionein—a feat of spectroscopy. In, Bertini I, Luchinat C, Maret W, and Zeppezauer M, Eds., *Progress in Inorganic Biochemistry and Biophysics, Vol. I, Zinc Enzymes,* Birkhäuser-Verlag, Basel, p. 595.

Waalkes MP, Garvey JS, and Klaassen CD (1985): Comparison of methods of metallothionein quantification: cadmium radioassay, mercury radioassay, and radioimmunoassay. *Toxicol. Appl. Pharmacol.* 79: 524.

Westhof E, Altschuh D, Moras D, Bloomer AC, Mondragon A, Klug A, and Van Regenmortel MHV (1984): Correlation between segmental mobility and the location of antigenic determinants in proteins. *Nature* 311: 123.

Wikner M, Nordberg GF, Nordberg M, and Garvey JS (1988): Copper and cadmium binding proteins from liver and kidney of moose and reindeer. *Arctic Med. Res.* 47: 179.

Winge DR and Garvey JS (1983): Antigenicity of metallothionein. *Proc. Nat. Acad. Sci. U.S.A.* 80: 2472.

Winge DR, Gray WR, Zelazowski A, and Garvey JS (1986): Sequence and antigenicity of calf metallothionein II. *Arch. Biochem. Biophys.* 245: 254.

Zelazowski AW, Garvey JS, and Hoeschele JD (1984): *In vivo* and *in vitro* binding of platinum to metallothionein. *Arch. Biochem. Biophys.* 229: 246.

Zimmerman AW, Garvey JS, Banta JV, and Horak E (1985): Urinary zinc and metallothionein in children with spina bifida. *Pediatric Neurol.* 1: 23.

Chapter 4

Chemistry of Mammalian Metallothionein

Jeremias H.R. Kägi and Milan Vašák
Institute of Biochemistry
University of Zurich
Zurich, Switzerland

INTRODUCTION

Metallothionein (MT) is a generic term for a variety of cysteine-rich, metal-containing polypeptides (Kägi and Vallee, 1960; Kägi and Kojima, 1987) which are believed to play essential roles in regulating the intracellular concentrations of the ionic forms of Zn and Cu and in protecting cells and organisms against the harmful influences of toxic elements such as Cd and Hg.

DEFINITION AND CLASSIFICATION

The classical mammalian forms have been characterized as having a molecular weight of 6000 to 7000 Da containing some 60 amino acid residues, among them 20 Cys, and binding a total of seven equivs of divalent metal ions. Aromatic amino acids are absent. All Cys occur in the reduced form and are coordinated to the metal ions through mercaptide bonds, giving rise to spectroscopic features characteristic of metal-thiolate clusters. In view of these conspicuous compositional and physicochemical features, the Committee on the Nomenclature of Metallothionein has recommended that any protein or polypeptide resembling mammalian MTs in several of these criteria be named an MT (Fowler et al., 1987). By considering structural differences, this phenomenologically defined "superfamily" of MTs is subdivided into three classes. Class I includes mammalian MTs and MTs from other phyla with related primary structure. Class II comprises MTs lacking such correspondence. Class III subsumes atypical polypeptides containing repetitive γ-glutamyl cysteinyl units. Representative examples are given in Figure 1.

AMINO ACID SEQUENCES

Following our early sequence studies in equine MT, the primary structure of over 80 MTs has now been determined, either completely or in part. The most conspicuous structural feature of all forms is the occurrence of multiple Cys-X-Cys tripeptide sequences, where X stands for an amino acid residue other than Cys. The hallmark of the class I MTs is the correspondence in the alignment of Cys along the chain (Figure 1). In the 37 mammalian MT structures known, 56% of all residues are totally conserved in evolution. They include all 20 Cys and nearly all Lys (or Arg), pointing to crucial roles of these residues. Most amino acid substitutions are conservative both with respect to the chemical and the space-filling properties of the residues. 60% of the substitutions are located in the amino-terminal half of the protein (residues 1–30), indicating fewer evolutionary constraints on this portion of the chain (Kägi and Kojima, 1987). No obvious sequence relationships are discernible among members of class II MTs (Figure 1). An interesting case is sea urchin MT which has nearly the same abundance of Cys-X-Cys and of Cys-Cys sequences as the mammalian MTs but with a reversed arrangement of these segments within the chain (Nemer et al., 1985). We attribute this skewed structural correspondence to convergent evolution imposed by the requirements of metal complexation and other as yet unidentified functional constraints. The class III MTs thus far characterized are homologous, atypical oligo- and polypeptides of the general structure $(\gamma Glu-Cys)_n X$, where $n = 2-8$ and X being most often Gly or β-alanine (Figure 1). They are homologs of glutathione or homoglutathione and are generated in tissues and cell cultures of higher plants and certain eukaryotic microorganisms exposed to heavy metal salts (Grill et al., 1986a; Reese et al., 1988).

METAL-BINDING SITES

The abundance of Cys predisposes MT for binding of "soft" metal ions through thiolate coordination. In mammalian MTs the 20 Cys collectively

Class I

	1[b]	20	40	60	
Human (MT-2)[c]	MDP	NCSCAAGDSCTCAGSCKCKECKCTSCKKSCCSCCPVGCAKCAQGCICKGASD		KCSCCA	Kissling & Kägi, 1977
Pigeon (MT-2)	MDPQDCTCAAGDSCSCAGSCKCKNCRCQSCRKSCCSCCPASCSNCAKGCVCKEPSSSKCSCCH				Lin et al., 1990
Trout (tMT-B)	MDP	CECSKTGSCNCGGSCKCSNCACTSCKKSCCPCCPSDCSKCASGCVCKGKTC	DTSCCQ		Bonham et al., 1987
Crab (MT-2)	PDP	C C NDKCDCKEGECKTGCKCTSCRCPPCEQCSSGC	KCANKEDCRKICSKPCSCCP		Lerch et al., 1982
Fungus		GDCGCSGASSCNCGSGCSCSNCGSK			Lerch, 1979

Class II

	1	20	40	60	
Sea urchin (Mtb)	MPDVKCVCCKEGNECACTGQDCCTIGKCCKDGTCCGKCSNAACKTCADGCTCGSGCSCTEGNCPC				Wilkinson & Nemer, 1987
Yeast	QNEGHECQCQCGSCKNNEQCQKSCSCPTGCNSDKCPCGNKSEETKKSCCSGK				Winge et al., 1985
Wheat germ (E_c protein)	GCNDKCGCAVPPGGTGCRCTSARSGAAAGEHTTCGCEHCGNPCACGGEGTPSGCAN[d]....				Lane et al., 1987
Cyanobacterium	TSTTLVKCACEPCLCNVDPSKAIDRNGLYYCCE=ACADGHTGGSKGCCHTGCNC				Olafson et al., 1988

Class III

	1	10	
S. pombe (cadystin B[f])	eCeCG[e]		Kondo et al., 1984
R. canina (phytochelatin, PC7)	eCeCeCeCeCeCG		Grill et al., 1986a
P. vulgaris (homophytochelatin, h-PC6)	eCeCeCeCeC-β-alanine		Grill et al., 1986b

[a] Open positions denote deletions introduced for optimal alignment of class I metallothioneins

[b] Numeration refers to the sequence determined for human metallothionein-2

[c] Specified subform of metallothionein

[d] Partial sequence

[e] "e" indicates glutamic acid residue linked by γ-glutamyl bond

[f] Also designated "phytochelatin PC2" (Grill et al., 1986a)

Figure 1. Classification of metallothioneins: amino acid sequences of representative forms.[a]

accommodate the seven bivalent metal ions. The details of metal coordination have been elucidated by a large variety of spectroscopic methods (Figure 2). For many of these studies, homogenously substituted derivatives had to be prepared in which the naturally bound and predominantly spectroscopically silent metal ions [Zn(II), Cd(II), Cu(I)] were replaced by spectroscopically active metal ions suitable for the chosen method. In particular, replacement studies with Co(II) proved useful in establishing the coordination geometry of metal binding (Vašák, 1980; Vašák and Kägi, 1981). The spectroscopic characterization of the Co(II) derivative documented that all metal ions are bound quite uniformly to four thiolate groups of Cys side chains in tetrahedral symmetry (MeS_4). Spectroscopic and magnetic studies showed, moreover, that in reconstituted $Co(II)_7$-MT these complexes do not exist in separation but are joined to oligonuclear structures, in which some of the thiolate ligands are shared by two adjacent metal ions. Such an arrangement or clustering of the metal ions is required if the tetrahedral tetrathiolate coordination geometry of the metal complex is to be reconciled with the measured stoichiometry of less than three thiolate ligands per di-

Method	Metal derivative studied	Reference
Ultraviolet absorption spectroscopy	Cd(II), Zn(II), Hg(II) Co(II) Fe(II)	cited in Kägi and Kojima (1987) Vašák and Kägi (1981) Good and Vašák (1986)
Circular dichroism spectroscopy	Cd(II), Zn(II), Hg(II)	cited in Kägi and Kojima (1987)
Magnetic circular dichroism spectroscopy	Cd(II), Zn(II), Hg(II) Fe(II), Co(II)	cited in Kägi and Kojima (1987)
Luminescence spectroscopy	Cu(I)	cited in Kägi and Kojima (1987)
Nuclear magnetic resonance spectroscopy (NMR)	^{113}Cd(II)	Otvos and Armitage (1980)
Electron paramagnetic resonance spectroscopy (EPR)	Co(II)	Vašák and Kägi (1981)
Extended x-ray absorption fine structure measurements (EXAFS)	Zn(II) Cu(I)	Abrahams et al. (1986) Smith et al. (1986)
Mössbauer spectroscopy	^{57}Fe(II)	Ding et al. (1987)
X-ray photoelectron spectroscopy	Cd(II), Zn(II), Hg(II)	cited in Vašák and Kägi (1983)

Figure 2. Spectroscopic methods employed in the study of metal-thiolate complexes in metallothionein.

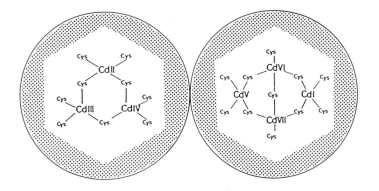

Figure 3. Domain structure of mammalian Cd_7-MT. Left: amino-terminal domain. Right: carboxyl-terminal domain.

valent metal ion. In mammalian MTs, the ratio of 20 Cys to seven metal ions demands that eight Cys serve as doubly coordinated bridging thiolate ligands and twelve as singly coordinated terminal thiolate ligands (Vašák and Kägi, 1983).

METAL-THIOLATE CLUSTERS

The first unambiguous experimental evidence for the existence of discrete metal-thiolate clusters has come from ^{113}Cd NMR studies of MT substituted with the stable NMR active isotope ^{113}Cd, i.e., $^{113}Cd_7$-MT, which revealed ^{113}Cd-^{113}Cd scalar coupling via the bridging thiolate ligands (Otvos and Armitage, 1980). Analogous indications of the spatial vicinity of the metal ions were provided by the observation of antiferromagnetic coupling between metal centers in EPR and magnetic susceptibility studies of Co(II)-substituted derivatives (Vašák and Kägi, 1981) and in Mössbauer studies of a Fe(II)-substituted derivative (Ding et al., 1988).

In mammalian MTs the seven Cd(II) were shown by ^{113}Cd-^{113}Cd homonuclear decoupling studies to be arranged in two topologically separate clusters, one made up of three metal ions and nine Cys, $Me(II)_3Cys_9$, having a cyclohexane-like structure, and one made up of four metal ions and eleven Cys, $Me(II)_4Cys_{11}$, having a bicyclo (3.3.1) nonane-like structure (Otvos and Armitage, 1980). As subsequently shown by Winge and Miklossy (1982), these two clusters are associated with separate domains formed by the amino-terminal and carboxyl-terminal halves of the protein, respectively (Figure 3).

SPATIAL STRUCTURE

This two-cluster, two-domain model has now been affirmed splendidly by the spatial structure derived from 2D NMR spectroscopic analysis of several mammalian MTs (Arseniev et al., 1988; Schultze et al., 1988; Messerle et al., 1990). A unique and essential step in this structure determination in aqueous solution was the unambiguous allocation of the 28 coordination bonds connecting the seven [113]Cd(II) with the 20 Cys by heteronuclear [1]H[113]Cd NMR correlation spectroscopy, a procedure specially developed for the study of [113]Cd[7]-MT (Frey et al., 1985). This method monitors heteronuclear coupling of each [113]Cd nucleus with the ^{1}H nuclei of the coordinated Cys (Figure 4) and thus allows the direct observation of the scalar connectivities of the seven [113]Cd resonances well separated in the [113]Cd NMR spectrum with the ^{1}H resonances of the ligated Cys which beforehand had been localized in the ^{1}H NMR spectrum by homonuclear 2D ^{1}H ^{1}H NMR measurements (Wagner et al., 1986; Wörgötter et al., 1987). The resulting Cd-Cys bonds, as determined in [113]Cd-substituted rat liver MT-2, are displayed in Figure 5. The arrangement shows that of the 20 Cys coordinated to the metal ions, Cys 7, Cys 15 and Cys 24 are the bridging ligands of the three-metal cluster, and residues Cys 34, Cys 37, Cys 44, Cys 50, and Cys 60 those of the four-metal cluster. Exactly the same organization of Cys-Cd connectivities was found in the NMR structures of rabbit liver MT-2a (Arseniev et al., 1988) and human MT-2 (Messerle et al., 1990).

From the interresidue distances given by the geometric requirements of the established 42 intramolecular Cys-Cd-Cys crosslinks and from the long-range through-space proton-proton distance constraints (<5Å) provided by 2D ^{1}H ^{1}H NMR NOESY measurements, the best spatial fold of the polypeptide chain of rat liver [113]Cd[7]-MT-2 satisfying these data was calculated, using a distance geometry algorithm developed for tertiary protein structures (Braun and Gō, 1985). A stereo view of this computed structure is shown

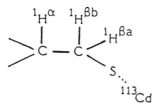

Figure 4. Complexation of [113]Cd(II) to Cys. Disposition of spin $I = 1/2$ nuclei ([1]H [113]Cd) allowing for heteronuclear through-bond coupling. a and b distinguish between the two Cys β-protons.

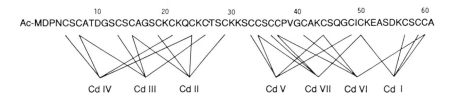

Figure 5. Cd-Cys bonds in rat liver MT-2 determined by heteronuclear $^1H^{113}Cd$ NMR correlation spectroscopy. Roman numerals refer to Cd topology of Otvos and Armitage (1980). (Adapted from Vašák et al., 1987.)

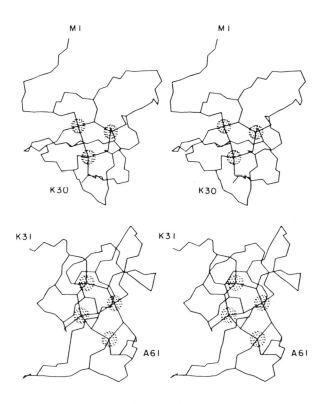

Figure 6. Two-dimensional NMR solution structure of amino-terminal domain (top) and carboxyl-terminal domain (bottom) of rat liver Cd_7-MT-2. Stereo view of polypeptide backbone, Cys side chains and metal positions (dotted spheres) as determined by two-dimensional $^1H^{113}Cd$ heteronuclear and two-dimensional $^1H^1H$ homonuclear NMR correlation spectroscopy. The domains are connected by a hinge region made up of the conserved Lys 30–Lys 31 segment in the middle of the polypeptide chain. Because of the paucity of interdomain contacts recognizable by NMR spectroscopy, the mutual orientation of the domains is not as yet defined. (Adapted from Figure 3 of Schultze et al., 1988.)

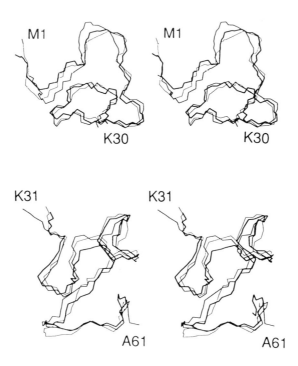

Figure 7. Stereo view of a superposition of the 2D NMR structures of the polypeptide backbone of rat MT-2 (thinnest line, Schultze et al., 1988), rabbit MT-2a (medium thickness line, Arseniev et al., 1988), and human MT-2 (thickest line, Messerle et al., 1990). Top: amino-terminal domain. Bottom: carboxyl-terminal domain. (Adapted from Messerle et al., 1990.)

in Figure 6. For the sake of clarity, the model is simplified to show only the course of the polypeptide backbone, the orientation of the Cys side chains, and the positions of the seven ^{113}Cd(II). It documents that the protein is composed of two about equally sized globular domains. Their structures which in reality are connected through the Lys 30–Lys 31 segment are drawn separately, since their mutual orientation is not sufficiently defined by the available 2D NMR data. Each domain contains in its interior the appropriate metal-thiolate cluster as a "mineral core" wrapped by two large helical turns of the polypeptide chain. In the amino-terminal domain, the spiral of the chain fold is right-handed, in the carboxyl-terminal, it is left-handed.

Although rat liver MT-2 differs from the two other mammalian forms in as much as 25% of their noncysteine amino acid residues (Kägi and Kojima, 1987), it displays a remarkably similar chain fold. A comparison of the best NMR-derived backbone structures of the two domains of the human, rabbit and rat proteins is shown in Figure 7. The close similarity of their folds which has now also been confirmed by a recent determination of the crystal structure of rat MT-2 (Stout et al., 1989) also extends to the secondary structure elements unique to the MTs and in particular to the steric organization of the metal-thiolate clusters. It strongly supports our suggestion that both the cluster geometries and the global peptide folds are dictated by the conserved arrangement of the 20 Cys in the chains (Kägi and Kojima, 1987).

REFERENCES

Abrahams IL, Bremner I, Diakun GP, Garner CD, Hasnain SS, Ross I, and Vašák M (1986): Structural study of the copper and zinc sites in metallothioneins by using extended X-ray-absorption fine structure. *Biochem. J.* 236: 585.

Arseniev A, Schultze P, Wörgötter E, Braun W, Wagner G, Vašák M, Kägi JHR, and Wüthrich K (1988): Three-dimensional structure of rabbit liver [Cd₇]metallothionein-2a in aqueous solution determined by nuclear magnetic resonance. *J. Mol. Biol.* 201: 637.

Bonham K, Zafarullah M, and Gedamu L (1987): The rainbow trout metallothioneins: molecular cloning and characterization of two distinct cDNA sequences. *DNA* 6: 519.

Braun W and Gō N (1985): Calculation of protein conformations by proton-proton distance constraints. A new efficient algorithm. *J. Mol. Biol.* 186: 611.

Ding X, Bill E, Good M, Trautwein AX, and Vašák M (1988): Mössbauer studies on the metal-thiolate cluster formation in Fe(II)-metallothionein. *Eur. J. Biochem.* 171: 711.

Fowler BA, Hildebrand CE, Kojima Y, and Webb M (1987): Nomenclature of metallothionein. *Experientia, Suppl.* 52: 19.

Frey MH, Wagner G, Vašák M, Sørensen OW, Neuhaus D, Wörgötter E, Kägi JHR, Ernst RR, and Wüthrich K (1985): Polypeptide-metal cluster connectivities in metallothionein 2 by novel ¹H-¹¹³Cd heteronuclear two-dimensional NMR experiments. *J. Am. Chem. Soc.* 107: 6847.

Good M and Vašák M (1986): Iron(II)-substituted metallothionein: evidence for the existence of iron-thiolate clusters. *Biochemistry* 25: 8353.

Grill E, Winnacker E-L, and Zenk MH (1986a): Synthesis of seven different homologous phytochelatins in metal-exposed *Schizosaccharomyces pombe* cells. *FEBS Lett.* 197: 115.

Grill E, Gekeler W, Winnacker EL, and Zenk HH (1986b): Homo-phytochelatins are heavy metal-binding peptides of homo-glutathione containing fabales. *FEBS Lett.* 205: 47.

Kägi JHR and Vallee BL (1960): Metallothionein, a cadmium- and zinc-containing protein from equine renal cortex. *J. Biol. Chem.* 235: 3460.

Kägi JHR and Kojima Y (1987): Chemistry and biochemistry of metallothionein. *Experienta, Suppl.* 52: 25.

Kissling MM and Kägi JHR (1977): Primary structure of human hepatic metallothionein. *FEBS Lett.* 82: 247.

Kondo N, Imai K, Isobe M, Goto T, Murasugi A, Wada-Nakagawa C, and Hayashi Y (1984): Cadystin A and B, major unit peptides comprising cadmium binding peptides induced in a fission yeast—separation, revision of structures and synthesis. *Tetrahedron Lett.* 25: 3869.

Lane B, Kajioka R, and Kennedy T (1987): The wheat-germ E_c protein is a zinc-containing metallothionein. *Biochem. Cell Biol.* 65: 1001.

Lerch K (1979): Amino-acid sequence of copper-metallothionein from *Neurospora crassa. Experientia, Suppl.* 34: 173.

Lerch K, Ammer D, and Olafson RW (1982): Crab metallothionein. Primary structures of metallothioneins 1 and 2. *J. Biol. Chem.* 257: 2420.

Lin L, Lin WC, and Huang PC (1990): Pigeon metallothionein consists of two species. *Biochem. Biophys. Acta* 1037: 248.

Messerle BA, Schäffer A, Vašák M, Kägi JHR, and Wüthrich K (1990): The three-dimensional structure of human [$^{113}Cd_7$]-metallothionein-2 in solution determined by nuclear magnetic resonance spectroscopy. *J. Mol. Biol.* 214: 765.

Nemer M, Wilkinson DG, Travaglini EC, Sternberg EJ, and Butt TR (1985): Sea urchin metallothionein sequence: key to an evolutionary diversity. *Proc. Natl. Acad. Sci. U.S.A.* 82: 4992.

Olafson RW, McCubbin WD, and Kay CM (1988): Primary- and secondary-structural analysis of a unique prokaryotic metallothionein from a *Synechococcus sp.* Cyanobacterium. *Biochem. J.* 251: 691.

Otvos JD and Armitage IM (1980): Structure of the metal clusters in rabbit liver metallothionein. *Proc. Natl. Acad. Sci. U.S.A.* 77: 7094.

Reese RN, Mehra RK, Tarbet EB, and Winge DR (1988): Studies on the γ-glutamyl Cu-binding peptide from *Schizosaccharomyces pombe. J. Biol. Chem.* 263: 4186.

Schultze P, Wörgötter E, Braun W, Wagner G, Vašák M, Kägi JHR, and Wüthrich K (1988): Conformation of [Cd_7]-metallothionein-2 from rat liver in aqueous solution determined by nuclear magnetic resonance spectroscopy. *J. Mol. Biol.* 203: 251.

Smith TA, Lerch K, and Hodgson KO (1986): Structural study of the Cu sites in metallothionein from *Neurospora crassa. Inorg. Chem.* 25: 4677.

Stout CD, McRee DE, Robbins AH, Collett SA, Williamson M, and Xuong XH (1989): Metallothionein in the crystal. Abstracts, International Chemical Congress of Pacific Basin Societies, Honolulu, Hawaii, USA, Vol. I, 04/57.

Vašák M (1980): Spectroscopic studies on cobalt(II) metallothionein: Evidence for pseudotetrahedral metal coordination. *J. Am. Chem. Soc.* 102: 3953.

Vašák M and Kägi JHR (1981): Metal-thiolate clusters in cobalt(II)-metallothionein. *Proc. Natl. Acad. Sci. U.S.A.* 78: 6709.

Vašák M and Kägi JHR (1983): Spectroscopic properties of metallothionein. *Met. Ions Biol. Syst.* 15: 213.

Vašák M, Wörgötter E, Wagner G, Kägi JHR, and Wüthrich K (1987): Metal coordination in rat liver metallothionein-2 prepared with or without reconstitution of the metal clusters, and comparison with rabbit liver metallothionein-2. *J. Mol. Biol.* 196: 711.

Wagner G, Neuhaus D, Wörgötter E, Vašák M, Kägi JHR, and Wüthrich K (1986): Sequence-specific ^{1}H-NMR assignments in rabbit-liver metallothionein-2. *Eur. J. Biochem.* 157: 275.

Wilkinson DG and Nemer M (1987): Metallothionein genes MTa and MTb expressed under distinct quantitative and tissue-specific regulation in sea urchin embryos. *Mol. Cell Biol.* 7: 48.

Winge DR and Miklossy K-A (1982): Domain nature of metallothionein. *J. Biol. Chem.* 257: 3471.

Winge DR, Nielson KB, Gray WR, and Hamer DH (1985): Yeast metallothionein. Sequence and metal-binding properties. *J. Biol. Chem.* 260: 14464.

Wörgötter E, Wagner G, Vašák M, Kägi JHR, and Wüthrich K (1987): Sequence-specific ¹H-NMR assignments in rat-liver metallothionein-2. *Eur. J. Biochem.* 167: 457.

Chapter 5

Regulation of Human and Yeast Metallothionein Gene Transcription by Heavy Metal Ions

Petra Skroch, Carla Inouye, and Michael Karin
Department of Pharmacology
University of California, San Diego
La Jolla, California

ABSTRACT

Organisms from yeast to mammals express low molecular weight metal binding, cysteine-rich proteins, the metallothioneins (MTs). The metal-dependent expression of MTs is controlled transcriptionally. No transacting factor conferring metal-inducibility upon mammalian MT-genes has been isolated thus far. Recently, however, the product of the yeast CUP2 gene was identified as a sequence specific Cu-dependent activator of the yeast MT gene, CUP1. The N-terminal DNA-binding domain of the CUP2 protein resembles CUP1 in its cysteine-content and arrangement. Study of *in vitro* synthesized wild-type and mutant CUP2 proteins demonstrated the effect of metal-binding on specific DNA-affinity and the importance of single amino acid residues in this process.

INTRODUCTION

Organisms as diverse as yeast, *drosophila* and mammals express heavy metal binding proteins, metallothioneins. These cysteine-rich, low molecular weight proteins play a key role in trace metal ion homeostasis and detoxification. By regulating the levels and availability of intracellular Zn and Cu, they contribute indirectly to the regulation of various Zn requiring enzyme systems, some of which are involved in replication, transcription and DNA repair (Karin, 1985a; Hamer, 1986). The major form of regulation of MT activity occurs by increased synthesis of these proteins in response to elevated heavy metal ion concentrations and various steroid and polypeptide hormones. The activation of the metallothionein genes by heavy metal ions and hormones occurs on the transcriptional control level, but whereas the highly conserved cis and trans-acting DNA elements involved in the response to hormone have been characterized and studied in detail, the trans-acting factors conferring metal inducibility could not be defined for a long time. Only recently a protein conferring Cu inducibility upon the yeast metallothionein gene CUP1 was isolated by a genetic approach and its function and structure could be studied in detail.

HUMAN METALLOTHIONEIN GENES AND REGULATION

The human genome contains 12 distinct MT genes, out of which six or seven code for functional proteins, whereas the rest are nonfunctional pseudogenes (Karin and Richards, 1982; Hunziker and Kägi, 1983; Richards et al., 1984; Klauser and Kaegi, 1985; Schmidt et al., 1985; Heguy et al., 1986). The MTIIA gene is the major human MT gene, accounting for 50% of the MTs expressed in cultured human cells and in liver (Karin and Herschman, 1980a). In addition to heavy metal ions the expression of the MTIIA gene is induced by glucocorticoid and progesterone hormones, interferon, interleukin I, serum factors, phorbol ester tumor promoters such as TPA and DNA damaged by UV-irradiation (Karin et al., 1980b; Friedman and Stark, 1985; Karin, 1985b; Imbra and Karin, 1986; Angel et al., 1986).

The cis-acting DNA elements involved in regulation of the MTIIA gene have been studied using *in vitro* mutagenesis and gene transfer experiments (Haslinger and Karin, 1985; Serfling et al., 1985; Karin et al., 1987a). The trans acting factors that bind these elements have been defined by the DNase I footprinting procedure and gel retardation assays. A GC-box located between nucleotides -57 to -68 relative to the start side of transcription is recognized by the specific transcription factor SP1. Interestingly, SP1 is a zinc-finger DNA-binding protein (Kadonaga et al., 1987) which raises the possibility that MT might indirectly control its activity. A TPA responsive element (TRE), another common regulatory DNA element, spans the region from -96 to -105 (Lee et al., 1987). It is recognized by the transcription factor AP1 (Angel et al., 1987). AP1 was demonstrated to be composed of both homodimeric and heterodimeric complexes involving the cJun and cFos protooncoproteins (Chiu et al., 1988). Further upstream, transcription factor AP2 binds to three relatively divergent sequences in the MTIIA promoter (Imagawa et al., 1987). The element that confers glucocorticoid responsiveness upon the MTIIA gene is located between positions -240 and -270 and was shown to serve as a binding site for the glucocorticoid receptor (Karin et al., 1984a). The same element also confers a response to progesterone (Slater et al., 1988). Because of its unusual responsiveness to a large number of hormonal and environmental cues, the MTIIA gene is an excellent system for analyzing the molecular mechanisms involved in a signal transduction to the transcriptional machinery. The activity of multiple synthetic copies of the MTIIA high-affinity AP2 binding site increases after treatment of cells with phorbol ester or cAMP-elevating agents. In contrast, a synthetic enhancer specifically recognized by AP1 is activated only by phorbol ester. Therefore, in contrast to AP1, AP2 appears to mediate transcriptional activation in response to two different signal transduction pathways, one involving the phorbol ester- and diacylglycerol-activated protein kinase C, the other involving cAMP-dependent protein kinase A. Steroid hormones bind to and activate a specific cytoplasmic receptor and lead to its migration into the nucleus, where it binds to a specific site on steroid responsive genes (Evans, 1988).

Interspersed between the basal promoter elements are four metal response elements (MREs) (Karin et al., 1987a). MREs are short (12 to 17 basepairs long) repetitive sequences that are highly conserved within one species and also between different species. In spite of their high sequence homology different MREs differ in their abilities to confer metal inducibility when assayed individually. Culotta and Hamer (1989) showed, that one out of the five distinct MRE sequences present in the mouse MT-I gene, confers a stronger metal induction to a heterologous promoter then the others. Two copies of this individual MRE cloned in front of its authentic promoter led to a 10 to 20 fold induction, whereas a single copy enhanced the metal dependent transcription only 2 to 4 fold. This suggests a cooperative effect, which coincides with the occurrence of multiple MREs in natural MT gene promoters. For example each of the MREs of the MTIIA gene is adjacent to another cis element (Karin et al., 1987a) and competition experiments have demonstrated that several of these elements promote binding of metal-dependent transcription factors to the MREs. This is likely to occur by protein-protein interactions as originally suggested by Scholer et al. (1986). Metal ion induced transcription of the MT genes is positively regulated, and the Zn induced transcription of MT mRNA in HeLA cells is insensitive to cycloheximide, which shows that the induction is not dependent on *de novo* protein synthesis (Karin et al., 1980c). These results are consistent with a model according to which a metal-responsive factor (MRF) exists in the cell prior to induction and its activated by metal ions. At elevated metal ion concentrations the factor might acquire an increased affinity for MREs as a prerequisite for transcriptional activation. As mentioned above, binding of the MRF may also depend on interactions with adjacent factors such as SP1 or AP1.

Generating a series of synthetic oligonucleotides containing point mutations, Culotta and Hamer (1989) defined a core region in which single base pair exchanges destroyed the activity of the element and a flanking GC-rich region which proved to be less critical for function. This region exhibits significant homology to the core binding site for mammalian transcription factor SP1, but a partially purified mouse SP1 preparation did not exhibit strong binding to this site. In addition purified human SP1 was never found to bind any of the MTIIA MREs (Lee et al., 1987). Using the exact same DNA sequence Westin and Schaffner (1988), showed evidence that this individual mouse MT1 MRE is recognized by SP1 as well as by another protein, possibly the one conferring metal inducibility. However, the two factors were reported to compete for the same binding site rather than act synergistically. The basis for these descriptions is not clear, but it is certain that under normal conditions SP1 does not interact with the MRE. In the human MTIIA gene, one or two MREs are present adjacent to each of the basal level enhancer elements. Just as the MRE sequences appear to work in a cooperative manner when multimerized (Searle et al., 1987; Culotta and Hamer 1989), a possible cooperation between the basal level enhancer elements and the MREs was also demonstrated (Karin et al., 1987a). *In vivo* competition experiments demonstrated that, in the presence of heavy metal ions, the MTIIA enhancer is able to compete more efficiently with the SV40 enhancer for binding of cellular factors. It is likely that the positively acting factor that binds to the MRE in the presence of heavy metal ions is acting by stabilizing the binding of adjacent trans-acting factor via protein-protein interactions (Scholer et al., 1986). Thus the cooperative interaction between basal factors and the MRF appears to operate both ways.

Extracts were prepared from Cd-induced and uninduced HeLa cells and partially purified, but failed to show any differences in their DNase I protection pattern on the MTIIA promoter. Actually the only upstream elements over which no protection was observed were the MREs (Karin et al., 1987b). However a DNA probe containing only a tandemly duplicated MRE sequence showed a footprint over the entire MRE sequence after incubation with either induced or uninduced HeLa cell extracts (Skroch, unpublished). Seguin and Hamer (1987) observed partial protection of some MRE sequences in footprinting experiments with the mouse MTI promoter using nuclear extracts from Cd-treated mouse L cells. However, other groups including ours have failed to reproduce these experiments. Mueller et al.

(1988) could demonstrate a change in protein-DNA contacts on the mouse MTI promoter by *in vivo* footprinting when cells are shifted from basal level expression to metal induced expression. The non-induced footprint pattern consists of interactions of factors such as SP1 and AP1 with the basal elements that are thought to be responsible for the moderate expression of this gene in the absence of added metal. By exposing the L-cells to Zn or Cd a new set of metal dependent footprints appeared over all five genetically defined MREs. These experiments provide further support to the existence of a positively regulated MRF interacting with the MREs.

Although several reports claiming detection of a protein with some of the features expected from the MRF have been published, none of them provided a conclusive proof that the detected factor was indeed the MRF. For example, the binding of some of these factors was affected only by Zn and not by Cd (Westin and Schaffner, 1988) or vice versa (Seguin and Hamer, 1987). The authentic MRF should respond to both of these metal ions. Furthermore, no purification and isolation of these factors has been reported. Our own attempts to detect an authentic MRF activity have failed (Skroch, unpublished). Since we could detect all of the other factors that bind to the MTIIA promoter we believe that the MRF is either extremely labile or present in very low amounts within the cell.

METALLOTHIONEIN GENE REGULATION IN YEAST

A convenient eukaryotic system for studying MT gene function and regulation is provided by the brewer's yeast *Saccharomyces cerevisiae*. Resistance to toxic effects of copper ions in *S. cerevisiae* is mediated by the inducible synthesis of a low molecular weight, cysteine-rich, metal-binding protein, known as copper chelatin or yeast metallothionein (Fogel and Welch, 1982; Butt et al., 1987). Various naturally occurring yeast strains differ over a 20-fold range in their resistance to the inhibitory effects of copper on growth. Increased resistance correlates with over-production of yeast MT (Welch et al., 1983). Enhanced resistance reflects gene amplification as a consequence of sister chromatic exchange and gene conversion events. The 1.95kb repeat units containing the yeast MT gene CUP1 are tandemly arrayed and copper resistant strains contain as many as 15 reiterated repeats was determined. The predicted amino acid composition derived from the DNA sequence shows, that the yeast CUP1 protein bears only limited primary sequence homology to the mammalian MTs (Karin et al., 1984). However, the two types of protein are similar in their small size (60 to 61 amino acids) and unusual composition: CUP1 contains 20% cysteines while mammalian MTs contain 30% cysteines. Also it has been shown that over-production of monkey MT can functionally substitute for the CUP1 gene, when transfected into yeast cells deleted of their CUP1 locus (Thiele et al., 1986a). The purified protein product of the CUP1 gene contains eight monovalent copper ions liganded by 12 cysteine residues, but it can bind *in vitro* also to eight silver ions or to four divalent zinc or cadmium ions (Winge et al., 1985). However, unlike the mammalian MT genes, transcription of the yeast gene is not affected by other ions such as cadmium, zinc or mercury (Karin et al., 1984b).

The regulatory region of the yeast CUP1 gene was studied in detail. By deletion analysis and construction of synthetic hybrid promoters the *cis*-acting control elements that confer copper dependent transcription have been narrowed down to nucleotides -105 to -180. This region contains at least two functional elements and consists of two related sequences of 32 and 34 nucleotides, denoted UASp and UASd respectively (Butt et al., 1984; Thiele and Hamer, 1986b). A series of overlapping oligonucleotides that span the complete region was synthesized and introduced into yeast after fusion to a deleted CYC1 promoter driving expression of the *Escherichia coli* galK reporter gene. Galactokinase activity was tested in the presence and absence of copper. The region between -105 and -148 spanning the UASp region showed the best result, activating transcription 7.5 fold. The precise nucleotides that are responsible for copper induced transcription were identified by systematic point mutagenesis of the UASp. UASd alone was not able to confer copper inducibility under these conditions. (Fuerst et al., 1988). Transcription of the 0.5kb CUP1 gene itself is stimulated 10 to 20 fold in response to elevated copper concentrations (Karin et al., 1984b).

To identify putative trans-acting regulatory genes whose products may interact with the copper responsive elements of the CUP1 promoter to mediate copper induction and resistance, a collection of copper sensitive mutants, induced by ethyl methane sulfonate (EMS) treatment of a wild-type multicopy CUP1r strain, was screened for possible regulatory gene mutations. In one recessive isolate, a mutation designated cup2, the phenotypic copper resistance was dramatically reduced by two orders of magnitude. This cup2 strain thus exhibited an even more pronounced sensitivity than a cup1s strain, which contains only a single CUP1 gene. The results of RNA blot analysis indicate that in cup2 cells, despite its presence in 11 copies, the CUP1 gene is expressed only at a very low basal level and is refractory to induction by exogenous copper ions. Consequently, cup2 was selected for extensive analysis based on the assumption that it is defective in production of a functional protein CUP2, which was supposed to act as a trans-acting factor for the metal dependent expression of the CUP1 locus. The mutant cup2 strain was transformed with a genomic wild-type DNA library cloned into a yeast expression shuttle vector. Transformants were isolated and tested for copper resistance. The wild-type allele of the CUP2 gene was rescued by retransformation of *E. coli* by plasmids extracted from four independent Cu-resistent yeast colonies (Welch et al., 1989).

To determine whether the effect on CUP1 expression in the cup2 strain was attributable to an altered interaction of regulatory proteins with the CUP1 promoter, nuclear protein extracts were prepared from wild-type (CUP1r, X2180) and the otherwise isogeneic cup2 strain. Incubation of a DNA probe spanning the copper responsive elements of the CUP1 promoter with the cup2 extract resulted in the formation of three different protein-DNA complexes. The same complexes formed after incubation with the wild-type extract, but now an additional distinct protein-DNA complex appeared. This result suggested, that mutant cup2 is defective in one of the DNA-binding activities which recognize the CUP1 promoter. Since introduction of a wild-type CUP2 allele into the cup2 strain restores copper resistance and CUP1 induction and leads to the appearance of the wild-type-specific protein-DNA complex, it was concluded that CUP2 encodes a regulatory protein required for Cu-dependent activation of CUP1 (Welch et al., 1989). Thiele (1988) used essentially the same approach to isolate a yeast gene named ACE1 that shows the identical features to CUP2: it restores copper resistance after reintroduction into a yeast strain that fails to grow in elevated copper concentrations. Sequencing of the cloned DNAs demonstrated the identity of the ACE1 and CUP2 genes.

The CUP2 coding sequences have the potential to form a 225 amino acid protein with a predicted molecular weight of 24 kDa. When expressed in *E. coli*, however, the protein migrates with an apparent molecular weight of 33 kDa. Examination of the distribution of charged amino acids encoded by the gene suggests, that CUP2 is a two domain protein. The amino terminal portion of the molecule, from amino acid 1 to 108, is unusually poor in hydrophobic and aromatic residues but is extremely rich in basic residues and has a predicted positive charge of +16. This part of the protein also contains 12 cysteine residues, ten of which are arranged in the CysXCys and CysXXCys configurations characteristic of yeast metallothionein itself and mammalian MTs as well. This highly charged domain could be responsible for the abnormal migration of the CUP2 protein. In contrast, the carboxy-terminal portion of the molecule has a predicted negative charge of −14, and thus resembles several highly acidic sequences known to act as transcriptional activation domains in yeast (Fuerst et al., 1988; Welch et al., 1989). The bacterially expressed CUP2 protein appears to be partially cleaved by an endogenous protease to yield two fragments corresponding to the two predicted domains (Buchman et al., 1989).

Although the primary sequences of the N-terminal domain of CUP2 and various MT sequences differ a lot, it is important to realize, that MTs themselves are highly divergent when comparing distantly related species, and that the primary sequence of the protein can vary considerably without exerting large effects on its metal binding properties and *in vivo* function. Based on the predicted structural similarities between CUP2/ACE1 and metallothionein, Fuerst et al. (1988) devised a preliminary model for how its relatively small N-terminal domain could combine specific DNA binding and metal binding properties. They proposed that the core structure of the CUP2/ACE1 N-terminal domain is a cuboidal Cu8-S12 cluster in which paired cysteine residues coordinate common copper ions, as it has been suggested recently for the CUP1 protein.

To analyze the properties of the CUP2 protein we cloned it into a bacterial expression vector and first expressed it as a trpE fusion protein. Extracts prepared from transformed *E. coli* cells grown in the presence of 1 m*M* CuSO$_4$ were assayed by gel retardation and were found to form one or two specific protein-DNA complexes with a CUP1 DNA probe containing the Cu responsive UASs. Expression of the N-terminal 122 amino acids of the protein followed by gel retardation analysis demonstrated that this domain alone is sufficient for binding to the CUP1 promoter. To examine the importance of copper for DNA binding of CUP2, *E. coli* cells expressing CUP2 were grown in the absence of copper and protein extracts were prepared. They were found to contain substantial amounts of CUP2 protein as shown by SDS polyacrylamide gel analysis, but hardly any DNA-binding activity was detected. Copper added to these extracts in the form of Cu$^+$ restored the DNA binding activity of the protein (Buchman et al., 1989). Cu$^+$ was chosen in these experiments instead of the Cu^{++} ion used for *in vivo* induction, as Cu$^+$ is the natural ligand of yeast MT (Winge et al., 1985). Indeed, while the DNA-binding activity of the trpE CUP2 fusion was also restored by Ag$^+$, which is electronically similar to Cu$^+$, the addition of Cu^{++} was much less efficient in restoring activity. Additionally, treatment of CUP2 protein with KCN, a chelator capable of removing Cu$^+$ ions from yeast MT led to loss of DNA binding activity, which could be restored upon addition of excess Cu$^+$ or Ag$^+$, whereas Zn^{++}, Cd^{++} or Hg^{++} were not effective (Buchman et al., 1989).

The two mutant yeast strains cup2 and ace1-1, that led to the identification of CUP2/ACE1 were isolated independently as ethyl-methanesulfonate-induced copper sensitive mutants from their copper resistant parental strains (Thiele, 1988; Welch et al., 1989). To determine the molecular basis for the failure of these strains to induce CUP1 in response to Cu, we isolated molecular clones of the two mutant alleles after their amplification by the polymerase chain reaction (Mullis and Faloona, 1987). Sequence analysis revealed, that each of the mutants differed from the wild type allele only by a single point mutation. The cup2 allele contained a G to A transition converting Gly37 to a glutamic acid residue, while in the ace1-1 strain Cys11 was converted to a tyrosine residue also by a G to A transition. To examine the effect of these mutations on CUP2 protein function, both alleles were cloned into bacterial expression vectors. The mutant trpE fusion proteins appeared to be as stable as the wild-type protein and showed identical mobility on SDS polyacrylamide gels. In a gel retardation analysis using the UASs as a DNA probe, trpE·ace1-1 had reduced DNA-binding activity, whereas trpE·cup2 did not exhibit any detectable binding to the CUP1 promoter. The activity of the N-terminal half of CUP2 is highly dependent on Cu^+ or Ag^+ ions suggesting that these specific ions interact with the cysteine residues to direct the folding of the DNA-binding domain. The reduced ability of the ace1-1 protein to bind to DNA, suggests, that Cys11 could be directly involved in formation of the Cu^+-coordinated DNA-binding domain. The reason for the dramatic effect of the cup2 mutation on DNA-binding is less obvious. One possibility is, that the Gly37 to Glu change introduced a negatively charged residue into a cluster of positively charged amino acids and thereby affected interaction with phosphate groups in the DNA-backbone. The other possibility is that the Gly to Glu change led to loss of conformational flexibility and interfered with proper folding of the DNA-binding domain. Unlike the Cys11 to Tyr mutation, the Gly37 to Glu mutation is not expected to affected Cu^+ binding per se (Buchman et al., 1989).

While the DNA-binding activity of the CUP2 protein is highly regulated by Cu, expression of the CUP2 gene is constitutive (Szczypka et al., 1989). Taken collectively, these findings suggest the following scheme for regulation of CUP1 expression. Cells grown with low levels of copper already contain a substantial amount of CUP2, but because of the low intracellular levels of Cu^+, most of it is in the inactive apoprotein form and, hence, is incapable of binding to the UASs of CUP1. Once the intracellular level of Cu^+ is elevated by exposure to extracellular Cu, CUP2 becomes rapidly activated, binds to the UASs and leads to transcriptional activation of the CUP1 gene. Over-expression of CUP1 will lead to chelation of all available Cu^+ within the cell and thereby decrease the DNA-binding activity of the CUP2 protein. This will result in dissociation of CUP2 from the CUP1 promoter and inactivation of CUP1 transcription. This concerted mechanism would lead to very precise regulation of CUP1 synthesis and maintenance of Cu-homeostasis.

More detailed analysis of CUP2 wild-type and mutant proteins was possible after they were expressed as non-fusion proteins in *E. coli* (Buchman et al., submitted). In mobility shift assays all proteins recognized the CUP1 promoter whereas the trpE·cup2 fusion protein has previously failed to do so, possibly due to interference caused by fusing the hydrophobic N-terminal half of trpE to the weak DNA binding domain of cup2. Methylation interference and footprinting analyses show that CUP2 protects a much larger region, covering the entire UAS, than does ace1 and that two molecules of either protein are bound to the Cu-responsive UAS. A CUP2 monomer binds first to the 5' half-site of the UAS between −140 and −128, followed by a second molecule binding to the 3' half site between −119 and −107. The data indicates that both CUP2 molecules lie on top of the minor groove and contact two adjacent segments of the major groove which are separated by one turn of the double helix. In contrast, an ace1 monomer first binds to the innermost part of the 3' half-site and the second molecule binds to the innermost part of the 5' half-site, leaving the outermost parts of the UAS unprotected. The results are consistent with CUP2 having a bipartite DNA binding domain with each DNA-binding element recognizing one portion of the half-site of the UAS. Each element of the DNA-binding domain can be considered as a Cu-knuckle, because of the important role that Cu ions play in organizing the polypeptide chain into a functional DNA-binding element.

CUP2 synthesized in *E. coli* (Buchman et al., submitted) activated transcription in a UASc-dependent manner in a mammalian extract. cup2 was transcriptionally inactive, an expected result given that it was 200-fold less active in DNaseI footprinting experiments. Surprisingly, ace1 which only showed a 10-fold decrease in DNA-binding activity was also transcriptionally inactive. However, the altered mode of DNA-binding by ace1 may also cause a defect in transcriptional activation. These results are consistent with the *in vivo* experiments in which cup2 and ace1 mutants are defective in CUP1 gene activation upon exposure to exogenous copper (Thiele, 1988; Welch et al., 1989). Cu-dependent transactivation of CUP1 by CUP2/ACE1 *in vitro* was also seen by Culotta et al. (1989). Interestingly, these authors also saw transactivation by the truncated protein containing the DNA-binding amino terminal half of CUP2. These findings suggest that the DNA-binding domain of CUP2 may be involved in interactions with the transcriptional machinery, in addition to its role in DNA binding.

CONCLUSIONS

Organisms, that are as far apart in evolution as yeast and mammals use similarly designed proteins to fulfill their need for metal ion homeostasis. These proteins are unusually abundant in cysteine residues which are mainly arranged in a CysXCys or CysXXCys configuration and accomplish the association with the metal ions. The activation of MT genes in response to metal ions is regulated at the transcriptional level by pre-existing trans-acting factors. The gene for transcription factor CUP2 that confers Cu-inducibility to its MT gene has been cloned from the brewer's yeast *S. cerevisiae*. The primary sequence of the metal-and DNA-binding domain of this factor shows a stunning similarity to the yeast CUP1 gene itself. Cu ions are complexed by cysteine residues arranged in CysXCys and CysXXCys motifs and the resulting conformational change increases the affinity of the factor to its DNA binding site, thereby leading to transcriptional activation of the CUP1 gene. It is very likely that mammals use the same regulatory mechanism to activate their MT genes. The affinity of a trans-acting factor to its binding site on the MT promoter is greatly increased by the interaction of this factor with metal ions, so its metal-binding domain might share the high content of cysteines and their specific arrangement with both the mammalian and the yeast MTs and the yeast MT-specific activator protein CUP2. It is very unlikely though, that the yeast and the mammalian factors share any primary sequence homology beside the cysteine-motifs. The difficulties in isolation of a mammalian metal responsive trans-acting factor or its coding gene can be taken as a hint for a relatively low DNA-binding affinity even in the activated form or for its very low abundance. In addition, the mammalian MRF may be regulated by a novel mechanism involving an interaction with another protein as a prerequisite for DNA-binding. Such a labile interaction, which is disrupted upon preparation of extracts of cellular proteins may have prevented its characterization up to now.

ACKNOWLEDGMENTS

This work was supported by grants from the National Institute of Environmental Health Sciences and the Environmental Protection Agency.

REFERENCES

Angel P, Poeting A, Mallick U, Rahmsdorf HJ, Schorpp M, and Herrlich P (1986): Induction of metallothionein and other mRNA species by carcinogens and tumor promoters in primary human skin fibroblasts. *Mol. Cell Biol.* 6: 1760.

Angel P, Imagawa M, Chiu R, Stein B, Imbra RJ, Rahmsdorf HJ, Jonat C, Herrlich P, and Karin M (1987): Phorbol ester-inducible genes contain a common cis element recognized by a TPA-modulated transacting factor. *Cell* 49: 729.

Buchman C, Skroch P, Welch J, Fogel S, and Karin M (1989): The CUP2 gene product, regulator of yeast metallothionein expression, is a copper-activated DNA-binding protein. *Mol. Cell. Biol.* 9: 4091.

Buchman C, Skroch P, Dixon W, Tullius TD, and Karin M: The metal-dependent transcription factor, CUP2, has a bipartite DNA-binding domain. Submitted for publication.

Butt TR, Sternberg EJ, Herd J, and Crooke ST (1984): Copper metallothionein of yeast, structure of the gene, and regulation of expression. *Gene* 27: 23.

Chiu R, Boyle W, Meek J, Smeal T, Hunter T, and Karin M (1988): The c-fos protein interacts with c-jun/AP1 to stimulate transcription of AP-responsive genes. *Cell* 54: 541.

Culotta V and Hamer D (1989): Fine mapping of a mouse metallothionein gene metal response element. *Mol. Cell. Biol.* 9: 1376.

Culotta VC, Hsu T, Hu S, Fuerst P, and Hamer D (1989): Copper and the ACE1 regulatory protein reversibility induce yeast metallothionein gene transcription in a mouse extract. *Proc. Natl. Acad. Sci. U.S.A.* 86: 8377.

Evans RM (1988): The steroid and thyroid hormone receptor superfamily. *Science* 240: 889.

Fogel S and Welch JW (1982): Tandem gene amplification mediates copper resistance in yeast. *Proc. Natl. Acad. Sci. U.S.A.* 79: 5342.

Friedman RL and Stark GR (1985): Alpha-interferon-induced transcription of HLA and metallothionein genes containing homologous upstream sequences. *Nature* 314: 367.

Fuerst P, Hu S, Hackett R, and Hamer D (1988): Copper activates metallothionein gene transcription by altering the conformation of a specific DNA binding protein. *Cell* 55: 705.

Hamer DH (1986): Metallothionein. *Ann. Rev. Biochem.* 55: 913.

Haslinger A and Karin M (1985): Upstream promoter element of the human metallothionein IIA gene can act like an enhancer element. *Proc. Natl. Acad. Sci. U.S.A.* 82: 8572.

Heguy A, West A, Richards RI, and Karin M (1986): Structure and tissue specific expression of the human metallothionein IB gene. *Mol. Cell. Biol.* 6: 2149.

Hunziker PE and Kaegi JHR (1983): Isolation of five human isometallothioneins. *Proc. 15th Meet. Fed. Eur. Biochem. Soc.* Brussels.

Imagawa M, Chiu R, and Karin M (1987): Transcription factor AP-2 mediates induction by two different signal-transduction pathways: protein kinase C and cAMP. *Cell* 51: 251.

Imbra RJ and Karin M (1986): Metallothionein gene expression is regulated by serum factors and activators of protein kinase. C. *Mol. Cell. Biol.* 7: 1358.

Kadonaga JT, Carner KR, Masiarz FR, and Tjian R (1987): Isolation of cDNA encoding transcription factor Sp1 and functional analysis of the DNA binding domain. *Cell* 51: 1079.

Karin M and Herschman HR (1980a): Characterization of the metallothioneins induced in HeLa cells by dexamethasone and zinc. *Eur. J. Biochem.* 107: 395.

Karin M, Herschman HR, and Weinstein D (1980b): Primary induction of metallothionein by dexamethasone in cultured rat hepatocytes. *Biochem. Biophys. Res. Commun.* 92: 1052.

Karin M, Andersen RD, Slater E, Smith K, Herschman HR (1980c): Metallothionein mRNA induction in HeLa cells in response to zinc or dexamethasone is a primary induction response. *Nature* 286: 295.

Karin M and Richards RI (1982): Human metallothionein genes: primary structure of the metallothionein II gene and a related processed pseudogene. *Nature* 299: 797.

Karin M, Haslinger A, Holtgreve H, Richards RI, Krautner P, Westphal HM, and Beato M (1984a): Characterization of DNA sequences through which cadmium and glucocorticoid hormones induce human metallothionein-IIA gene. *Nature* 308: 513.

Karin M, Najarian R, Haslinger A, Valenzuela P, Welch J, and Fogel S (1984b): Primary structure and transcription of an amplified genetic locus: the CUP 1 locus of yeast. *Proc. Natl. Acad. Sci. U.S.A.* 81: 337.

Karin M (1985a): Metallothioneins: proteins in search of function. *Cell* 41: 9.

Karin M, Imbra RJ, Heguy A, and Wong G (1985b): Interleukin I regulates human metallothionein expression. *Mol. Cell. Biol.* 5: 2866.

Karin M, Haslinger A, Heguy A, Dietlin T, and Cooke T (1987a): Metal-responsive elements act as positive modulators of human metallothionein enhancer activity. *Mol. Cell. Biol.* 7: 606.

Karin M, Imagawa M, Imbra RJ, Chiu R, Heguy A, Haslinger A, Cooke T, Sundramurthi S, Jonat C, and Herrlich P (1987b): Hormonal and environmental control of metallothionein gene expression. In *Transcriptional Control Mechanisms,* Alan R. Liss, New York, p. 295.

Klauser S and Kaegi JHR (1985): Characterization of isoprotein patterns in tissue extracts and isolated samples of metallothioneins by reversed-phase high pressure liquid chromatography. *Biochem. J.* 209: 71.

Lee W, Haslinger A, Karin M, and Tjian R (1987): Activation of transcription by two factors that bind promoter and enhancer sequences of the human metallothionein gene and SV40. *Nature* 352: 368.

Mueller PR, Salser S, and Wold B (1988): Constitutive and metal-inducible protein: DNA interactions at the mouse metallothionein I promoter examined by *in vivo* and *in vitro* footprinting. *Genes Dev.* 2: 412.

Mullis KB and Faloona FA (1987): Specific synthesis of DNA *in vitro* via a polymerase-catalyzed chain reaction. *Methods Enzymol.* 155: 335.

Richards RI, Heguy A, and Karin M (1984): Structural and functional analysis of the human metallothionein IA gene: differential induction by metal ions and glucocorticoids. *Cell* 37: 263.

Schmidt CJ, Jubier MF, and Hamer DH (1985): Structure and expression of two human metallothionein I isoform genes and related pseudogene. *J. Biol. Chem.* 280: 7731.

Scholer H, Haslinger A, Heguy A, Holtgreve H, and Karin M (1986): *In vivo* competition between a metallothionein regulatory element and the SV40 enhancer. *Science* 232: 76.

Szczypka MS and Thiele DJ (1989): A cysteine rich nuclear protein activates metallothionein gene transcription. *Mol. Cell. Biol.* 9: 421.

Searle PF, Stuart GW, and Palmiter RD (1987): Metal regulatory elements of the mouse metallothionein-I gene. *Exper. Suppl.* 52: Metallothionein II; Birkhäuser-Verlag, Basel, p. 407.

Seguin C and Hamer D (1987): Regulation of *in vitro* metallothionein gene binding factors. *Science* 235: 1383.

Serfling E, Luebbe A, Dorsch-Haesler K, and Schaffner W (1985): Metal-dependent SV40 viruses containing inducible enhancers from the upstream region of metallothionein genes. *EMBO J.* 4: 3851.

Slater E, Cato A, Karin M, Baxter J, and Beato M (1988): Progesterone induction of metallothionein-IIA expression. *Mol. Endo.* 2: 485.

Thiele D, Walling MJ, and Hamer D (1986): Mammalian metallothionein is functional in yeast. *Science* 231: 854.

Thiele D and Hamer D (1986): Tandemly duplicated upstream control sequences mediate copper-induced transcription of the *Saccharomyces cerevisiae* copper-metallothionein gene. *Mol. Cell. Biol.* 6: 1158.

Thiele D (1988): *Mol. Cell. Biol.* 8: 2745.

Welch JW, Fogel S, Cathala G, and Karin M (1983): Industrial yeast display tandem gene iteration at the CUP1 region. *Mol. Cell Biol.* 3: 1353.

Welch J, Fogel S, Buchman C, and Karin M (1989): The CUP2 gene product regulates the expression of the CUP1 gene, coding for yeast metallothionein. *EMBO J.* 8: 255.

Westin G and Schaffner W (1988): A zinc-responsive factor interacts with a metal-regulated enhancer element (MRE) of the mouse metallothionein-I gene. *EMBO J.* 7: 3763.

Winge D, Nielson K, Gray W, and Hamer D (1985): Yeast metallothionein. *J. Biol. Chem.* 260: 14464.

Function and Regulation of Yeast Cu-Metallothionein

Dean Hamer, Valeria Culotta,
Peter Fürst, Rebecca Hackett, Tsao Hsu,
Stella Hu, and Ravi Kambadur
Laboratory of Biochemistry
National Cancer Institute
National Institutes of Health
Bethesda, Maryland

ABSTRACT

The yeast *Saccharomyces cerevisae* has been used to study the function and regulation of Cu-metallothionein in a simple, genetically accessible eukaryotic organism. Studies of a mutant that cannot synthesize metallothionein show that the sole function of metallothionein in yeast is to detoxify Cu by maintaining low levels of the free ion. Metallothionein is *not* obligatorily involved in Cu transport, accumulation, or the synthesis of Cu enzymes in this organism. The ability of yeast metallothionein gene transcription to be induced by Cu ions is directly controlled by the *ACE1* regulatory protein. Cu(I) ions bind to the amino-terminal domain of ACE1, change its conformation, and thereby activate its ability to bind to the MT gene control DNA sequences. Once bound, the carboxy-terminal domain of ACE1 activates transcription by stimulating the formation of a committed transcription complex. We hypothesize that Cu(I) ions bind to the 12 cysteine residues of ACE1 to form an MT-like, polynuclear "copper fist" which forms the core for several DNA-binding "knuckles."

INTRODUCTION

Copper plays a dual role in biology. On the one hand, small amounts of copper are essential because of their participation in oxidation, electron transfer and many other enzymatic reactions. On the other hand, inappropriately high concentrations of copper are highly toxic and can cause cell death, developmental abnormalities and other deleterious effects. Thus all organisms must solve the problem of getting enough copper to survive, while at the same time protecting themselves from copper toxicity.

For some time, it has been speculated that metallothionein (MT) might play a critical role in the delicate balance between too much and not enough copper. Although MT was discovered as a Cd protein in horse kidney, it was soon realized that MT also binds avidly to Cu both *in vivo* and *in vitro*. In most higher eukaryotes, Cu-MT is observed only after experimental exposure to Cu, whereas in some fungi Cu-MT is the predominant natural form of the protein. The discovery that MT is transcriptionally regulated by Cu ions lent further fuel to the notion that MT might be involved in Cu homeostasis (reviewed in Hamer, 1986, and references therein).

Five years ago, this laboratory set out to answer two questions about MT and Cu. First, what exactly is the function of MT in Cu metabolism and detoxification? Second, how is MT gene expression regulated by Cu ions? The yeast *S. cerevisae*, because of its genetic manipulatability, proved ideal for answering both of these questions. The present manuscript describes our current understanding of these questions, and is mostly based on previously published papers. Portions of this manuscript are being concurrently published elsewhere (Imbert et al., 1989).

THE *CUP1* LOCUS

Yeast metallothionein is encoded by the *CUP1* locus, which is located on chromosome VIII, 42 centimorgans distal to the centromere. Yeast cells control the amount of intracellular MT by two distinct mechanisms, gene amplification and transcriptional control (for references, see Hamer, 1986). Most laboratory strains of yeast contain multiple copies of the *CUP1* locus, are resistant to 0.3 mM Cu in the medium, and are designated *CUP1*[R]. The Cu-MT structural gene is present in such strains as a 2 kilobase (kb) segment of DNA that is tandemly reiterated from 4 to 20 times. Other naturally occuring yeast strains contain a single copy of the *CUP1* locus, are sensitive to 0.3 mM Cu, and are designated *cup1*[s]. The reason for this variation in *CUP1* copy number amongst different strains is not understood.

The second mechanism for regulating MT concentration in yeast is transcriptional control. When yeast cells are grown in standard growth medium, which contains approximately 0.1 μ*M* Cu, the *CUP1* locus is transcribed at a low but detectable basal level. When excess Cu is added to the medium (between 1 and 500 μ*M*, depending on the strain), the transcription rate is increased by 10- to 50-fold, leading to the rapid accumulation of Cu-MT.

STRUCTURE OF CU-MT

The sequence of the cloned *CUP1* gene predicted a protein of 61 amino acids. We were therefore surprised, when we collaborated with Dennis Winge's lab to purify and characterize Cu-MT, to discover a protein of only 53 amino acids. Protein sequencing revealed that the first 8 amino acids of the protein were lacking, even when the protein was purified in the presence of various protease inhibitors or from a protease deficient strain (Winge et al., 1985). Interestingly, the removed sequence contains 5 hydrophobic residues, 2 of which are aromatic—an unusual type of sequence for an MT.

In an effort to understand the significance of this amino-terminal processing, which had not been observed in any other MT, we constructed two types of *CUP1* mutants. In one mutant, the complete "leader" sequence (except, of course, the initiator Met), has been deleted. Hence, in this mutant, the mature MT is directly synthesized without processing. In the second mutant, the cleavage site is changed from Asn Phe Gln to Arg Ile Gln. Protein sequencing showed that this mutant is not processed and accumulates predominantly as the full length, 61 amino acid species. Surprisingly, both mutant proteins were functional *in vivo*. Further studies showed that in the 61 amino acid protein, the amino-terminal peptide was selectively removed by various peptidases, suggesting that it does not participate in the tertiary fold. These results argue that the unusual amino-terminal peptide is not required for either the structural integrity or biological function of yeast MT (Wright et al., 1987).

The structure of the mature yeast Cu-MT has been studied both by genetic (this laboratory) and biochemical methods (in collaboration with Dennis Winge's laboratory). MT isolated from cells exposed to Cu during cell growth contains 8 Cu(I) ions ligated by 12 Cys residues. Reconstitution studies showed 8 mol eq of Cu(I) are required to fully reconstitute the apothionein and deplete the Zn content of Zn MT. Thus yeast MT has 8 binding sites for Cu(I). Ag(I) binds with the same stoichiometry. Yeast MT can also bind to Cd(II) and Zn(II) ions *in vitro,* even though it is not induced by them *in vivo*. Binding and displacement assays showed that these divalent ions associate with the protein with a maximal stoichiometry of 4 ions per molecule. Thus yeast MT, like mammalian MTs, exhibits two distinct binding configurations for Cu(I) and Ag(I) as compared to Cd(II) and Zn(II) (Winge et al., 1985). The contribution of various segments and Cys residues of yeast MT to metal binding have been investigated using truncated and mutated proteins (Bryd et al., 1988; Thrower et al., 1988; Wright et al., 1988).

The three-dimensional structure of yeast MT, and the precise arrangement of the Cu(I)-Cys cluster, are still not known. However, partial proteolysis experiments suggest that there is only a single cluster as compared to the two clusters found in higher eukaryotic MTs. An EXAFS study showed triganol coordination of each Cu(I) ion by S at a distance of 2.23 Å. Based on these data, it was proposed that the cluster structure for yeast Cu-MT is a distorted cube in which a Cu(I) occupies each corner and Cys sulfurs bridge each of the 12 edges (George et al., 1988).

FUNCTION OF YEAST CU-MT

The function of MT has been debated for more than 30 years. Fortunately, there is a powerful and simple method to determine the function of defined gene products in yeast. First, one uses recombinant DNA technology to delete the gene of interest. Second, one compares the wild-type and mutated strains for various functions in which the gene product is thought to be involved. Obviously, if the gene product is necessary for a given process, then the mutant strain should be deficient in that process.

To test the function of yeast MT, we constructed a strain in which the *CUP1* locus is deleted and replaced by the *URA3* gene. Analysis of protein synthesis showed that this strain does not make any MT. Nevertheless, it grows perfectly well on standard laboratory medium. It can also grow on various carbon sources and can go through all of the normal phases of the yeast life-cycle including haploid growth, mating, diploid growth, sporulation and germination. Moreover, the mutant took up Cu from the medium with the same kinetics as wild type and accumulated normal amounts of a copper enzyme, copper-zinc dismutase. Therefore, Cu-MT is a nonessential protein that is not required for Cu accumulation or the activation of a Cu enzyme under normal laboratory conditions (Hamer et al., 1985).

Two differences between yeast that do and do not make MT were noted. First, the mutant strain is very sensitive to Cu toxicity; it dies at less than 75 μM Cu as compared to 125 μM for *cup1*[s] or 1 mM for *CUP1*[R]. Second, it has an elevated level of transcription from an episomal *CUP1* promoter when grown in standard medium containing 0.1 μM Cu (Hamer et al., 1985). Both of these phenotypes can be attributed to increased levels of free intracellular Cu in the mutant (Wright et al., 1988), and can be complemented by expression of a mammalian MT in yeast (Thiele et al., 1986). We conclude that the main function of MT in yeast is to maintain low levels of *free* intracellular Cu.

Yeast is, in many senses, a typical eukaryotic cell. Therefore, we believe that the results obtained in yeast will probably hold true for other cell types. Indeed, certain lines of mammalian cells that make no apparent MT are known to grow perfectly well (reviewed in Hamer, 1986). However, our experiments cannot speak to any possible role of MT in whole body metal metabolism, nor to the function of Cd,Zn-MT. The function of higher eukaryotic MTs will be revealed only when appropriate mutants and transgenics are available.

REGULATION OF THE *CUP1* GENE BY *ACE1*

We showed previously that the ability of the *CUP1* gene to be transcriptionally induced by Cu is controlled by a short UAS (*U*pstream *A*ctivation *S*equence) which is located upstream of the MT coding sequences and can be functionally subdivided into UASc and UASd elements (Thiele and Hamer, 1986). This UAS can confer Cu regulation to a heterologous gene, suggesting that it acts as a binding site for a transcriptional activator protein. A genetic approach was used to isolate mutants in, and subsequently clone the gene for, this activator protein. The rationale for the screen was that cells lacking the activator protein would be deficient in MT and therefore, by analogy with *CUP1*[▲] strains, would be sensitive to Cu toxicity (Thiele and Hamer, 1987). Analysis of one such mutant, *ace1-1*, showed that it is a recessive gene located on chromosome VII. The subsequent cloning of the wild-type gene and construction of a null allele showed that *ACE1* is a nonessential gene whose only obvious function is to transactivate *CUP1* (Thiele, 1988).

Recently, the isolation of a second allele of *ACE1* has been reported. This mutant was initially called *cup2* (Welch et al., 1989), but subsequent DNA sequencing demonstrated that the wild-type "*CUP2*" gene is in fact identical to *ACE1* (Buchman et al., 1989). Thus *ACE1* and *CUP2* are the same gene; they have simply been called different names by different groups.

ACE1 IS A TWO DOMAIN PROTEIN

The sequence of the *ACE1* gene revealed that it encodes a protein of 225 amino acids (Fürst et al., 1988). Inspection of the deduced protein sequence immediately suggested the presence of two discrete domains. The carboxyterminal 100 residues are very acidic and resemble the activation domains of other yeast transcription factors such as *GAL4* or *GCN4*. In contrast, the aminoterminal 122 amino acids contain 28 lysines plus arginines and 12 cysteines. Six of these cysteines are arranged as CyxXCys and four more as CysXXCys, very similar to the organization of cysteines in metallothionein itself. The sequence of the aminoterminal domain suggested that it might bind to metals and/or DNA (Fürst et al., 1988).

The two-domain nature of *ACE1* has been confirmed by a genetic analysis using *ACE1-GAL4* hybrids (S. Hu, P. Fürst and D. Hamer, manuscript submitted). A hybrid with the aminoterminal domain of *ACE1* and the activation domain of *GAL4* activates *CUP1* gene expression in response to copper and galactose. Conversely, a fusion of the carboxyterminal domain of *ACE1* to a *GAL4* DNA-binding domain is a specific activator of *GAL1* but not responsive to copper. The genetic separation of the DNA-binding and activation domains of *ACE1* is confirmed by the biochemical analyses described below.

ACE1 IS CONSTITUTIVELY SYNTHESIZED

In principle, copper could activate MT gene transcription by two quite different mechanisms. First, copper could increase the expression of the *ACE1* locus and thereby increase the concentration of *ACE1* protein. Second, *ACE1* could be produced constitutively and affected by copper through a post-translational modification. To distinguish between these mechanisms, we used immunoblotting to measure the levels of *ACE1* peptide in cells grown in the presence or absence of copper and showed that they are equivalent (R. Hackett and D. Hamer, unpublished results). This result indicates that the basic mechanism of regulation is alteration of preexisting *ACE1* protein by copper. A similar conclusion was reached based on the analysis of an *ACE1-lacZ* fusion protein (Szczypka et al., 1989).

ACE1 IS A CU-DEPENDENT
DNA-BINDING PROTEIN

To determine whether the *ACE1* protein directly binds to DNA, it was first necessary to produce the protein from the cloned gene. For this purpose, the *ACE1* locus was cloned into a SP64 vector, appropriately truncated, transcribed by SP6 polymerase and translated in a wheat germ extract. The resulting *ACE1* protein, which is radioactively pure but far from chemically pure, was then tested for DNA binding activity by gel retardation or footprinting assays using *CUP1* control DNA sequences as probe. The full length polypeptide as well as a truncation mutant at amino acid residue 122 both bind to a 32P-labeled UASc oligonucleotide in a copper dependent manner. The apoprotein does not bind to DNA in any assay. The binding activity is reconstituted by adding micromolar concentrations of copper or silver (see below). Point mutant oligonucleotides which fail to induce gene expression *in vivo* do not bind *in vitro*. Thus the aminoterminal domain of *ACE1* is a copper-dependent DNA binding protein (Fürst et al., 1988).

In extracts prepared from yeast cells that overproduce the *ACE1* protein, a DNA binding activity with the same retardation in a gel shift assay and the same sequence specificity as the *in vitro* made protein can be detected. This binding activity, however, appears to be constitutive, probably due to contaminating copper in the extract. The amount of activity roughly correlates with the copy number of the *ACE1* gene (Fürst et al., 1988).

Methylation interference experiments indicate that at least four guanosine residues, G-142, G-140, G-131, and G-128, make close contact to the *ACE1* protein produced in wheat germ extract or in yeast cells. Notably, three of these guanines correspond to positions in which a transition mutation causes a loss of transcriptional competence (Fürst et al., 1988). DNaseI footprinting on a *CUP1* promoter fragment reveals two prominent binding regions, one covering a large part of the sequences present in UASc and a second, lower affinity one corresponding to UASd (Fürst and Hamer, 1989). The precise contacts within UASc, and the possibility of multiple binding sites for ACE1, are currently under investigation.

METAL SPECIFICITY

ACE1 specifically binds to DNA in the presence of either Cu(I) or Cu(II). However, the reaction is reversed by KCN, an effective chelator of Cu(I), and not by the Cu(II) chelator EDTA. Furthermore, Ag(I) (silver nitrate), a good electronic analog of Cu(I), also induces DNA binding activity *in vitro* and gene transcription *in vivo*. These results indicate that Cu(I) is the active species binding to the apoprotein, analogous to the interaction of copper with metallothionein. Divalent cations such as Cd(II), Zn(II), Pb(II), and Sn(II), all fail to activate *ACE1* either *in vitro* or *in vivo* (Fürst et al., 1988).

A COOPERATIVE CONFORMATIONAL SWITCH

In order to investigate how copper and silver activate DNA binding, we used partial proteolysis to probe the conformation of the full length and aminoterminal *ACE1* peptides in the presence or absence of metals and DNA. Copper protects the otherwise highly susceptible aminoterminal domain of ACE1 from trypsin degradation, strongly indicating that the metal ion directly binds to the protein. The main protected product has a molecular weight of 9 kDa (Fürst et al., 1988). Copper titration experiments, measuring either trypsin proteolysis or DNA binding, reveal a high degree of cooperativity (Hill coefficient 4.2). No intermediate size peptide fragments are observed at low copper concentrations. This indicates an all or none conformational change in the binding domain upon copper binding. Specific DNA further stabilizes the Cu-enzyme without changing the overall affinity for copper (Fürst and Hamer, 1989).

Silver activates the *ACE1* protein with different characteristics than copper. Although low concentrations of Ag(I) induce DNA binding, a large excess is required for saturation and the reaction is considerably less cooperative than for copper (Hill coefficient approximately 1.5). Furthermore, silver alone hardly protects the peptide from proteolysis, although in the presence of DNA a 9 kDa molecular weight peptide is protected from trypsin digestion. These results suggest that the Ag(I)-ACE1 complex has a somewhat different 3-dimensional structure than the Cu-protein, presumably due to the different ionic radius of Ag(I) compared to Cu(I). The copper form of the protein is perfectly poised to bind DNA whereas the silver form must undergo a further conformational alteration (Fürst and Hamer, 1989).

The highly cooperative effect of copper on DNA binding could, in principle, be due to interaction with multiple subunits or with multiple sites within a single subunit. To distinguish between these possibilities, the subunit composition of *ACE1* bound to UASc was determined by gel shift experiments using mixtures of full length and truncated ACE1 peptides. At least at low protein concentrations, the primary binding form is a monomer. This shows that the cooperative conformational switch of the ACE1 protein is due to the interaction of several copper ions with a single peptide chain. This cooperative interaction allows the cells to respond to small changes in the free copper concentration with a large increase in metallothionein gene expression (Fürst and Hamer, 1989).

TRANSCRIPTIONAL ACTIVATION *IN VITRO*

The carboxyterminal domain of *ACE1* is not required for DNA binding but is required for transcriptional activation (Fürst et al., 1988). Thus *ACE1* resembles many other eukaryotic transcription factors which contain discrete and separable DNA recognition and transcriptional activation domains. The activation domain of *ACE1* resembles those of the yeast *GAL4* and *GCN4* activators in that it is highly acidic and has the potential to form α-helices. We have begun to analyze the requirements for transcriptional activation by *ACE1* using a heterologous *in vitro* transcription assay with either total or fractionated mouse nuclear extract (Culotta et al., 1989, and unpublished results). These experiments showed that efficient activation by *ACE1* requires the following: (1) both the activation and DNA-binding domains of

ACE1; (2) *ACE1* binding sites on the template; (3) a TATA sequence; (4) mouse extract to provide RNA polymerase II and additional general factors; (5) TFIID, the TATA-binding factor; and (6) Cu or Ag. Interestingly, the formation of a committed transcription complex by *ACE1* is reversible by Cu(I) chelators (Culotta et al., 1989). This may give the cell a mechanism to turn off *CUP1* gene transcription once the levels of intracellular Cu have fallen.

PRELIMINARY STRUCTURAL MODEL: THE COPPER FIST

The DNA-binding domain of *ACE1* bears several intriguing structural resemblances to MT itself, particularly to yeast Cu-MT: the ability to bind Cu(I) and Ag(I); the all-or-none nature of the metal binding reaction; the stability of the metalloprotein and the sensitivity of the apoprotein to proteases; the paucity of hydrophobic and aromatic residues; and, most important, the presence of 12 cysteine residues, 10 of which are arranged in pairs similar to those found in MT. Based on these similarities, we have proposed a copper cluster model for the aminoterminal domain of *ACE1* gene product (Figure 1). We emphasize that this is a highly speculative model which is not supported by any biophysical data; its sole purpose is to try to explain how a peptide of this size could bind both to metals and DNA.

According to our model, the 12 cysteines of the aminoterminal domain bind 8 copper atoms. We speculate that these form a Cu_8-S_{12} cuboidal cluster in which each copper ion is chelated by 3 sulfur ligands. In the structure shown in Figure 1B, these are arranged such that paired cysteines contact a common copper ion. This arrangement would allow the interspersed polypeptides, which are rich in basic aminoacid residues, to form loop structures that are appropriately poised to bind DNA. These loops could be projected away from the copper cluster by β-turns and could easily accommodate the DNA binding site (Fürst et al., 1988).

Although we do not yet have physical data to support this model, two observations from site-directed mutagenesis are at least consistent with our ideas. First, several Cys to Ser conversion mutants fail to undergo a copper-induced conformational switch. Second, two mutants in basic residues bind to metals normally but to DNA with greatly reduced affinity (S. Hu, P. Fürst and D. Hamer, manuscript submitted). Although this is only correlatory data, these mutants should prove useful for subsequent physical analyses.

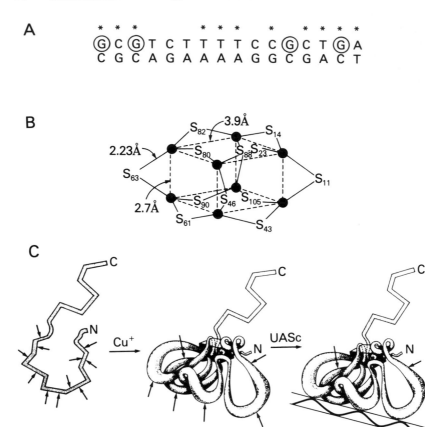

Figure 1. Preliminary structural model of the *ACE1* metalloregulatory factor. (A) The *ACE1* DNA binding site. Bases that were protected in the methylation interference assay are circled. Bases for which a transition causes lack of *in vivo* transcriptional activity are starred. (B) A possible coordination scheme for the proposed Cu_8S^{12} core of the amino-terminal domain. The sulfur atoms represent cysteine thiolates, and are numbered according to the position of the cysteine residues in the *ACE1* sequence. The bond distance are taken from an EXAFS analysis of copper metallothionein (George et al., 1988). (C) Proposed folding scheme. The arrows represent exposed trypsin sites. In the absence of copper (left section), the amino-terminal domain is a randomly folded configuration in which the basic residues are susceptible to trypsin. Addition of copper (middle section) causes folding of the amino-terminal domain around the Cu-S cluster according to the coordination scheme in part B. Binding of DNA to the basic loops (right section) results in further protection against trypsin. The twists at the beginning of loop I and at the ends of loops II and IV represent proposed β-turns. The carboxy-terminal domain is drawn without meaning to imply any particular structure. (From Fürst et al. [1988], *Cell* 55: 705. With permission.)

CONCLUSION

We now have a reasonably clear outline of how Cu ions induce yeast MT gene transcription. In either the absence or presence of copper, the cell constitutively expresses the *ACE1* locus and synthesizes *ACE1* protein. However, in the absence of added copper, the aminoterminal domain of the protein exists in a randomly folded conformation which cannot recognize DNA. When high amounts of metals are added to the cell, they bind to the aminoterminal domain and form a copper-sulfur cluster. The protein folds around this domain to form a structure which can specifically recognize the UAS control sequences, probably through basic loop structures. The cooperative nature of the folding reaction suggests that binding of the first atom(s) of metal to the protein folds it into a conformation that is ideally suited for binding additional metal ions and DNA. Once the protein is folded, one or more molecules bind to the *CUP1* upstream DNA sequences and activate transcription. Once the *CUP1* gene has been activated, the resulting mRNA is translated into apothionein, which tightly and cooperatively binds to Cu ions and thereby protects the cell from Cu toxicity.

Now that the broad outline of this mechanism is known, two questions remain outstanding. First, what is the three-dimensional structure of this unusual Cu and DNA-binding regulatory protein? And second, how does it activate transcription once bound to the DNA? These are topics of current research in this laboratory.

REFERENCES

Buchman C, Skroch P, Welch J, Fogel S, and Karin M (1989): The CUP2 gene product, regulator of yeast metallothionein expression, is a copper-activated DNA-binding protein. *Mol. Cell. Biol.* 9: 4091.

Byrd J, Berger RM, McMillin DR, Wright CF, Hamer D, and Winge DR (1988): Characterization of the copper-thiolate cluster in yeast metallothionein and two truncated mutants. *J. Biol. Chem.* 263: 6688.

Culotta VC, Hsu T, Hu S, Fürst P, and Hamer DH (1989): Copper and the ACE1 regulatory protein reversibly induce yeast metallothionein gene transcription in a mouse extract. *Proc. Natl. Acad. Sci. U.S.A.* 86: 8377.

Fürst P, Hu S, Hackett R, and Hamer D (1988): Copper activates metallothionein gene transcription by altering the conformation of a specific DNA binding protein. *Cell* 55: 705.

Fürst P and Hamer D (1989): Cooperative activation of a eukaryotic transcription factor: interaction between Cu(I) and yeast ACE1 protein. *Proc. Natl. Acad. Sci. U.S.A.* 86: 5267.

George GN, Byrd J, and Winge DR (1988): X ray absorption studies of yeast copper metallothionein. *J. Biol. Chem.* 263: 8199.

Hamer DH (1986): Metallothionein. *Ann. Rev. Biochem.* 55: 913.

Hamer DH, Thiele DJ, and Lemontt JE (1985): Function and autoregulation of yeast copperthionein. *Science* 228: 685.

Imbert J, Culotta V, Fürst P, Gedamu L, and Hamer DH: Regulation of metallothionein gene transcription by metals, in *Advances in Inorganic Biochemistry 8: Metal-Ion Induced Regulation of Gene Expression,* Eichhorn GL and Marzilli LG (1990), Eds, Elsevier, New York, pp. 139–164.

Szczypka MS and Thiele DJ (1989): A cysteine-rich nuclear protein activates yeast metallothionein gene transcription. *Mol. Cell. Biol.* 9: 421.

Thiele DJ (1988): ACE1 regulates expression of the *Saccharomyces cerevisiae* metallothionein gene. *Mol. Cell. Biol.* 8: 2745.

Thiele DJ and Hamer DH (1986): Tandemly duplicated upstream control sequences mediate copper-induced transcription of the *Saccharomyces cerevisiae* coppermetallothionein gene. *Mol. Cell. Biol.* 6: 1158.

Thiele DJ, Walling MJ, and Hamer DH (1986): Mammalian metallothionein is functional in yeast. *Science* 231: 854.

Thiele DJ and Hamer DH (1987): Cis and trans-acting genetic elements that regulate copper-metallothionein gene expression in yeast, in *RNA Polymerase and the Regulation of Transcription,* pp. 431-856. Elsevier, Amsterdam.

Thrower AR, Byrd J, Tarbet EB, Mehra RK, Hamer DH, and Winge DR (1988): Effect of mutation of cysteinyl residues in yeast cu-metallothionein. *J Biol. Chem.* 263: 7037.

Welch J, Fogel S, Buchman C, and Karin M (1989): The CUP2 gene product regulates the expression of the CUP1 gene coding for yeast metallothionein. *EMBO J.* 8: 255.

Winge DR, Nielson KB, Gray WR, and Hamer DH (1985): Yeast metallothionein. *J. Biol. Chem.* 260: 14464.

Wright CF, McKenney K, Hamer DH, Byrd J, and Winge DR (1987): Structural and functional studies of the amino terminus of yeast metallothionein. *J. Biol. Chem.* 262: 12912.

Wright CF, Hamer DH, and McKenney K (1988): Autoregulation of the yeast copper metallothionein gene depends on metal binding. *J. Biol. Chem.* 263: 1570.

Chapter 7

Native and Engineered Metallothioneins

P.C. Huang,[1] Chris Cody, Mary Cismowski, Mark Chernaik, In-Koo Rhee[2] and L.Y. Lin[3]
Department of Biochemistry
The Johns Hopkins University
School of Hygiene and Public Health
Baltimore, Maryland

ABSTRACT

Structural constraints on the functionality of native and engineered class I metallothioneins (MT) were examined. For the native molecules, a repertoire of known sequences was examined for variation in length, composition and isoforms. Unlike mammals which carry two basic isoforms of MT, avian and fish species may carry one or two depending on their origin. In one case, MTs from diverse species share the same amino acid sequence, with the exception of an added residue in each of the two domains and a unique histidine at the carboxyl terminus. Among the amino acids held invariant in native MTs from vertebrates, cysteine, serine and lysine have been selectively replaced by recombinant techniques in this study to see if

[1]To whom to address correspondence.
[2]Present address: Department of Agricultural Chemistry, Kyungpook National University, Taegu, Korea.
[3]Present address: Institute of Molecular Biology, Academia Sinica, Nankang 11529, Taipei, Taiwan, R.O.C.

these structural alterations affect MT properties. Using metal toxicity in transformed yeast systems as a biological marker, the ability of these variants to convey resistance to an otherwise lethal dosage of metals such as cadmium and copper were examined. Observed changes depend upon the site and nature of the mutation. Insertion mutagenesis with peptides of increasing length introduced into the interdomain hinge region rendered the resulting variants unstable. These results suggest that present day MT has evolved to assume a most stable configuration for its function with only a limited range for further mutation.

INTRODUCTION

A distinct structural feature of class I MTs (Fowler et al., 1987) is that each of them consists of two domains, coded respectively by separate exons (see review by Hamer, 1986). Models for their structure have been deduced by X-ray crystallographic (Furey et al., 1986) and 2-D nuclear magnetic resonance spectroscopic measurements (Wagner et al., 1986; Arseniev et al., 1988; Frey et al., 1988; Schultze et al., 1988). The assignments are consistent with MT being made up of two nearly spherical domains of identical size, 15 to 20 Å in diameter. As predicted earlier (Otvos and Armitage, 1980) there is a metal thiolate cluster in each of these domain centers. Thus, metal ions are partitioned into two metal-thiolate groups of three and four, respectively, in the amino terminal (beta domain) or the carboxyl terminal (alpha domain) halves of the polypeptide chains. While the domains are linked by a tripeptide lys-lys-ser hinge which may maintain the flexibility of the molecule, indirect evidence suggests that metal dependent folding of MT to create one cluster occurs independent of constraints or influences from the other; the two domains may thus form and function separately (Winge and Miklossy, 1982; Nielson and Winge, 1985; Nielson et al., 1985).

At least two questions may be generated from these general models:

1. What is the limit of variation for MTs as revealed by their native sequences?
2. What are certain amino acids held invariant in native MTs?

This study is undertaken to elucidate some of the answers pertaining to the structural constraints on the functionality of MTs.

VARIATIONS IN NATIVE METALLOTHIONEINS FROM VERTEBRATES

Thirty five class I MT amino acid sequences from mammals determined directly or deduced from cDNA are collected and compared (Figure 1). All mammalian MTs have 61 amino acids with the exception of canine MT which has its N-terminal methionine removed, probably due to lysosomal processing, and rabbit MT which has 62 amino acids. Two fragments, the N-terminal MDPNCSC and the interdomain sequence CKKSCCSCCP are entirely conserved. All 20 cysteinyl residues are invariant; three of the serines, S-6, S-32 and S-35 are also constant. The other serines, however, may be replaced by arginine, leucine, valine or, most commonly, threonine. Lysines K-22, K-30, K-31, K-51 and K-56 are invariant, but K-20, K-25, and K-43 may be substituted by arginine; K-20 may also be replaced by alanine, glycine, or threonine. Basic amino acids may replace glycine as shown where there is one example of a substitution by arginine at position 39. All mammalian MTs terminate with alanine at their carboxyl ends except human 1F MT, which ends with aspartic acid.

Birds and fish are the only phyla of lower vertebrates whose MTs have recently been examined. Like mammals, pigeon has two isoforms of MT (Lin et al., 1989). Chicken, on the other hand, has only one (McCormick et al., 1988; Wei and Andrew et al., 1988). The single duck MT has the same amino acid sequence as that from chicken (Lin et al., in preparation). Fish may have one or two isoforms of MT. Thus far only MTs in rainbow trout (Bonham et al., 1987), winter flounder (Chan et al., 1989) and plaice (Leaver and George, 1989) have been deduced from cDNA sequences. These MT sequences are shown in Figure 2. They differ from those of mammals in several aspects:

1.. Avian MTs carry two extra amino acids, one in each domain, for a total of 63 amino acids. Fish MTs, on the other hand, have a total of 60 amino acids, lacking an asparagine near the N-terminus.
2.. In contrast to the alanine in mammalian MTs, the carboxyl termini of avian MTs are either lysine or histidine; all fish MTs have either glutamine or asparagine at their carboxyl ends.
3.. Arginine or asparagine can replace lysine at residue 30 of the interdomain sequence CKKSCCSCCP in avian and fish MTs, respectively. Proline can replace serine at position 35 in fish MTs.
4.. In both avian and fish MTs, serine is present in place of proline, lysine, glycine, alanine, glutamine and/or aspartic acid at various sites, resulting in MT sequences containing up to 14 serines.
5.. In trout MTs, plaice MT, and flounder MT there is an extra cysteine in position 55.

```
Equine 1A MDPNCSCPTGGSCTCAGSCKCKECRCTSCKKSCCSCCPGGCARCAQGCVCKGASDKCSCCA
   L-54   ------------------------------------------------------L-------
   R-39   ------------------------------------------R-------------------
      1B  -------VA-E-----------Q---A----------------------------------

Human 1   -------AT-V--------------K--------------V---K-----I---T-E------
      1A  -------A--------T--------K-N------------M---K-----I-----E-----
      1B  -------T-----A----------K--------------V---K-----------E-----
      1E  -------A----------------K--------------V---K-----------E-----
      1F  -------AA-V-------------K--------------V--SK-----------E----D
      1G  -------AA-V-----S-------K--------------V---K-----I-----E-----
      1PG -------SPD---A----------T--------------V---K-S---I---T--------
      1H  -------AA-V-------------K--------------V---K-----I-----E-----
      1J  -------AA-V-------------K--------------V---K-----I-----E-----
      1K  -------AA-V-----S-------K--------------V---K-----I-----E-----
      1L  -------SPV---A----------K--------------V---K-----I---T--------
      2   -------VA-D-------------K--------------M---K-----I------------
      2A  -------AA-D-------------K--------------V---K-----I------------
      2PG -------AASD-------------K--------------V---K-----I-----A------

CHO   1   -------S-GST---SS--G--D-K--------------V--SK--------------T---
      2   -------A-D---S----------K--T-----------V---K-S------E---------

Bovine 2  -------TA-E------------D-K-A-----------V---K-----------------
 fetal 1  ----------------------A---P------------V---K-----------------

Rat   1   -------S-------SS--G--N-K--------------V--SK--------------T---
      2   -------A-D---S----------Q-K------------V---K-S---I--E---------

Mouse 1   -------S-------TS--A--D----------------V--SK--------------T---
      2   -------ASD---S---A----Q-K--------------V---K-S---I--E---------

Monkey 1  -------A--V-----D-------K--------------V---K-----------E--N---
      2   -------VA---------------K--------------V---K-----I--------N---

               AA              -
Canine    ------S----------------K--------------V---K------------------

Sheep     --------------S-----T--A---P-----------V---K------------------

Rabbit 1  -------AAD------T--R----K--------------A--TK-----I-----------
      2   -------AAD------T-----------------------S---K-----I-----------
      2A  -------^A-D-----N--T--A-K--------------P---K-----I-----------
      2B  -------A--D-----S-------K--------------A--TK-----I-----------

Dolphin   -------TA----A-P--------K--------------V---K-----I-----------
```

Figure 1. Mammalian metallothionein sequences. From Kägi and Kojima (1987), except dolphin. Rhee I (1988), personal communications.

```
Equine 1A MDP NCSCPTGGSCTCAGSCKCKECRCTSCKKSCCSCCPGGCARCAQGCVCKGASDK CSCCA  a

Chick/Duck---QD-TCAA-D--S--------N---R--R--------A--NN--K-----EPASSK----H  b

Pigeon 1  ---QD-P-AA--T---GAN----N---------------A---K---------PPSAK----K  c
       2  ---QD-T-AA-D-----------N---Q--R--------AS-SN--K-----EP-SSK----H

Plaice 1  ---  -E-SKT---N-G---T--N-S----N----P---S--PK--S-----KTCD T---Q  d

Trout  A  ---  -E-SKT---N-G-----SN-A---------P---SD-SK--S------KTAT ----Q  e
       B  ---  -E-SKT---N-G-----SN-A---------P---SD-SK--S------KTCD T---Q

Flounder  ---  -E-SKT---N-G---T--N-S----N----P---S--PK--S------KTCD TT--N  f
```

Figure 2. Comparison of equine, avian, and fish metallothioneins. From a, see Figure 1; b, chicken: Wei and Andrew (1988), McCormick et al. (1988); duck: Lin and Huang (unpublished); c, Lin et al. (1989); d, Leaver and George (1989); e, Bonham et al. (1987); f, Chan et al. (1989).

> 6.. At least three lysine residues are replaced in fish MTs by either threonine or asparagine, but at other sites lysine replaces threonine, arginine or alanine; the net basic charge remains similar.

As a whole, MTs in vertebrates show limited variation. With the exceptions noted above, the interdomain spacing and the number and position of the cysteines and some of the serine residues are invariant.

ENGINEERED METALLOTHIONEINS

With recombinant DNA techniques, mutant MTs have been generated to examine whether the conserved structural features in native MTs can be altered without the impairment of function. Two repertoires of mutants were examined, in which the interdomain hinges were perturbed, and specific amino acids were substituted.

Materials and Basic Methodology

Chinese hamster (CHO) MT2 cDNA (Griffith et al., 1983) was used throughout as the starting material; alterations were made by insertion and substitution mutagenesis. Insertions were made in the interdomain hinge by taking advantage of the presence of an Alu-1 endonuclease cleavage site which bisects the coding sequence into two halves, corresponding to the beta and the alpha domains of MT (Figure 3). A second Alu-1 site at nucleotide position 174 was eliminated by oligonucleotide directed mutagenesis, changing the ser codon from AGC to AGT. Defined sequences of oligomers pCCCGGG or pTCCCCCGGGGGA were inserted between the domains to generate a series of chimeric plasmids carrying inserts of one

(MTX61) or two (MTX62) hexamers or a single (MTX121) or multiple (MTX122, MTX123 and MTX124) dodecamers (Rhee et al., 1989).

Site directed mutagenesis was carried out in two ways. For most of the cysteine and serine replacement mutants, bisulfite induced changes in the positive and negative strands of CHO MT2 cDNA were used to yield two repertoires of random mutants altered in single or multiple amino acids (Pine and Huang, 1987). Other amino acid replacement mutants, such as S-35, K-30 and K-31, however, were generated by oligonucleotide directed mutagenesis (Kunkel et al., 1987). All mutations were confirmed by direct DNA sequencing. The specific sites of mutation used in this study are summarized in Figure 4.

A series of single and high copy yeast episomal plasmids were constructed from M13 RF DNA carrying the appropriate MT cDNA or its variants and two *Escherichia coli*-yeast shuttle vectors, pYSK102 and pYSK54 (Smith, Kline, and French) using standard recombinant DNA methods (Maniatis et al., 1982). Plasmid DNA mediated transformation of yeast was carried out with lithium chloride (Ito et al., 1983) and transformants were selected by growth on tryptophan-deficient (trp$^-$) plates. The recipient host AB-DE1 (Mat a, arg4–8, leu2–3, leu2–112, his7–2, trp1–289, ade5, cup1^{del}) is devoid of its endogenous thionein gene, which allowed a direct assay for the ability of the introduced MT cDNA to convey metal resistance (Ecker et al., 1986). The promoter from the yeast triose phosphate isomerase

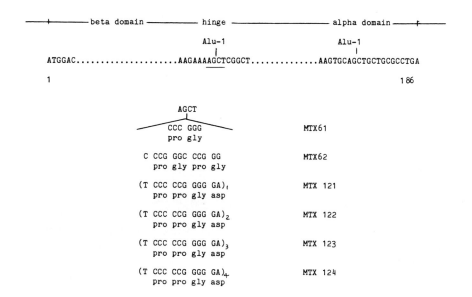

Figure 3. Insertion mutagenesis of CHO MT2 at the interdomain hinge region.

PARENTAL SEQUENCE

MDPNCSCATDGSCSCAGSCKCKECKCTTCKKSCCSCCPVGCAKCSQGCVCKEASDKCSCCA

A. Cysteine mutants

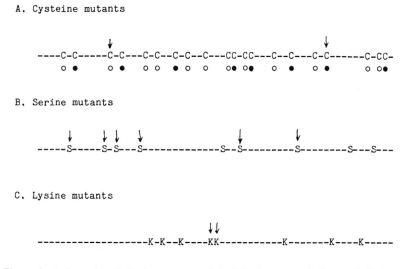

B. Serine mutants

C. Lysine mutants

Figure 4. Amino acid substitution mutants of CHO MT2. Arrows indicate substitution sites of mutants included in this study. (○) denotes terminal cysteine and (●) bridging cysteine as assigned by 2-D NMR analyses (Arseniev et al., 1988; Schultze et al., 1988).

gene, which is not affected by exogenous metal ions, was used to direct the expression of the MT coding sequences.

Transformed cells were also examined for their copy number of the chimeric plasmids carrying MT cDNA or its variants and for the level of mRNA (Ohi et al., 1981; Morris and Huang, 1987, 1989) as well as for MT accumulation. MT and its variants were characterized by high cysteine content, reactivity with iodoacetamide, size and net charge density. Quantitative preparations (Cismowski et al., 1988) of some of these mutants were subjected to measurements for metal affinity by atomic absorption spectrometry.

Interdomain Perturbation

The two domains of native mammalian MTs are separated by a tripeptide lys-lys-ser. The conserved nature of this hinge region may reflect a structural constraint for folding or stability of MTs. In this study we have generated mutants of MT by inserting dipeptide or tetrapeptide codons of varying lengths between the interdomain space, cloned them into a high copy number yeast shuttle vector, and used the vector to transform cup1[del] yeast cells. Using metal resistance as a biological marker, the constructs were shown to be functional in rendering the host cells resistant to either copper or cadmium. The level of activity, however, diminished with the length of the insert. As many as sixteen amino acid codons could be placed between the two metal-thiolate domain clusters without affecting the ability of these proteins to detoxify; larger variants were metal sensitive.

The reduced tolerance seen in the larger inserts may be due to the fact that MT cDNA sequences introduced failed to replicate, transcribe, or translate. A plasmid containing repetitive sequences may form internal hairpin loops or undergo intramolecular recombination. Exogenous sequences in mRNA may present signals which cause abortive transcription. Novel proteins may not survive cellular surveillance systems and degrade rapidly. To rule out these possibilities, determinations were made for copy number of the chimeric plasmids and MT mRNA levels in the transformed cells. Results showed that the replicational and transcriptional capacity of the long and short constructs were equivalent (Rhee et al., 1989). Differences may exist, however, in the fidelity of translational and/or post-translational processes as less MT protein could be detected in cells transformed with MT containing long inserts. Therefore, the length of insertion in the hinge region may be a constraint on the stability of the protein constructs, as longer interdomain insertions apparently render the protein less stable.

The inserted sequences (pro-gly)$_{1-2}$ or (pro-pro-gly-asp)$_{1-4}$ are not known to be targets for a specific endopeptidase. They could provide additional flexibility, which is minimal in native MT. Although both domains are linked with a tripeptide lys-lys-ser, the distance between the domains can not be estimated here. We may speculate that long inserts may slow down translation by the presence of possible secondary structure. Alternatively, we may envision that extensive spacing between domains in MT renders the molecule more flexible in the hinges and more vulnerable to protease attack. We note that MTs in their fully metallated states are highly resistant to protease digestion. While sensitivity of some of our constructs may provide a clue to the mechanism with which cells exclude unnatural proteins, the functionality of the others reveals the extent of engineering which MT can structurally tolerate.

Cysteine Mutants

Nuclear magnetic resonance and X-ray spectroscopic studies have established that cysteine in MT is involved in metal binding. In mammalian MTs the binding involves the formation of tetrahedryl metal-thiolate clusters. Two types of linkage exist; terminal cysteines bind only one metal while bridging cysteines link two metals. In this regard, a discrepancy exists over the assignment by 2-D NMR and by X-ray crystallography of specific cysteine residues to specific metal atoms (see Kägi and Schaffer, 1988). By NMR, C-13 is assigned as terminal and C-50 is bridging. By X-ray data, the reverse is suggested. One would predict *a priori* that the disruption of a bridging cysteine would be more detrimental to the structure and metal binding capacity of MT than would disruption of a terminal one.

In this study, mutants were chosen from a mutant library constructed earlier (Pine et al., 1985). The mutants chosen for study consist of a single cysteine to tyrosine replacement at position 13 in the beta domain (C13Y), or at position 50 in the alpha domain (C50Y), or at both sites (C13,50Y). Using a high copy-number yeast vector, these mutant cDNAs and the corresponding wild type cDNA were cloned and expressed constitutively in a yeast cup1^{del} strain. Each MT sequence was able to confer at least a 40-fold increased resistance to cadmium compared to the host transformed with the expression vector alone. The rate of growth in rich media for all four MT producing strains is indistinguishable from that of the controls. In the presence of 20 μM CdCl$_2$, however, there was a slight retardation in the growth of C13Y and the native MT, and a marked inhibition in C50Y and C13,50Y. The latter two also failed to reach saturation in the presence of 20 μM cadmium.

The wild type and three mutant MTs were purified from cadmium containing liquid cultures. The purified proteins were subjected to NMR analysis (to be reported elsewhere). Atomic absorption spectrometry measurements show that wild-type Cd-MT bound 7 metal ions/molecule, with cadmium being the predominant metal species and zinc and copper present in trace amounts. The mutant MTs bound less cadmium but somewhat higher amounts of zinc than the wild type, with a total of approximately 6 metal ions/molecule.

We have thus shown that wild type CHO MT2 and its mutants containing specific, single or double cysteine to tyrosine replacements are functional in yeast in cadmium detoxification. This is consistent with earlier work with monkey MTs (Thiele et al., 1986). However, two mutants, C50Y and C13,50Y, which share a cys to tyr replacement at position 50 have a markedly lower ability to confer resistance to cadmium in the recipient cells. The reduced capacity to impart resistance can not be explained by lowered copy number of the vector nor by lowered steady-state MT mRNA or protein levels. It also cannot be attributed to the introduction of a large aromatic side chain, as a cysteine to serine replacement at position 50, but not at position 13, also confers lowered resistance to cadmium in liquid medium (unpublished observations). Hence the reduction is probably due to the specific loss of a cysteine residue at position 50. Our work is consistent with recent studies on the class II yeast MT (Thrower et al., 1988; George et al., 1988; Winge et al., 1985; Byrd et al., 1988) which showed that some

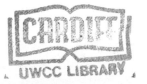

cysteine residues are more important than others in conveying resistance to copper toxicity.

Results from our studies indicate that there is no simple correlation between the stable cadmium binding capacity of MT and its ability to confer resistance to cadmium *in vivo*. The stoichiometries of bound cadmium, zinc and copper in wild type and mutant MTs differ by approximately one atom, yet the ability of these proteins to detoxify *in vivo* varies greatly. We postulate that this differential resistance is due to the disruption of the normally static alpha domain by the mutation at C-50. Differential modification studies with iodoacetamide (Bernhard et al., 1986) and ^{113}Cd saturation transfer NMR experiments (Otvos et al., 1987) show that cadmium bound to the beta domain is dynamic while cadmium bound to the alpha domain is static. Although all cadmium atoms of wild type MT are stably bound, cadmium bound to the beta domain is more labile, as can be seen by selective removal of the metals with chelators such as EDTA (Stillman and Zelazowski 1987, 1988). That the two domains of MT may contribute to different extents in cadmium detoxification has been further tested with additional mutants at positions 13 and 50, replacing the cysteines with serine instead of tyrosine, with similar results (Chernaik et al., unpublished). Replacing cysteines at other sites in these domains is being attempted.

Serine Mutants

The invariance of half of the serines in mammalian MTs and the extraordinarily rich serine content in fish and avian MTs prompted the inquiry into its importance in MT structure and function. Presumably, serines could be responsible for maintaining the three dimensional structure of MT.

CHO MT2 has a total of nine serine residues at positions 6, 12, 14, 18, 32, 35, 45, 54, and 58. By substitutional mutagenesis we have created a set of mutants with a single replacement of serine by phenylalanine at residue 6, 12, 18, 35 or 45. These mutants are designated S6F, S12F, S14F, S18F:I9T and S45F, respectively; all possess a single amino acid substitution except S18F:I9T which also has the isoleucine at position 9 replaced by threonine. These 5 mutants have all been subcloned into the single copy yeast vector. Transformation of AB-DE1 with these variant metallothioneins confers resistance to 30 μM copper or cadmium on trp$^-$ plates; wild type MT confers the same level of metal resistance.

S6F and S45F have been characterized in depth. These variant metallothioneins have been further subcloned into the high copy number, yeast vector. When AB-DE1 is transformed by this vector containing wild type or phenylalanine variant MTs, the transformants will grow on trp$^-$ plates supplemented with 300 μM cadmium or copper. In rich media supplemented with 20 μM cadmium, transformants of either variant will grow at the same rate as the wild type MT2 transformant with a doubling time of 2.7 h.

Both the variants express a protein characteristic of MT. The high copy yeast vector transformants express a cysteine-rich protein which can be visualized by labeling with ^{35}S-cysteine. These variant proteins can be visualized on 18% native polyacrylamide gels or, upon treatment with iodoacetamide, on 15% SDS gels. The mobility of the phenylalanine variants on either type of gel is similar to that of wild type MT2.

Our data suggest that replacement of a single serine with phenylalanine does not result in a gross distortion of MT as evidenced by conference of metal resistance to yeast AB-DE1 and protein expression. We are currently investigating whether metallothionein can be perturbed by replacing serine with amino acids other than phenylalanine.

Lysine Mutants

The interdomain hinge region in all class I metallothioneins is conserved; two basic amino acids are flanked by sequences rich in serine and cysteine, SCKKSC. Lysines have been implicated in neutralizing the negative charges generated by the cysteine residues (Pande et al., 1986). Furthermore, we speculate that the positively charged lysines in the hinge may be involved in allowing the protein to fold properly. With this in mind, we have constructed metallothionein variants that substitute glutamic acid or glutamine for either lysine residue 30 or 31.

Mutants have been constructed by site-directed mutagenesis (Kunkel et al., 1987), replacing lysine 30 with glutamic acid (K30E) and replacing lysine 31 with glutamic acid (K31E) or with glutamine (K31Q). All three mutants have been subcloned into the high copy yeast vector and all confer metal resistance to yeast AB-DE1. Transformants can all grow on trp⁻ plates supplemented with 300 μM copper or cadmium. Additionally, these three transformants grow in rich media supplemented with 20 μM cadmium with a doubling time of 2.7 h like wild type MT transformants. Hence, the lysine variants appear to confer the same level of metal resistance to AB-DE1 as the wild type protein.

[35]S-cysteine labeled lysine variants have been visualized on native and SDS gels. The lysine variants can only be visualized on SDS gels following iodoacetamide treatment and migrate at the same position as wild type MT2. An interesting observation is made when zinc MT2 and zinc lysine variants are run on an 18% native gel. Mobility is seen to vary with charge density; K30E and K31E, which have the highest net negative charge density, migrate the furthest. Wild type MT2, which has the highest positive charge density, migrates the least distance, as expected. K31Q has an intermediate charge density and migrates more slowly than the glutamate variants but faster than wild type MT.

Since lysine residues 30 and 31 occupy essentially equivalent positions in the tripeptide composing the interdomain hinge, replacement of either lysine with glutamate would be expected to result in MT variants with the same charge density. K30E, however, migrates faster than K31E. This implies that the substitution of the lysine residue K-30 perturbs MT to a different extent than substituting K-31, perhaps by weakening the binding to zinc. The nature of such a difference is being studied.

CONCLUSIONS

In summary, we have identified the highly conserved features of mammalian MTs studied to date and contrasted them with those derived from two phyla of lower vertebrates, fish and birds. The genetic polymorphism of MT appears to be limited to variations that do not perturb the two distinct metal binding domains. Using the ability to convey resistance to otherwise sensitive cells, MT mutants altered at some of the conserved sites were examined. By insertion mutagenesis, we showed that addition of peptides up to 12 amino acids between two domains had no apparent effect, but MTs with longer inserts were unstable *in vivo*. While a number of alterations showed no functional changes, replacement of a single cysteine in either the alpha or beta domain caused reduction in metal binding. Furthermore, two adjacent highly conserved lysines in the interdomain region of MT may contribute differently to the structure. This was reflected in differential change in charge and/or configuration of the mutant MT. A general picture thus emerges from these initial observations that modern MTs are evolved with strong structural constraints for their unique function in metal detoxification and presumably also in metal homeostasis. Further studies with the purified mutant proteins including metal affinity, protease sensitivity, thiol group reactivity and NMR spectroscopy would be informative and are being pursued.

ACKNOWLEDGMENT

This study was supported in part by U.S. NIH Grant GM32606 to P.C. Huang.

REFERENCES

Arseniev A, Schultze P, Wörgötter E, Braun W, Wagner G, Vašák M, Kägi JHR, and Wuthrich K (1988): Three-dimensional structure of rabbit liver Cd-7 metallothionein-2a in aqueous solution determined by nuclear magnetic resonance. *J. Mol. Biol.* 201: 637–657.

Bernhard WR, Vašák M, and Kägi JHR (1986): Cadmium binding and metal cluster formation in metallothionein: a differential modification study. *Biochemistry* 25: 1975–1980.

Bonham K, Zafarullah M, and Gedamu L (1987): The rainbow trout metallothioneins: molecular cloning and characterization of two distinct cDNA sequences. *DNA* 6: 25–59.

Byrd J, Berger RM, McMillin DR, Wright CF, Hamer D and Winge DR (1988): Characterization of the copper-thiolate cluster in yeast metallothionein and two truncated mutants. *J. Biol. Chem.* 263: 6688–6694.

Chan KM, Davidson WS, Hew CL, and Fletcher G (1989): Molecular cloning of metallothionein complementary DNA and analysis of metallothionein gene expression in winter flounder tissues. *Can. J. Zool.* 67: 2520–2527.

Cismowski M, Chernaik M, Rhee I-K and Huang PC (1988): Expression of a Chinese hamster metallothionein coding sequence and its variants in *S. cerevisiae*. In *Metal Ion Homeostasis: Molecular Biology and Chemistry*, (Winge D and Hamer D, Eds.), UCLA Symposia on Molecular and Cellular Biology, Alan R. Liss, New York, New Series, 98: 237–246.

Ecker DJ, Butt TR, Sternberg EJ, Neeper MP, Debouck C, Gorman JA, and Crooke ST (1986): Yeast metallothionein function in metal ion detoxification. *J. Biol. Chem.* 261: 16895–16900.

Fowler BA, Hildebrand CE, Kojima Y, and Webb M (1987): Nomenclature of metallothionein. In *Metallothionein II, Experientia Supplementum* 52: 19–22.

Frey MV, Wagner G, Vašák M, Sorensen OW, Neuhaus D, Wörgötter E, Kägi JHR, Ernst RR, and Wüthrich K (1988): Polypeptide-metal cluster connectivities in metallothionein-2 by novel ^{1}H-^{113}Cd heteronuclear two dimensional NMR experiments. *JACS* 107: 6847–6851.

Furey, WF, Robbins AH, Clancy LL, Winge DR, Wang BC, and Stout CD (1986): Crystal structure of CD,Zn metallothionein. *Science* 23: 704–710.

George GW, Byrd J, and Winge DR (1988): X-ray absorption studies of yeast copper metallothionein. *J. Biol. Chem.* 263: 8199–8203.

George S, Leaver M, Frerich N, and Burgess D (1989): Fish metallothioneins: molecular cloning studies and induction in cultured cells. *Mar. Environ. Res.* 28: 173–178.

Griffith BB, Walters RA, Enger MD, Hildebrand CE, and Griffith JK (1983): cDNA cloning and nucleotide sequence comparison of Chinese hamster metallothionein I and II mRNA. *Nucl. Acids Res.* 11: 901–910.

Hamer DH (1986): Metallothionein. *Ann. Rev. Biochem.* 55: 913–951.

Ito H, Fukuda Y, Murata K, and Kimura A (1983): Transformation of intact yeast cells treated with alkali cations. *J. Bacteriol.* 153: 163–168.

Kägi JHR and Kojima Y (1987): Chemistry and biochemistry of metallothionein. In *Metallothionein II, Experientia Supplementum* 52: 25–61.

Kägi JHR and Schaffer A (1988): Biochemistry of metallothionein. *Biochemistry* 27: 8509–8515.

Kunkel TA, Roberts JD, and Zakour R (1987): Rapid and efficient site-specific mutagenesis without phenotypic selection. In *Methods of Enzymology*, Wu R, Grossman L, and Moldave K, Eds., 154: 367–382.

Leaver M and George S (1989): Characterization of a metallothionein cDNA clone from the plaice, *Pleuronectes platessa,* and comparison with other fish metallothionein. *Fish Physiol. Biochem.* (in press).

Lin LY, Lin WC, and Huang PC (1989): Pigeon metallothionein consists of two species. *Biochim. Biophys. Acta* 1037: 248–255.

Maniatis T, Fritsch EF, and Sambrook J, Eds., (1982): *Molecular Cloning, a Laboratory Manual,* 545 pp. Cold Spring Harbor Laboratory, NY.

McCormick CC, Fullmer CS, and Garvey JS (1988): Amino acid sequence and comparative antigenicity of chicken metallothionein. *Proc. Natl. Acad. Sci. U.S.A.* 85: 309–311.

Morris S and Huang PC (1987): Transient response of amplified metallothionein genes in CHO cells to induction by alpha interferon. *Mol. Cell. Biol.* 7: 600–605.

Morris S and Huang PC (1989): Intracellular metallothionein concentration and the rate of zinc or cadmium influx and MT mRNA accumulation in a CHO Cd^r variant. *Expt. Cell Res.* 185: 166–175.

Nielson KB, Atkin CL, and Winge DR (1985): Distinct metal-binding configurations in metallothionein. *J. Biol. Chem.* 260: 5342–5350.

Nielson KB and Winge DR (1985): Independence of the domains of metallothionein in metal binding. *J. Biol. Chem.* 260: 8698–8701.

Ohi S, Cardenosa G, Pine R, and Huang PC (1981): Cadmium-induced accumulation of metallothionein mRNA in rat liver. *J. Biol. Chem.* 256: 2180–2184.

Otvos JD and Armitage IM (1980): Structure of the metal clusters in rabbit liver metallothionein. *Proc. Natl. Acad. Sci. U.S.A.* 77: 7094–7098.

Otvos JD, Engeseth HR, Nettesheim DG, and Hilt CR (1987): Interprotein metal exchange reactions of metallothionein. In *Metallothionein II, Experientia Supplementum* 52: 171–178.

Pande J, Vasak M, and Kagi JHR (1985): Interaction of lysine residues with the metal thiolate clusters in metallothionein. *Biochemistry* 24: 6717–6722.

Pine, R, Cismowski M, Liu S, and Huang PC (1985): Construction and characterization of a library of metallothionein coding sequence mutants. *DNA* 4: 115–126.

Rhee IK, Lee KS, and Huang PC (1989): Metallothioneins with interdomain hinges expanded by insertion mutagenesis. *Protein Engineering* 3: 205–213.

Schultze P, Wörgötter E, Braun W, Wagner G, Vašák M, Kägi JHR, and Wüthrich K (1988): Conformation of Cd_7 metallothionein-2 from rat liver in aqueous solution determined by nuclear magnetic resonance spectroscopy. *J. Mol. Biol.* 203: 251–268.

Stillman MJ, Cai W, and Zelazowski AJ (1987): Cadmium binding to metallothioneins. *J. Biol. Chem.* 262: 4538–4548.

Stillman MJ and Zelazowski AJ (1988): Domain specificity in metal binding to metallothionein. *J. Biol. Chem.* 263: 6128–6133.

Theile DJ, Walling MJ and Hamer, DH (1987): Mammalian metallothionein is functional in yeast. *Science* 231: 854–856.

Thrower AR, Byrd J, Tarbet EB, Mehra RK, Hamer DH, and Winge DR (1988): Effect of mutation of cysteinyl residues in yeast Cu-metallothionein. *J. Biol. Chem.* 263: 7037–7042.

Wagner G, Neuhaus D, Wörgötter E, Vašák M, Kägi JHR, and Wüthrich K (1986): Sequence-specific ¹H-NMR assignments in rabbit-liver metallothionein-2. *Eur. J. Biochem.* 157: 275–289.

Wei A and Andrews GK (1988): Molecular cloning of chicken metallothionein, detection of the complete amino acid sequence and analysis of expression using cloned cDNA. *Nucl. Acids Res.* 16: 537–553.

Winge DR and Miklossy K-A (1982): Domain nature of metallothionein. *J. Biol. Chem.* 257: 3471–3476.

Winge DR, Nielson KB, Gray WR, and Hamer DH (1985): Yeast metallothionein: sequence and metal-binding properties. *J. Biol. Chem.* 260: 14464–14470.

Molecular Biology of the Chicken Metallothionein Gene*

Glen K. Andrews and Lawrence P. Fernando
Department of Biochemistry and Molecular Biology
University of Kansas Medical Center
Kansas City, Kansas

ABSTRACT

Chicken metallothionein (cMT) cDNA encodes a cysteine-rich protein of 63 amino acids that shares extensive homology with mammalian MTs. Southern blot analysis of genomic DNA from the chicken, pheasant, turkey and quail indicates that in each of these birds the *MT* gene is not a part of a large family of related sequences, but rather is likely to be a unique gene sequence. Analyses of purified chicken MT protein, cloned *cMT* cDNAs and genes has established that the chicken has a single *MT* gene which encodes a single MT isoform. This gene consists of three exons, separated by two intervening sequences, and the number and placement of the introns in the *cMT* gene is precisely the same as that in the mammalian *MT* genes. The promoter contains three metal regulatory elements (MREs) with 100% homology to the MRE core consensus sequence (at -47, -488, and -577-bp), and three regions with 90% or greater homology to the 10-bp Sp1 binding site consensus sequence. The proximal and distal MREs are pal-

*This work was supported by a Grant from the U.S. Department of Agriculture (No. 88-37266-4117) to G.K.A.

indromes and their 5′-flanking sequences are highly homologous. In the proximal MRE, this immediate 5′-flanking sequence is a potential Sp1 binding site. In transient expression assays, both the distal and proximal MRE regions could independently confer metal ion responsiveness on the fire fly luciferase (*Luc*) cDNA. Furthermore, the 68-bp DNA fragment (spanning bases -623 to -555) containing the distal MRE region functions as a metal responsive enhancer element. Therefore, in the chicken MT promoter a single MRE, in the context of its immediate surrounding promoter region is sufficient for metal ion regulation.

INTRODUCTION

In the chicken, levels of hepatic MT are upregulated in response to many of the same factors that influence expression of mammalian *MT* genes (Wei and Andrews, 1988; Fernando et al., 1989), such as essential and toxic metal ions, glucocorticoids, and bacterial endotoxin (for reviews see Karin, 1985; Hamer, 1986; Kägi and Schaffer, 1988). However, in contrast to the mammals, which have at least two isoforms of MT (designated MT-I and MT-II), one form of MT protein predominates in the chicken, as well as in some other birds, reptiles and amphibians (Richards, 1984; McCormick et al., 1988; Suzuki and Kawamura, 1984; Bell and Lopez, 1985). This suggests that, in the chicken, a single form of MT must fulfill all of the functional roles of this protein, and that this *MT* gene must have a promoter which is structurally adapted to respond to a wide array of signaling mechanisms. Although the mammalian *MT* genes have been studied extensively, and a few *MT* gene promoters have been analyzed for structure-function relationships (Karin, 1985; Hamer, 1986), little is known about the avian *MT* genes. This manuscript summarizes some of the findings from this laboratory regarding the molecular biology of an avian *MT* gene, and its regulation by metal ions (Wei and Andrews, 1988; Fernando et al., 1989; Fernando and Andrews, 1989).

METHODS

Animals

White-Leghorn chickens at 4 to 5 weeks of age (400 to 600 g) were housed with a continuous supply of feed and water, and with 12 h light and dark cycles. Fertile eggs were incubated at 38°C in 85% relative humidity with rotation every 2 h. Under these conditions the eggs hatched during day 21 of incubation. Pheasant, quail, and turkeys were purchased from Peterson Game Farm (Madison, KS).

Chickens were injected subcutaneously with $ZnCl_2$ (50 mg/kg) and livers were removed after 5 h and frozen at $-70°C$. These served as a source of mRNA for a cDNA library.

Northern Blot Analysis of RNA

Total RNA was isolated and northern blot hybridization accomplished as described by Wei and Andrews (1988) and Andrews et al. (1987).

Southern Blot Analysis of Genomic DNA

High molecular weight DNA was isolated from crude nuclear pellets and restriction enzyme cleavage and Southern blot hybridizations of DNA were performed as described by Andrews et al. (1982).

Screening of a Chicken Liver cDNA Library

The methods for construction and screening of the chicken liver cDNA library were described in detail previously (Wei and Andrews, 1988). Briefly, Poly-A$^+$ RNA was converted to double-stranded cDNA according to the procedure of Okayama and Berg (1982) as modified by Gubler and Hoffman (1983), and double-stranded cDNA was blunt-end ligated into the Sma I site in the polylinker region of the plasmid pSP65 (Promega Biotec, Madison, WI). Approximately 4000 transformants were screened as described by Maniatis et al. (1984). Filters were hybridized with anti-sense RNA (cRNA) synthesized from mouse MT-I cDNA provided by Dr. Richard Palmiter, University of Washington (Seattle, WA), and hybrids were detected by autoradiography.

Screening of a Charon 4A Chicken Genomic DNA Library

Details of these methods are presented in Fernando and Andrews (1989). Briefly, a partial EcoRI Charon 4A chicken genomic DNA library (a generous gift of Dr. J. Robbins, University of Cincinnati School of Medicine, OH) was screened using the a full-length high-specific activity *cMT* cRNA probe (Wei and Andrews, 1988) prepared according to the method of Melton et al. (1984). DNA fragments from positive phage were analyzed by Southern blot hybridization as described above, and appropriate *cMT* gene containing fragments were subcloned for subsequent analysis.

DNA Sequence Analysis of Chicken Metallothionein cDNA and Genomic DNA Clones

Nucleotide sequence analyses were performed according to Maxam and Gilbert (1980) using 5′ and 3′ end-labeled fragments of DNA, and by using the dideoxy chain termination method (Sanger et al., 1977) as modified by Chen and Seeberg (1985), and pSP6, T7 or synthetic oligodeoxyribonucleotide primers designed from sequence data of the *MT* gene. A series of nested deletions were created from 3′ and 5′ ends of the subcloned gene, as well as from subcloned internal restriction fragments of the *MT* gene, using a combination of exonuclease III and S1 nuclease as described by Wu and Guo (1983). DNA fragments were sequenced on both strands at least twice.

Construction of a Chicken MT Promoter-Luc Fusion Gene

The construction of the *cMT*-fire fly *Luc* cDNA (*cMT-Luc*) fusion gene was described in detail by Fernando and Andrews (1989). Briefly, the *cMT* gene 5′-flanking sequence (685 bp), including the cap site (+1) and 62 bp of untranslated sequence was ligated to the fire fly *Luc* cDNA (de Wet et al., 1987). Directional 5′ promoter deletion mutants of *cMT-Luc* were created by treatment with exonuclease III and S1 nuclease as described by Wu and Guo (1983). The extent of deletion was determined by nucleotide sequence analysis.

Cell Culture and Transient Expression Assay

Chick embryo fibroblasts (CEF) were prepared from day 12 chicken embryos essentially as described by Hunter (1979), except that the cells were dispersed by stirring for 10 min at room temperature in 0.05% trypsin, 0.02% EDTA. CEF (1.5×10^6 per 100 mm dish) were plated in Ham's F-12 medium plus 10% FBS, and cultured at 37°C for 24 h before transfection (Fernando and Andrews, 1989). CEFs were transfected with DNA-calcium phosphate coprecipitates prepared according to the procedure of Wigler et al. (1977). Following 3 h of incubation with the DNA-calcium phosphate coprecipitate, the cells were shocked for 1 min with 15% glycerol, and cultured for 24 h in DMEM-high glucose plus 10% FBS before exposure for 18 h to 100 μM $ZnCl_2$. Cells were harvested for Luc assay in 100 mM phosphate buffer pH 7.0, 5 mM DTT or frozen at -70°C for RNA extraction. In addition to the *cMT-Luc* fusion genes, CEF were cotransfected with a plasmid which constitutively expresses bacterial chloramphenicol acetyltransferase (CAT) under the control of the Rous sarcoma virus enhancer (RSV-CAT) (Gorman et al., 1982) as an internal standard, to correct for transfection efficiencies.

Luciferase and CAT Enzyme Activity Assays

Transfected cell lysates were prepared, and analyzed for Luc activity according to the procedure of de Wet et al. (1987), using a Monolight 2001 luminometer (Analytical Luminescence Laboratory, Inc.). The peak height of the light emitted during the reaction was recorded. CAT enzyme assay were carried out as described by Sleigh (1986). An aliquot of the cell extraction was heated for 10 min at 65°C to inactivate potential endogenous acetylations, and the heat-treated extract was assayed in a mixture containing 1.6 mM chloramphenicol, 0.15 M Tris-HCl, pH 7.8, 90 μM ^{14}C-acetyl-CoA (1 μCi/ml), by incubating at 37°C for 1 h. The total reaction was extracted with ethyl acetate, and the ethyl acetate phase, containing acetylated chloramphenicol, was collected, and the amount of radioactivity determined by liquid scintillation counting. The protein content of the cell lysate supernatant was determined using the Bio-Rad protein assay kit (Bio-Rad, Richmond, CA). Data were calculated as the amount of Luc activity per μg protein and corrected for CAT activity per μg protein.

RESULTS

Deduction of the Amino Acid Sequence of Chicken MT and its Homology with Mammalian MTs

Eight positive chicken *MT* cDNA clones were obtained from chicken liver cDNA libraries, and the longest (376-bp) contained an open reading frame of 189 bases, and coded for a protein of 63 amino acids (Wei and Andrews 1988; Fernando et al. 1989). Only a single protein coding sequence was found in all of the cDNA clones isolated, and the single full-length cDNA clone was able to completely hybrid arrest translation of MT in a cell-free translation system (Fernando et al., 1989). These data are consistent with a single form of cMT. A comparison of the amino acid sequence of cMT with the previously published amino acid sequences of several mammalian MTs indicates that cMT is highly homologous to all of the mammalian MTs (Table I), and more closely related to the mammalian MT-II isoforms. The nucleotide sequence of the coding region of *cMT* cDNA is approximately 70% homologous to the consensus sequence for the mammalian MTs (Wei and Andrews, 1988).

A comparison of the amino acid sequence of cMT with that of the human or monkey MT-II (Figure 1) shows that the placement of cysteine residues is precisely conserved, and the majority of amino acid substitutions are conservative. However, cMT contains two additional amino acids (63 total) which are located near the amino and carboxyl termini (Figure 1).

TABLE I.
Amino Acid Sequence Homology Between
Chicken MT and Mammalian MTs

	Percent amino acid identity[a]	
	Isoform	
Species	I	II
Rat	64.5	—
Mouse	64.5	67.7
Hamster	62.9	71.0
Monkey	69.4	74.2
Human	—	74.2

[a]Homologies determined by the FASTP program (Lipman and Pearson, 1985) represent identity in amino acid overlap. Amino acid sequences were obtained from the following references: rat (Andersen et al., 1986), hamster (Griffith et al., 1983), mouse (Durnam et al., 1980; Searle et al., 1984), human (Karin and Richards, 1982), and monkey (Schmidt and Hamer, 1983). Reprinted with permission from Wei and Andrews (1988), *Nucl. Acids Res.* 16: 537.

```
Chicken Metallothionein (63 aa)

     * *     * *   * * * *   *  ** **   *   *   * *       * **
MDPQDCTCAAGDSCSCAGSCKCKNCRCRSCRKSCCSCCPAGCNNCAKGCVCKEPASSKCSCCH
::: .:.::::::::::::::: ::.:::::::::...::.::.::. ::.::::
MDP-NCSCAAGDSCTCAGSCKCKECKCTSCKKSCCSCCPVGCAKCAQGCICKG-ASDKCSCCA

Human and Monkey Metallothionein-II (61 aa)
```

Figure 1. Comparison of chicken MT, and human and monkey MT-II amino acid sequences. The amino acid sequence of cMT was deduced from the nucleotide sequence of cloned cDNA (Wei and Andrews, 1988), and is compared here with the amino acid sequence of human and monkey MT-II (Karin and Richards, 1982; Schmidt and Hamer, 1983). With optimal alignment (Lipman and Pearson, 1985) the sequence homology between cMT, and human and monkey MT-II is 74.2%. (*) Denotes cysteine residues. (:) Denotes conserved amino acids; (·) Denotes conservative changes in amino acids. (Reprinted with permission from Wei and Andrews [1988], *Nucl. Acids Res.,* 10:537.)

Organization of the MT Gene in Chicken and Three Other Avian Species

The gross organization of *MT* genes in the chicken, and in the turkey, quail, and pheasant was analyzed by Southern blot hybridization. Genomic DNA was extracted from liver, and cleaved with the restriction enzyme BgII. This enzyme cleaves the *cMT* cDNA very near the center (in exon 3 of the gene; Figure 3), and thus divides the cDNA into two halves of about

150 bp each (Wei and Andrews, 1988). Radioactive cRNA probes to each half of the *cMT* cDNA were prepared, and Southern blots of the digested genomic DNAs were hybridized with these 3'- and 5'-region specific cRNA probes. Hybridization with either probe gave a single band (Figure 2). The 3'-specific probe hybridized with a DNA fragment of about 0.5 to 0.7 kb in the DNA samples from these four birds, whereas the 5'-specific probe hybridized with a DNA fragment which varied in length (2.2 to 4.8 kb) among these four birds. These data, and a variety of other restriction enzyme analyses, establish that the *MT* gene is well conserved among these birds, and suggest the presence of a single copy *MT* gene in turkey, quail, pheasant and chicken.

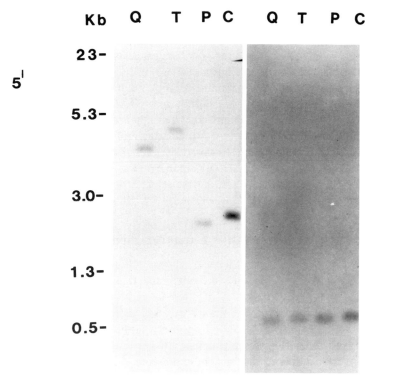

Figure 2. Southern blot analysis of quail (Q), turkey (T), pheasant (P), and chicken (C) DNA using chicken *MT* cRNA probes specific to 5'- or 3'-regions of the *cMT* cDNA. DNA was recovered from livers, and digested with the restriction endonuclease BglI which cleaves in exon three of the *cMT* gene (Figure 3), and near the center of the cloned cDNA (Wei and Andrews, 1988). The digested DNA was analyzed by Southern blot hybridization using ^{32}P-labeled *cMT* cRNA probes produced from the 5' or 3'-half of *cMT* cDNA. Hybridization was carried out in 0.60 *M* NaCl at 55°C, and filters were subjected to a final wash in 0.30 *M* NaCl at 55°C.

Structure of the Cloned Chicken MT Gene

The *cMT* gene was isolated from a λ Charon 4A-chicken genomic library (Fernando and Andrews, 1989). All positive plaques identified contained the same 20-kb EcoRI fragment of genomic DNA. Sequence analysis of the cloned *cMT* gene established that the mRNA coding sequence is interrupted by two intervening sequences of 87 and 1047 bp (Figure 3). The transcription start point (*tsp*) was determined by S1 nuclease mapping (62-bp 5′ to the translation start codon), and this G residue was designated + 1 (Fernando and Andrews, 1989).

Structure of the Chicken MT Promoter

Several interesting structural features of this G + C rich promoter are evident. The pentanucleotide sequence **CACGG** is repeated 13 times in the *cMT* promoter region, and 12 of these repeats are located between nucleotides − 79 and − 196 with respect to the *tsp*. This suggests that an insertional event may have occurred in the *cMT* promoter.

Three regions of homology with the MRE core consensus sequence (Stuart et al., 1985) are found at − 47, − 488, and − 577, and the proximal and distal MREs are palindromes (Figure 3). The sequences directly flanking the proximal and distal MREs also show a high degree of homology (Figure 4). These flanking sequences are closely related to the 10-bp consensus binding site for Sp1 (Briggs et al., 1986; Kadonaga et al., 1987). A similar sequence also overlaps the distal MRE, and a perfect Sp1 consensus binding site is located at − 160.

Identification of Metal Responsive Enhancer Elements in the Chicken MT Promoter

A fusion gene between the *cMT* promoter and the firefly *Luc* cDNA (de Wet et al., 1987) was created as detailed in Fernando and Andrews, 1989 (Figure 5A). Progressive 5′-promoter deletion mutants of this fusion gene were constructed, and transfected into primary cultures of chick embryo fibroblasts (CEFs). The effects of metal ions on *Luc* mRNA, and Luc enzyme activity were determined in transient expression assays. Northern blot analysis detected a *Luc* transcript of approximately 1.9 kb in CEFs transfected with fusion gene constructs containing at least 107-bp of *cMT* promoter, but not with those containing only 30-bp (TATA box, but no MRE) (Figure 5B). Proper transcription of the transfected fusion gene was confirmed by S1 nuclease mapping (Fernando and Andrews, 1989). The level of the *Luc* transcript was increased following exposure of the transfected cells to Cd (Figure 5B). Assays of Luc activity in transfected CEFs showed that Zn induced a 15-fold increase in activity in cells transfected with the

```
                    CTG CAGCCACGCG GCTCCCGGCT
                        Pst I
-600 CTCAGCACGG CCCCACGCTG TGCGCACCGC CTCGCAGCGC GGCCCGGGGG
                                                    Sma I
-550 GGTGGCGGGG GTGGGAGCAG CAGTGGCGCA ATGACCCCTC CGGGTCACAT
-500 TCCCGCAACC GAGCGCAGAG TGCGTGGCCG GGAAATTCCC CCCCCCCAAT
-450 TCGCCTTTCG GCAGCCAAAG CGGGAGGGGG GGAGTGAGGA GGGTCAGGCA
-400 CGTTGGGGTC CGTGCCGTGT TCTGGCAAAG TGTCGTGTTT GGGGGGGGGG
-350 GGGAGCAAGG AAGGGAGGCG AGGGGTGAGG ACACAAAGCA AAAGCGCCCT
-300 AAATCTGTTG GCACACATGG CCATCCCACA GCTGTATCCC CCTGCTTTGG
                        Bal I       Pvu II
-250 GGGAACCCCA ACACCCAGGGC TGGCCCCGCG GTGAGGCTCC CCCCAGGCAG
-200 GGGGCACGGC CGTGACCCCG CTGAGCACGG CACGGCGCTG CCCCGCCCCG
        Xma III
-150 CTGAGCACGG CACGGCACGG CACGGCACGG CCCCCCGAGC ACGGCTCAGC
-100 ACGGCACGGC GCTCAGCACG GCACGGATCG GCACCGCCCC GCCGTGCGCT
 -50 GCGCGCAGCA CCACCCCGGC CCTATAAATA CAGGGCGGGC AGCGGGACTC
     Bss HII
 +1 GGGACTGCTA CGAGCCCACC CGAGCTGACC CTGCGTGAGC CGAACCGACC +50

                     MetAspPro GlnAspCysT hrCysAlaAl aG
     CGAACAGAAC CATGGACCCT CAGGACTGCA CTTGTGCTGC TGGTAAGTGG +100
                 Nco I
     ACGCGACAGG ACTCGGTCTG GCTCGGCTCG GCTCGGTTCG GCCCGGCTCG +150

                          l yAspSerCys SerCysAlaG
     TGTCGCTGAC GGCTTCTTTC CTGTCCCAGG TGACTCCTGC TCCTGTGCTG +200
     lySerCysLy sCysLysAsn CysArgCysA rgSerCysAr gLysS
     GGTCGTGCAA GTGCAAGAAC TGCCGCTGCC GGAGCTGCCG CAAGAGTGAG +250

     TTGGGGGCTG CGGGGTCCCT GACCCAGGGG TGCTTTGGGG GTCCCTGCCC +300
     CGTGGTCCTC TGTCCTTCCC CTATGGGACT CTCATGGAGA CCTCTTTCCC +350
     TCCTTCTGCT CGTGGGAAAC ACTCTTCTCC CTGCTCCTGC TGGATCCCCT +400
                                                    Bam HI
     CCCACTTGCT CCCGTAGGAA CCCCTATGGA CACCCCCTCA CCGTCTCTGA +450
     TGTGCTCTTG TAGGACCCCC TTTGGACAGC CCTCCCACCT CCAATTTTTC +500
     CTGTAGAACC CCCTATCCAT ACCCCTCCC TGCCCTCCAC TTACTCCTTT +550
     AGGAACCCCA ATGAACACCC CCTCCTTGTC CCTGGCTTAC TCTGGTAGGA +600
     CCCCCTATGG ACACCCCCCT GGTCCCCGAC TTACTCCTGT TGGACCCCCT +650
     TTGGACAGCC CCCCCCCCCT TCCCTGACTT GCTCCTGTAG GACTCCGTAT +700
     GGACACTCCC CTGCCCCTGA CATGTTCCTG TAGGTCTTCC TATGGACAGC +750
     CCCCCAGCTG CCACTTGCTC CTGCAACACC CCTATGGACA CCCTCTCCCT +800
          Pvu II
     ACCCTCCACT TGCTCCTGTT GGACCTGCTA TGGACACTCC CCCATCTATT +850
     TGCTCCTTTC AAACCCGCTA TGGATAGCCC CCCTCCAACT TGCTCCCTGT +900
     AGGACTCCCC TATGTACAGC TTCCTGCCCC TGACTTGCTC TGTAGGTCCT +950
     ACAGCCCCCA TTTCCCCTGT CCACTTGCTC CTGTAGGACC CATGGCACACA +1000
                                               Nco I
     AACCCCCAAC TCTCCTGGAG GTGCCTATCC TATCCTGTAG CACTGCTCCG +1050
     TGTACACCAT AGAGCCCCAT GATTCCTACC TTCTCCCTGG AACCCCCCCT +1100
     CGCTCCTCCC CTATGGAGAG AGAAGGGGAG AATCTCCAAC ACATGGGACC +1150
     CTCATGGACT CTCCCCACCC CCATTGGAAC CACAGCCCTG CACCATGGGG +1200
                                               Nco I
     ATTCCCATTC CCACGATGCC CCTTGATCCT TCCCCATATA CTGCGTCTCC +1250

                  erCysC
     ACCCCCATCC TTCCCCACCCC CTAACTCTTG TGTTCTCCCC CTAGGCTGCT +1300
     ysSerCysCy sProAlaGly CysAsnAsnC ysAlaLysGl yCysValCys
     GCTCCTGCTG CCCCGCCGGC TGCAACAACT GTGCCAAGGG CTGTGTCTGC +1350
                 Bgl I
     LysGluProA laSerSerLy sCysSerCys CysHisStop
     AAGGAACCGG CCAGCAGCAA GTGCAGCTGC TGCCACTGAG CCGCCCGCCT +1400
                          Pvu II
     CGCCTGTAAA TAGCTGCCAT GCTTCGGGAA CAGGGTGGGG GGTGACAGGG +1450
     ACCACGAAAA GCTTATTTTA CATGTTTGTA CCTTCCATAC CGATGAAGGA +1500
                 Hind III
     AATAAATGAG TTTGGCTGAA GCTG
```

Figure 3. Nucleotide sequence of the chicken *MT* gene. The *cMT* gene was isolated from a lambda phage charon 4A-chicken genomic DNA library (EcoRI), and the nucleotide sequence was determined on both strands using the dideoxy chain termination method (Sanger et al., 1980) and double-stranded DNA templates. Shown here are 623 bp of 5'-flanking sequence, and the sequence of the exonic and intronic DNA regions. The site of initiation of transcription was determined by S1 mapping (Berk and Sharp, 1977) as presented in Fernando and Andrews (1989). Putative regulatory consensus sequences shown in bold and/or underlined are: metal regulatory elements, −577, −488, and −47; TATA box, −21; cap site, +1; splicing junctions (GT-AG); polyadenylation signal (AAATAAA), +1500. (Reprinted with permission from Fernando and Andrews [1989], *Gene* 81:177.)

```
                                        55-00000-976775
MRE consensus sequence                  CTNTGCRCNCGGCCC

                        GCACGGCCCC    ACGCTGTGCGCACCGCCT    CGCAGCGC

                        GCACCGCCCCGCCGTGCGCTGCGCGCAGCA    CCACCCCG

Sp1 consensus           GCTCCGCCCC
sequence                ATCA      TA
```

Figure 4. Comparison of the proximal and distal MRE core and flanking regions in the chicken *MT* promoter. The proximal (lower) and distal (upper) MREs in the *cMT* promoter are aligned with the MRE consensus sequence (Stuart et al., 1985). The core regions shown in bold type (TGCRC; R = A or G) in the proximal and distal MREs were a perfect match with the MRE consensus sequence core, and formed the cores of the palindrome. The consensus nucleotide frequency at each position in the MRE consensus sequence indicated above is 5 = 50%, 6 = 60%, 7 = 70%, 9 = 90%, and 0 = 100% (Stuart et al., 1985); N = any base. Regions 5' to or within the *cMT* MREs which share homology with the 10-bp consensus binding site for Sp1 transcription factor are underlined (Briggs et al., 1986; Kadonaga et al., 1987), and the 5'-flanking regions are optimally aligned with each other and the Sp1 consensus sequence. Alternate bases in the Sp1 binding site are shown below the underlined consensus sequence.

cMT-Luc plasmid containing only 107-bp of the *cMT* promoter (Figure 5C). These results establish that the proximal MRE region (core plus flanking sequence) is functional. Specific deletion of the 23-bp region (-39 to -61) encompassing the proximal MRE core, while leaving the Sp1 binding site intact, completely abolished metal ion responsiveness of the -107 *cMT-Luc* fusion gene (Fernando and Andrews; manuscript in preparation). Therefore, as expected, the proximal MRE core sequence is essential for metal ion responsiveness.

That the distal MRE core (centered at -577) plus flanking sequence also functions in metal ion regulation was established by ligating the 68-bp DNA fragment, which spans bases -623 to -555 in the *cMT* promoter, immediately upstream of the TATA box in the -30 *cMT-Luc* fusion gene (containing only the first 30-bp of the *cMT* promoter). This DNA fragment conferred metal ion responsiveness on -30 *cMT-Luc* in transient expression assay (Figure 6). In fact, the distal MRE region functioned regardless of orientation or distance from the TATA box (Figure 6). Other experiments established that this DNA region also confers metal ion regulation on a heterologous promoter (Fernando and Andrews, manuscript in preparation). Therefore, the distal MRE plus flanking sequence functions as bona fide metal ion responsive enhancer element.

Experiments are underway to better define those sequences required for metal ion responsiveness in the distal MRE enhancer. Preliminary results suggest that the distal MRE core (-564 to -591) alone is insufficient for metal ion regulation, and optimal metal ion responsiveness requires both the MRE core sequence, and the 5'-flanking region with homology to the Sp1 binding site (80% homology) (Fernando and Andrews, unpublished results).

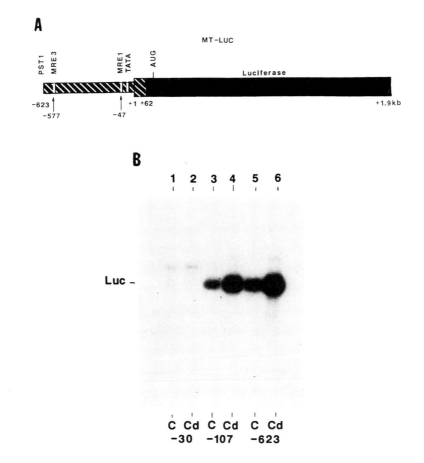

Figure 5. Transient expression of the chicken *MT* Promoter-*Luc* Fusion gene in chick embryo fibroblasts cells. **Part A:** The *cMT* promoter was fused with firefly *Luc* cDNA as described in detail by Fernando and Andrews (1989). The *cMT* gene provides the promoter, and transcription initiation site, and the *Luc* cDNA provides the translation initiation codon and polyadenylation signal. Putative regulatory sequences shown are; MRE 1 (proximal MRE core) and MRE 3 (distal MRE core); TATA, TATA box; AUG, translation initiation codon. Deletion mutants of the *MT* promoter were created using exonuclease III, and the extent of each deletion was determined by sequence analysis. **Part B:** Chick embryo fibroblasts (CEF) were prepared from day 12 chicken embryos, and the cells were cotransfected with *cMT-Luc* fusion gene plasmids and RSV-CAT as a control for the efficiency of transfection. Transfected cells were exposed for 18 h to 7.5 μM CdCl$_2$, and RNA was extracted from the transfected cells, and analyzed by Northern blot hybridization using a *Luc* cRNA probe. -30, -107, and -623, refer to the length (bp) of the 5′-flanking sequence in the *cMT* promoter in each construct. **Part C:** Primary cultures of CEF were transfected using the calcium phosphate method, with the *cMT-Luc* fusion gene containing 30-bp, 107-bp, or 623-bp of 5′-flanking sequence. Transfected cells were exposed for 18 h to 100 μM ZnCl$_2$, and cell lysates were prepared, and analyzed for Luc activity according to the procedure of de Wet et al. (1987). CAT enzyme assay were carried out as described by Sleigh (1986). The protein content of the cell lysate

C

Plasmid Transfected	Fold Induction by Zinc
-623	18.1 ± 5.0
-107	15.3 ± 2.8
-30	1.1 ± 0.7

Figure 5. (continued.)

supernatants was determined using the Bio-Rad protein assay kit (Bio-Rad, Richmond, CA). Data were calculated as the amount of Luc activity per μg protein and corrected for CAT activity per μg protein and are expressed as the fold-induction of Luc activity in metal-treated relative to control cultures plus or minus the standard error of the mean (n = 8). (Reprinted with permission from Fernando and Andrews [1989], *Gene* 81:177.)

DISCUSSION

It has been suggested that in response to metal ions the chicken liver (Weser et al., 1973), in contrast to the mammalian liver, synthesizes a single form of MT. Apparently, the same form of chicken MT is found in liver, pancreas, kidney, and intestinal mucosa (Oh et al., 1979; McCormick, 1984), and in the liver of the embryo and newborn chick (Sandrock et al., 1983; Chakraborty et al., 1987). Despite these interesting findings, until recently no genetic evidence was available to support or refute this hypothesis. The cloning and sequence analysis of *cMT* cDNA (Wei and Andrews, 1988) and the *cMT* gene (Fernando and Andrews, 1989), allowed the deduction of the amino acid sequence of this protein, and has provided several lines of evidence which support the concept of a single *cMT* gene and gene product. The structural similarities and high degree of sequence conservation between the mammalian MTs and chicken MT (Wei and Andrews, 1988; McCormick et al., 1988; Fernando et al., 1989), are consistent with a critical function(s) for this protein.

Whether, among avian species, the existence of a single *MT* gene is unique to the chicken remains to be determined. Two "isoforms" of MT have been described in quail (Yamamura and Suzuki, 1984). However, in the turkey, a single form of MT is detected (Richards, 1984). Apparent heterogeneity in MT can be generated by virtue of the type of metal ion bound to the protein (McCormick et al., 1988). Analysis of MT "isoforms" using reverse-phase chromatography often resolves multiple components. Although these components have been termed "isoforms" of MT, in many species direct evidence for differences in primary sequence among the fractions is lacking. Southern blot hybridization of genomic DNA from chicken, quail, pheasant, and turkey, using *cMT* cDNA probes, suggests that the nucleotide sequence of the cDNA coding region of this gene is highly con-

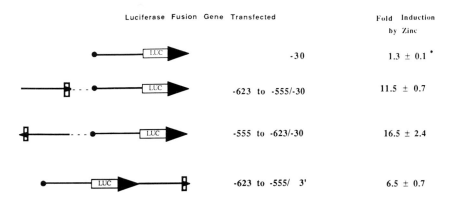

Figure 6. Delineation of a metal responsive enhancer element in the *cMT* promoter. The *cMT* promoter region −623 to −555 (which contains the distal MRE core sequence, and the 5′-flanking sequences homologous to those found near the proximal MRE; Figure 4), was isolated (as a PstI/SmaI fragment; Figure 3) and ligated into the −30 *cMT-Luc* plasmid which contains only 30-bp of the *cMT* promoter. This 68-bp region was inserted in the normal, as well as in the reverse orientation, and also at the 3′-end of the *Luc* cDNA. These plasmids were transfected into CEFs along with RSV-CAT plasmid as an internal control. The cells were treated with Zn, and processed for Luc and CAT activities as described in the legend to Figure 5. The normalized luciferase activity with respect to the CAT activity was calculated per μg of protein. The fold-induction of luciferase activity (± S.E.M.) was statistically analyzed by one factor anova followed by Fisher PLDS and Scheffe F-test (at $\alpha = 0.05$ level). (*) indicates zinc induction was not significantly different from control (at 0.05 significance level). *Luc* cDNA is indicated by the large arrow with a solid head. Symbols are as follows: [], potential Sp1 binding site; small arrows, MRE core sequences (and the head of the arrow indicates the orientation of the MRE); (●), TATA box; (---), 23-bp of the polylinker region of the vector.

served among the birds, and that the *MT* gene family in each of these birds is simple, perhaps consisting of a single gene. A dual MT gene system has been documented genetically in an insect (*Drosophila*; Mokdad et al., 1987), a fish (Rainbow trout; Bonham et al., 1987), and in all mammals examined (Hamer, 1986). However, based on protein fractionation studies, the existence of a single isoform of MT has been reported in some amphibians (Suzuki and Kawamura, 1984; Flos et al., 1986), reptiles, (Bell and Lopez, 1985; Suzuki et al., 1983) and in other fishes (Shears and Fletcher, 1985). Although this suggests the possibility of a single *MT* gene in many of the lower eukaryotes, detailed studies of the organization of the *MT* genes in other birds, amphibians, reptiles and fishes are required to determine whether the presence of a single isoform of this protein is the rule or the exception.

Comparison of the structural organization of the *cMT* gene with that of mammalian *MT* genes (Hamer, 1986) and a Rainbow trout *MT* gene (Zafarullah et al., 1988) establishes that the tripartite structure of these genes has been conserved during evolution. In fact, the introns interrupt the coding sequences of all of these *MT* genes at precisely the same locations. In the chicken this is at amino acids 11 and 33 (Fernando and Andrews, 1989).

The promoter sequences of all *MT* genes contain multiple copies of DNA sequences with homology to the MREs of the mouse *MT* promoter (Stuart et al., 1985). These sequences are thought to be binding sites for transacting proteins which exhibit metal-dependent DNA-binding activity (Seguin and Hamer, 1987; Anderson et al., 1987; Mueller et al., 1988; Westin and Schaffner, 1988), as has been documented to occur during activation of the yeast *MT* gene (Buchman et al., 1989; Huibregtse et al., 1989; Fürst and Hamer, 1989). The *cMT* promoter is functional in mammalian cells (Fernando and Andrews, 1989) which suggests that *trans*acting factors which regulate metal ion responsiveness of the *MT* genes in mammalian cells can interact productively with the MREs in the *cMT* promoter. Thus, the metal responsive system has been conserved during evolution.

The chicken *MT* promoter is unique in that only three regions of similarity to the MRE core sequence are present, and only one is present within the first 400-bp of the promoter. Furthermore, the proximal and distal MRE core sequences are palindromes, and are flanked by regions of similarity to the Sp1 binding site. The transcription factor Sp1 has been shown to bind to specific sites in the promoter regions of mouse, rat and human *MT* genes (Andersen et al., 1987; Lee et al., 1987; Mueller et al., 1988). The MREd of mouse *MT-I,* and the MRE4 of human *MT-IIA* overlap with potential binding sites for Sp1 (Westin and Schaffner, 1988) as does the distal MRE in the *cMT* promoter (Fernando and Andrews, 1989). In contrast, the trout *MT-B* gene apparently has no Sp1 binding sites (Zafarullah et al., 1988).

Both the proximal and distal MREs were shown to be functional elements in the *cMT* promoter, and a 68-bp region, encompassing the distal MRE, functions as a metal responsive enhancer element. Thus a single MRE (proximal or distal) from the chicken *MT* promoter is sufficient for metal ion regulation. The distal MRE core region alone apparently does not provide optimal metal ion responsiveness under these assay conditions, but requires the flanking sequences (Fernando and Andrews, unpublished results). In the mouse, multiple copies of the natural or synthetic MREs are required for optimal metal ion responsiveness (Stuart et al., 1985; Searle, et al., 1985; Culotta and Hamer, 1989), and multiple copies of the MREd from the mouse *MT-I* gene can function as a metal-regulated enhancer element (Westin and Schaffner, 1988). However, the mouse *MT-I* MREa can function synergistically with the thymidine kinase distal promoter element (Searle et al., 1985), and in the human *MT-IIa* gene, deletion of the basal level enhancer, which flanks a proximal MRE, leads to loss of metal responsiveness (Karin et al., 1987). This suggests that the cooperative interactions of regulatory proteins, perhaps including Sp1-like factors, may account for metal responsive enhancer activity of the metallothionein genes in several distantly related species. Many transcription factors can interact synergistically with steroid hormone receptors (Schule et al., 1988), and the cooperativity of two different protein binding motifs in the SV40 enhancer has been documented (Fromental et al., 1988).

ACKNOWLEDGMENTS

This work was supported by a Grant from the U.S. Department of Agriculture (No. 88-37266-4117) to G.K.A. We wish to thank Mrs. Cathy O'Rourke for expert technical assistance, and Mr. Deyue Wei for his initial contributions to these studies.

REFERENCES

Andersen RD, Birren BW, Taplitz SJ, and Herschman HRC (1986): Rat Metallothionein-I structural gene and three pseudogenes, one of which contains 5′-regulatory sequences. *Mol. Cell Biol.* 6: 302.

Andersen RD, Taplitz SJ, Wong S, Bristol G, Larkin B, and Herschman HR (1987): Metal-dependent binding of a factor *in vivo* to the metal responsive elements of the metallothionein I gene promoter. *Mol. Cell. Biol.* 7: 3574.

Andrews GK, Dziadek M, and Tamaoki T (1982): Methylation of the mouse alpha-fetoprotein gene in embryonic, adult and neoplastic tissue. *J. Biol. Chem.* 257: 5148.

Andrews GK, Lehman LD, Huet YM, and Dey SK (1987): Metallothionein gene regulation in the preimplantation rabbit blastocyst. *Development* 100: 463.

Bell JU and Lopez JM (1985): Isolation and partial purification of a cadmium-binding protein from the liver of alligators exposed to cadmium. *Comp. Biochem. Physiol.* 89: 123.

Berk AJ and Sharp PA (1977): Sizing and mapping of early adenovirus mRNAs by gel electrophoresis on S1 endonuclease-digested hybrids. *Cell* 12: 721.

Bonham K, Zafarullah M, and Gedamu L (1987): The rainbow trout metallothioneins: molecular cloning and characterization of two distinct cDNA sequences. *DNA* 6: 519.

Briggs MR, Kadonaga JT, Bell SP, and Tjian R (1986): Purification and biochemical characterization of the promoter-specific transcription factor, Sp1. *Science* 234: 47.

Buchman C, Skroch P, Welch J, Fogel S, and Karin M (1989): The CUP2 gene product, regulator of yeast metallothionein expression, is a copper-activated DNA-binding protein. *Mol. Cell. Biol.* 9: 4091.

Chen EY and Seeberg PH (1985): Supercoil sequencing: a fast and a simple method of sequencing plasmid DNA. *DNA* 4: 165.

Culotta VC and Hamer D (1989): Fine mapping of a mouse metallothionein gene metal response element. *Mol. Cell. Biol.* 9: 1376.

de Wet JR, Wood KV, Deluca M, Helinski DR, and Subramani S (1987): Firefly luciferase gene: structure and expression in mammalian cells. *Mol. Cell. Biol.* 7: 725.

Durnam DM, Perrin F, Gannon F, and Palmiter RD (1980): Isolation and characterization of the mouse metallothionein-I gene. *Proc. Natl. Acad. Sci. U.S.A.* 77: 6511.

Fernando LP and Andrews GK (1989): Cloning and expression of an avian metallothionein-encoding gene. *Gene* 81: 177.

Fernando LP, Wei D, and Andrews GK (1989): Structure and expression of chicken metallothionein. *J. Nutr.* 119: 309.

Flos R, Bas J, and Hidalgo J (1986): Metallothionein in the liver of the small lizard *Podarcis muralis. Comp. Biochem. Physiol.* 83: 93.

Fromental C, Kanno M, Nomiyama H, and Chambon P (1988): Cooperative and hierarchial levels of functional organization in the SV40 enhancer. *Cell* 54: 943.

Fürst P and Hamer D (1989): Cooperative activation of a eukaryotic transcription factor: interaction between Cu(I) and yeast ACE1 protein. *Proc. Natl. Acad. Sci. U.S.A.* 86: 5267.

Gorman C, Merlino G, Willingham M, Pastan I, and Howard BH (1982): The rous sarcoma virus long terminal repeat is a strong promoter when introduced into a variety of eukaryotic cells by DNA-mediated Transfection. *Proc. Natl. Acad. Sci. U.S.A.* 77: 6777.

Griffith BB, Walters RA, Enger MD, Hildebrand CE, and Griffith JK (1983): cDNA cloning and nucleotide sequence comparison of Chinese hamster metallothionein I and II mRNAs. *Nucl Acids Res.* 11: 901.

Gubler U and Hoffman BJ (1983): A simple and very efficient method for generating cDNA libraries. *Gene* 25: 263.

Hamer DH (1986): Metallothionein. *Ann. Rev. Biochem.* 55: 913; Huibregtse JM, Engelke DR, and Thiele DJ (1989): Copper-induced binding of cellular factors to yeast metallothionein upstream activation sequences. *Proc. Natl. Acad. Sci. U.S.A.* 86: 65.

Hunter E (1979): Biological techniques for avian sarcoma viruses. *Meth. Enzymol.* 58: 380.

Kadonaga JT, Carner KR, Masiarz FR, and Tjian R (1987): Isolation of cDNA encoding transcription factor Sp1 and functional analysis of the DNA binding domain. *Cell* 51: 1079.

Kägi JHR and Schaffer A (1988): Biochemistry of metallothionein. *Biochemistry* 27: 8509.

Karim M and Richards DI (1982): Human metallothionein genes: primary structure of the metallothionein-II gene and a related processed gene. *Nature* 299: 797.

Karin M (1985): Metallothioneins: proteins in search of function. *Cell* 41: 9.

Karin M, Haslinger A, Heguy A, Dietlin T, and Cooke T (1987): Metal-responsive elements act as positive modulators of human metallothionein-II$_A$ enhancer activity. *Mol. Cell. Biol.* 7: 606.

Lee W, Haslinger A, Karin M, and Tjian R (1987): Activation of transcription by two factors that bind promoter and enhancer sequences of the human metallothionein gene and SV40. *Nature* 325: 368.

Lipman DJ and Pearson WR (1985): Rapid and sensitive protein similarity searches. *Science* 227: 1435.

Maniatis T, Fritsch EF, and Sambrook J, Eds., (1984): *Molecular Cloning: A Laboratory Manual.* Cold Spring Harbor, New York.

Maxam A and Gilbert W (1980): Sequencing with base-specific chemical cleavages. *Meth. Enzymol.* 65: 499.

McCormick C, Fullmer CS, and Garvey JS (1988): Amino acid sequence and comparative antigenicity of chicken metallothionein. *Proc. Natl. Acad. Sci. U.S.A.* 85: 309.

Melton DA, Krieg PA, Rebagliati MR, Maniatis T, Zinn K, and Green MR (1984): Efficient *in vitro* synthesis of biologically active RNA and RNA hybridization probes from plasmids containing a bacteriophage SP6 promoter. *Nucl. Acids Res.* 12: 7035.

Mokdad R, Debec A, and Wegnez M (1987): Metallothionein genes in *Drosophila melanogaster* constitute a dual system. *Proc. Natl. Acad. Sci. U.S.A.* 84: 2657.

Mueller PR, Salser SJ, and Wold B (1988): Constitutive and metal inducible protein: DNA interactions at the mouse metallothionein I promoter examined by *in vivo* and *in vitro* footprinting. *Genes and Develop.* 2: 412.

Okayama H and Berg P (1982): High efficiency cloning of full-length cDNA. *Mol. Cell. Biol.* 2: 161.

Richards MP (1984): Synthesis of a metallothionein-like protein by developing turkey embryos maintained in long-term, shell-less culture. *J. Ped. Gastroent. Nutrit.* 3: 128.

Sanger F, Nicklen S, and Coulson AR (1977): DNA sequencing with chain-terminating inhibitors. *Proc. Natl. Acad. Sci. U.S.A.* 74: 5463.

Schmidt CJ and Hamer DH (1983): Cloning and sequence analysis of two monkey metallothionein cDNAs. *Gene* 24: 137.

Schule R, Muller M, Kaltschmidt C, and Renkawitz R (1988): Many transcription factors interact synergistically with steroid receptors. *Science* 242: 1418.

Searle PF, Davison BL, Stuart GW, Wilkie TM, Norstedt G, and Palmiter RD (1984): Regulation, linkage and sequence of mouse metallothionein-I and II genes. *Mol. Cell. Biol.* 4: 1221.

Seguin C and Hamer DH (1987): Regulation *in vitro* of metallothionein gene binding factors. *Science* 235: 1383.

Shears MA and Fletcher GL (1985): Hepatic metallothionein in the winter flounder *(Pseudopleuronectes americanus) Can. J. Zool.* 63: 1602.

Sleigh MJ (1986): A nonchromatographic assay for the expression of CAT gene in eukaryotic cells. *Anal. Biochem.* 156: 251.

Stuart GW, Searle PF, and Palmiter RD (1985): Identification of multiple metal regulatory elements in the mouse metallothionein-I promoter by assaying synthetic sequences. *Nature* 317: 828.

Suzuki KT, Tanaka Y, and Kawamura R (1983): Properties of metallothionein induced by zinc, copper and cadmium in the frog, *Xenopus laevis. Comp. Biochem. Physiol.* 75: 33.

Suzuki KT and Kawamura R (1984): Metallothionein present or induced in the three species of frogs *Bombina oreintalis, Bufo bufo japonicus* and *Hyla arborea japonica. Comp. Biochem. Physiol.* 79: 255.

Wei D and Andrews GK (1988): Molecular cloning of chicken metallothionein: deduction on the complete amino acid sequence and analysis of expression using cloned cDNA. *Nucl. Acids Res.* 16: 537.

Westin G and Schaffner W (1988): A zinc-responsive factor interacts with a metal-regulated enhancer element (MRE) of the mouse metallothionein-I gene. *EMBO J.* 7: 3763.

Wigler M, Silverstein S, Lee L, Pellicer A, Cheng Y, and Axel R (1977): Transfer of purified herpes virus thymidine kinase gene to cultured mouse cells. *Cell* 11: 223.

Wu R and Guo LH (1983): Exonuclease III: use for DNA sequence analysis and in specific deletions of nucleotides. *Meth. Enzymol.* 100: 60.

Yamamura M and Suzuki KT (1984): Induction and characterization of metallothionein in the liver and kidney of Japanese quail. *Comp. Biochem. Physiol.* 77: 101.

Zafarullah M, Bonham K and Gedamu L (1988): Structure of the rainbow trout metallothionein B gene and characterization of its metal-responsive region. *Mol. Cell. Biol.* 8: 4469.

Chapter 9

Species Differences in Metallothionein Regulation: A Comparison of the Induction of Isometallothioneins in Rats and Mice[1]

Lois D. Lehman-McKeeman,[2] William C. Kershaw[2]
and Curtis D. Klaassen[3]
Department of Pharmacology, Toxicology, and Therapeutics
University of Kansas Medical Center
Kansas City, Kansas

INTRODUCTION

It is now more than 30 years since the metal-binding protein, metal-lothionein (MT), was isolated (Margoshes and Vallee, 1957). Since that time, the structure, function and regulation of this unusual protein have been studied in detail by many scientists. It is generally recognized that the metal binding properties of MT result from its high sulfhydryl content, as 1 mole of MT can effectively sequester 7 moles of metal. Furthermore, the importance of MT in the homeostasis of essential metals and in the detoxifi-

[1]Supported by USPHS Grant ES-01142.
[2]Current Address: Miami Valley Laboratories, Procter & Gamble Co., Cincinnati, OH 45239.
[3]To whom all correspondence should be sent.

cation of non-essential heavy metals is well-documented. Induction of MT synthesis by heavy metals, glucocorticoid hormones and a variety of stressful environmental conditions and treatments has also been studied extensively. (For recent reviews, see Kägi and Schaffer, 1988; Klaassen and Lehman-McKeeman, 1989). More recently, cDNA clones of MT mRNA nucleotide sequences in several species, including humans have been isolated and much has been learned about molecular events that regulate MT (Hamer, 1986).

In all mammals, there are two major isoforms of MT, referred to as MT-I and MT-II. These proteins, which differ electrophoretically and chromatographically, have a similar number of cysteine residues and identical metal-binding capacities. In all species, MT-II is more acidic than MT-I (Cherian, 1974). In rats, the isoMTs differ by twelve amino acid substitutions, all of which are conservative changes (Winge et al., 1984). The presence of MT isoforms is most complex in human tissues, in which at least 5 variants of MT-I have been identified, whereas only one functional MT-II has been isolated (Kägi et al., 1984; Hunziker and Kägi, 1985).

Until recently, studies evaluating MT induction have focused on changes in total protein rather than quantitating specific changes in MT-I and MT-II. Therefore, a major objective of the work presented herein was to quantitate hepatic concentrations of MT-I and MT-II under basal and induced conditions. Specifically, induction by heavy metals (Cd and Zn) and by non-metal primary inducers (glucocorticoids) was determined. The concentration of isoMTs in immature animals, when constituent levels are very high, was also determined.

The second major objective of the work presented herein was to compare the induction of MT-I and MT-II in rats and mice. The primary structure of the isoforms are very similar between these commonly-used laboratory animals. For example, rat and mouse hepatic MT-I differ by only 5 amino acids (Winge et al., 1984; Huang et al., 1977). Despite this sequence homology, experiments describing the molecular regulation of the MT-I and MT-II genes in rats and mice have suggested that the pattern of induction of isoMTs may differ between rats and mice (Yagle and Palmiter, 1985; Lehman-McKeeman et al., 1987). To characterize further species differences in MT regulation, hepatic isoMT levels were determined in untreated adult and immature rats and mice, as well as adult rats and mice exposed to Cd, Zn, or dexamethasone.

METHODS

For all experiments, adult male Sprague-Dawley rats (225 to 275 g) and Cf-1 mice (20 to 25 g) were used. Immature animals were born and maintained in the animal facilities of the University of Kansas Medical

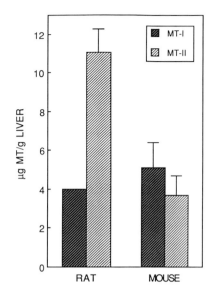

Figure 1. Constituent levels of hepatic MT-I and MT-II in adult male Sprague-Dawley rats and CF-1 mouse. Results represent the mean ± S.E.M. of 11 rats and 16 mice. [Adapted from Lehman-McKeeman and Klaassen (1987) and Kershaw et al. (1990).]

Center. $ZnCl_2$, $CdCl_2$ and dexamethasone were dissolved in 0.9% saline and administered s.c. in a volume of 10 ml/kg.

MT isoforms were separated by anion-exchange, high-performance liquid chromatography (HPLC) and quantified as heat-stable, Cd-saturated proteins with direct, simultaneous detection by atomic absorption spectrophotometry. This method has been described in detail by Lehman and Klaassen (1986).

RESULTS

Hepatic concentrations of MT-I and MT-II in untreated adult rats and mice are shown in Figure 1. In rats, MT-II was more abundant than MT-I, whereas hepatic levels of MT-I and MT-II were similar in mice. The total hepatic concentration of MT was not different between the two species.

Exposure to Cd increased hepatic iso-MTs in a dose dependent manner (Figure 2). In rats, the lowest dosage of Cd that increased both MT-I and MT-II levels was 3 μmol/kg, whereas in mice, the lowest dosage of Cd that induced MT-I and MT-II was 5 μmol/kg. Rats tolerated high dosages of Cd much better than mice, suggesting that MT induction might differ between the two species. In rats, the highest dosage of Cd tested increased both MT-I and MT-II to maximum levels of nearly 300 μg/g liver (or 600 μg/liver for total MT). In mice, the maximum induction of the isoforms was lower than rats, reaching levels of approximately 200 and 100 μg/g liver for MT-I and MT-II (or only 300 μg/g liver for total MT). For all the Cd dosages tested in rats, the ratio of the isoforms (MT-I/MT-II) approached unity. In contrast, for all dosages administered to mice, Cd induced MT-I to much higher levels than MT-II, resulting in a MT-I/MT-II ratio of more than 2.

The pattern of induction of hepatic iso-MTs by Zn treatment was also very different in rats and mice (Figure 3). Administration of Zn in equimolar dosages (3 mmol/kg), resulted in significantly higher levels of MT in rats than in mice (635 vs. 480 μg/g total MT, respectively). In addition, a very

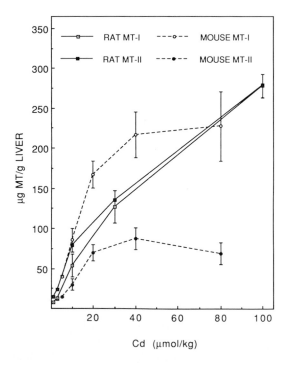

Figure 2. Induction of MT-I and MT-II following Cd treatment to rats (1 to 100 μmol/kg) and mice (5 to 80 μmol/kg). MT levels were determined 24 h after metal treatment. Results represent the mean ± SE of 6 rats and 4 to 8 mice. [Adapted from Lehman-McKeeman and Klaassen (1987) and Kershaw et al. (1990).]

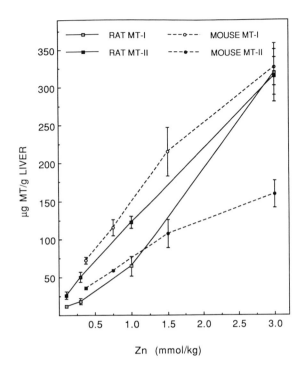

Figure 3. Induction of MT-I and MT-II following Zn treatment to rats (0.1 to 3 mmol/kg) and mice (0.38 to 3 mmol/kg). MT levels were determined 24 h after metal treatment. Results represent the mean ± S.E.M. of 6 rats and 4 to 8 mice. [Adapted from Lehman-McKeeman and Klaassen (1987) and Kershaw et al. (1990).]

different pattern of induction of the iso-MTs was also observed. In rats given dosages of 0.1, 0.3, or 1 mmol Zn/kg, the concentration of MT-II was approximately three-times higher than MT-I(MT-I/MT-II = 0.36). However, at higher dosages of Zn, the concentrations of MT-I and MT-II were similar. In contrast, at all dosages of Zn given to mice, the concentrations of MT-I were significantly higher than MT-II(MT-I/MT-II = 2).

Very distinct differences in MT induction by the synthetic glucocorticoid, dexamethasone, were noted between rats and mice (Figure 4). Unlike the metals which produced higher MT levels in rats, dexamethasone was a much more effective inducer in mice. Dexamethasone increased rat MT levels only 2.5 times control values, whereas mouse MTs increased more than 10 times control levels. In rats, dosages of 0.3 μmol/kg and higher increased MT levels. However, this induction was seen only with MT-II, as MT-I levels were unchanged by dexamethasone treatment. Dosages greater than 10 μmol/kg did not increase rat MT levels any further. Unlike rats,

MT levels increased in mice following dosages of 10 μmol dexamethasone per kg and higher. At dosages of 10, 30, and 100 μmol/kg the concentration of the isoforms were similar, whereas at higher dosages, the concentration of MT-I were significantly higher than MT-I(MT-I/MT-II = 1.5).

The ontogeny of the MT isoforms in developing rats and mice is shown in Figures 5 and 6, respectively. In both species, hepatic MT levels reached maximum levels on postnatal day 7. At this time, however, the total MT

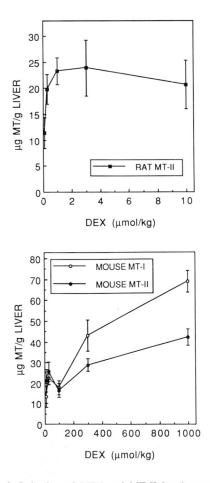

Figure 4. Induction of MT-I and MT-II by dexamethasone treatment in rats (0.3 to 10 μmol/kg) and mice (10 to 1000 μmol/kg). MT levels were determined 24 h after dexamethasone administration. Results represent the mean ± S.E.M. of 6 rats and 4 to 8 mice. (Adapted from Lehman-McKeeman et al. [1988a[and Kershaw et al. [1990].)

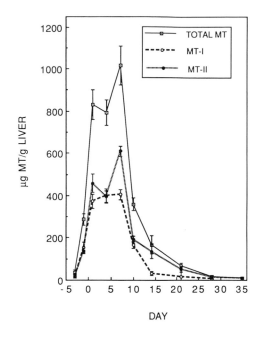

Figure 5. Concentration of total MTs (MT-I plus MT-II) and the MT isoforms in rat liver during development. Negative days represent days prior to parturition. Adult values represent MT levels in male rats approximately 75 days old. Results represent the mean ± S.E.M. of 6–8 rats. [Adapted from Lehman-McKeeman et al. (1988b).]

present in rat liver was approximately 3 times higher than that in mouse liver. Hepatic MT levels declined after day 7, with developing rats reaching adult values at 35 days of age and developing mice reaching adult values at 21 days of age. Differences in the hepatic concentrations of the isoforms were also noted between the two species. In rats, MT-II was more abundant than MT-I with significant differences noted on postnatal days 14 and 21. In mice, MT-I was significantly higher than MT-II(MT-I/MT-II = 2) from postnatal day 1 through day 14.

DISCUSSION

The purpose of the present work was to evaluate the basal and induced concentrations of hepatic iso-MTs and to compare the regulation of these proteins in rats and mice. The results indicate that induction of MT-I and MT-II is both inducer- and species-specific, as differences in both the magnitude of and pattern of induction of the isoforms in rats and mice were observed. The results also suggest that there are significant differences in the quantity of hepatic MT-I and MT-II in developing rats and mice. Specifically, the pattern of developmental changes in total hepatic MT levels was not different between rats and mice. However, MT-I was more abundant than MT-II in developing mice, whereas no large differences were observed in isoMT levels in developing rats. The major difference between developing rats and mice was that the peak total hepatic MT concentration was about 3 times higher in rats than in mice.

In rats, constituent levels of MT-II were higher than MT-I, and MT-II was also more abundant than MT-I in Zn and dexamethasone-treated animals. In mice, however, MT-I was typically more abundant than MT-II with all inducing agents.

Hepatic levels of MT-I and MT-II are determined by the transcription of their respective genes, translation of the mRNA and intracellular degradation. Studies undertaken to evaluate the molecular regulation of the MT genes have shown that the MT-I and MT-II genes are coordinately regulated in rats and mice (Yagle and Palmeter, 1985; Lehman-McKeeman et al., 1988a,b,c). In mice, there is a direct correlation between the relative abun-

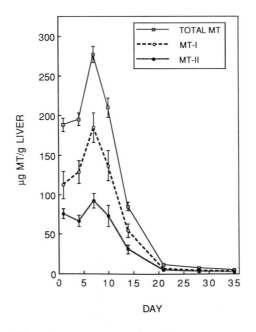

Figure 6. Concentration of total MTs (MT-I plus MT-II) and MT isoforms in mouse liver during development. Results represent the mean ± S.E.M. of 6 to 7 mice. [Adapted from Kershaw et al. (1990).]

dance of MT-I and MT-II mRNAs and their respective proteins. That is, MT-I mRNA has been reported to typically be 1.5 to 2 times more abundant than MT-II mRNA (Yagle and Palmiter, 1985) and similar ratios are seen for the isoproteins (Kershaw et al., 1990). In rats, however, this direct correlation between protein and message is not observed. For example, although dexamethasone treatment increased only hepatic MT-II content, both MT-I and MT-II mRNAs are increased by the glucocorticoid (Lehman-McKeeman et al., 1988a). This discrepancy suggests that there may be a translational component for rat MT regulation that is particularly important for glucocorticoid induction of MT-I. Translational regulation of rat MTs by glucocorticoids, along with differences in glucocorticoid hormone receptor content may explain why the amount of MT synthesized in rat liver is so much less than that synthesized by mice following dexamethasone treatment.

Protein degradation also appears to be an important determinant of rat MT-I and MT-II levels. It has been shown that Zn-induced MT-II has a significantly longer half-life than MT-I (Lehman-McKeeman et al., 1988c). Thus, the shorter half-life of MT-I helps to explain the difference in rat hepatic isoform levels following Zn treatment. To date, however, the importance of isoMT degradation in determining MT-I and MT-II in mice has not been established. For example, it is not known whether the significant differences between the maximum induction of MT in rats and mice are determined by differences in gene transcription, protein synthesis or rates of degradation of the isoforms.

Regulation of MT genes during development is not well defined. It has been suggested that both endogenous Zn (Gallant and Cherian, 1986) and glucocorticoids (Ouelletta, 1982; Quaife et al., 1986) contribute to the high constituent MT levels seen in immature animals. Furthermore, translational regulation of MT synthesis during development has been suggested (Piletz et al., 1983; Lehman-McKeeman et al., 1988b). The results of the present study have shown that there are significant differences in the amount of total hepatic MT synthesized by young rats and mice, as 1-week-old rats have nearly 3 times more MT than mice. These results suggest that there are significant differences in the factors that control MT synthesis in young rats and mice or that there may be major differences between these two species in the need for MT during development.

In summary, the results presented herein have uncovered differences in iso-MT levels in two commonly-used laboratory animals. The primary structure of MT-I and MT-II in rats and mice is very similar. However, the proteins are induced quite differently by metals and non-metals in these two species. Therefore it appears that differences in the induction of MT-I and MT-II in rats and mice result from species variation in the molecular regulation, synthesis and degradation of these proteins.

REFERENCES

Cherian MG (1974): Isolation and purification of cadmium binding proteins from rat liver. *Biochem. Biophys. Res. Comm.* 61: 920–926.

Gallant KR and Cherian MG (1986): Influence of maternal mineral deficiency on the hepatic metallothionein and zinc in newborn rats. *Biochem. Cell Biol.* 64: 8.

Goering PL and Klaassen CD (1984): Resistance to cadmium-induced hepatotoxicity in immature rats. *Toxicol. Appl. Pharmacol.* 74: 321–329.

Hamer DH (1986): Metallothionein. *Annu. Rev. Biochem.* 55: 913.

Huang I-Y, Yoshida A, Tsunoo H, and Nakajima H (1977): Mouse liver metallothioneins. Complete amino acid sequence of metallothionein-I. *J. Biol. Chem.* 252: 8217–8221.

Hunziker PE and Kägi JHR (1985): Isolation and characterization of six human hepatic isometallothioneins. *Biochem. J.* 231: 375–382.

Kägi JHR, Vasak M, Lerch K, Gilg DEO, Hunziker P, Bernhard WR, and Good M (1984): Structure of mammalian metallothionein. *Environ. Hlth. Perspect.* 54: 93–103.

Kägi JHR and Schaffer A (1988): Biochemistry of metallothionein. *Biochemistry.* 27: 8509.

Kershaw WC, Lehman-McKeeman LD, and Klaassen CD (1990): Hepatic isometallothioneins in mice: induction in adults and post-natal ontogeny. *Toxicol. Appl. Pharmacol.* 104: 267–275.

Klaassen CD and Lehman-McKeeman LD (1989): Induction of metallothionein. *J. Am. Coll. Toxicol.* 8: 1315.

Lehman LD and Klaassen CD (1986): Separation and quantitation of metallothioneins by high-performance liquid chromatography coupled wtih atomic absorption spectrophotometry. *Ana. Biochem.* 153: 305.

Lehman-McKeeman LD and Klaassen CD (1987): Induction of metallothionein-I and metallothionein-II in rats by cadmium and zinc. *Toxicol. Appl. Pharmacol.* 88: 195.

Lehman-McKeeman LD, Andrews GK, and Klaassen CD (1988a): Induction of hepatic metallothioneins determined at isoprotein and messenger RNA levels in glucocorticoid-treated rats. *Biochem. J.* 249: 429.

Lehman-McKeeman LD, Andrews GK, and Klaassen CD (1988b). Ontogeny and induction of hepatic isometallothioneins in immature rats. *Toxicol. Appl. Pharmacol.* 92: 10.

Lehman-McKeeman LD, Andrews GK, and Klaassen CD (1988c): Mechanisms of regulation of rat hepatic metallothionein-I and metallothionein-II levels following administration of zinc. *Toxicol. Appl. Pharmacol.* 92: 1.

Margoshes M and Vallee BL (1957): A cadmium protein from equine kidney cortex. *J. Am. Chem. Soc.* 79: 4813.

Ouellette AJ (1982): Metallothionein mRNA expression in fetal mouse organs. *Dev. Biol.* 92: 240.

Piletz JE, Andersen RD, Birren BW, and Herschman HR (1983): Metallothionein synthesis in fetal, neonatal and maternal rat liver. *Eur. J. Biochem.* 131: 389–495.

Quaife C, Hammer RE, Mottet NK, and Palmiter RD (1986): Glucocorticoid regulation of metallothionein during murine development. *Dev. Biol.* 118: 549–555.

Winge DR, Nielson KB, Zeikus RD, and Gray WR (1984): Structural characterization of the isoforms of neonatal and adult rat liver metallothionein. *J. Biol. Chem.* 259: 11419–11425.

Yagle MK and Palmiter RD (1985): Coordinate regulation of mouse metallothionein I and II genes by heavy metals and glucocorticoids. *Mol. Cell Biol.* 5: 291.

Chapter 10

Metallothionein and Sulfur Metabolism in Newborn Rat Liver

M. George Cherian
Department of Pathology
University of Western Ontario
London, Ontario, Canada

INTRODUCTION

The mammalian intracellular hepatic levels of cysteine and glutathione during development are regulated by various factors such as the transfer of nutrients from the mother to the fetus and also the development of synthetic pathways for these sulphur compounds (Heinonen, 1973; Tateishi et al., 1974; Kaplowitz et al., 1985; States et al., 1987). In both fetal and newborn rat livers, the synthetic pathway of glutathione is at a submaximal level and the concentration of GSH is lower than in adults (Taniguchi et al., 1974; Wirth and Thorgeirsson, 1978). Although, in late gestation, substantial concentrations of cysteine are transported to the fetus via, the placenta (Tateishi et al., 1980; Malloy et al., 1983), the free cysteine level in rat liver is low. Glutathione has been proposed to be involved in the hepatic storage of cysteine (Tateishi et al., 1977). However the newborn rat liver contains a high concentration of γ-glutamyltranspeptidase, the enzyme responsible for glutathione degradation (Tateishi et al., 1980; Taniguchi and Inoue, 1986). This enzyme activity in newborn liver is high during the first week and then rapidly decreases to reach adult low levels. Therefore glutathione may not serve to store cysteine in newborn rat liver.

In addition to glutathione there is another cysteine pool in fetal-neonatal rat liver, namely the high cysteine containing metalloprotein-metallothionein bound to zinc and copper (Bell, 1979; Wong and Klaassen, 1979; Panemangalore et al., 1983). In rats, the concentration of this protein is high in the liver from day 20 of gestation to about 12 to 14 days after birth. The factors involved in its induced synthesis in liver during certain periods in development and the physiological roles of this protein during mammalian development are not yet understood. It has been proposed that this protein may serve as a storage source for zinc and copper (Templeton et al., 1985; Gallant and Cherian, 1986, 1987), similar to ferritin which stores iron in fetal liver. In addition a cysteine storage role for metallothionein also has been proposed in human fetal liver (Zlotkin and Cherian, 1988) where the conversion of methionine to cysteine through the cystathionase or transsulfuration pathway is absent. The developmental pattern of cystathionase enzyme and its inverse relationship to metallothionein have been demonstrated in the livers of prematurely born children. Since it is extremely difficult to obtain fetal and newborn tissue samples from humans, we have recently undertaken experimental studies in newborn rat model (Gallant and Cherian, 1989; Taniguchi and Cherian, 1990) to elucidate a cysteine storage function for metallothionein. Potential interactions between the cysteine pools in newborn rat liver are shown in a proposed model in Figure 1.

This article will review some of the preliminary results and other new approaches used to study the interactions between glutathione and metallothionein, two distinct cysteine pools in newborn rat liver. However, it should be pointed out that synthetic pathways of this tripeptide (glutathione) and polypeptide (metallothionein) are controlled by two different mechanisms. While the glutathione synthesis is regulated by enzymatic pathways, metallothionein synthesis takes place on free polyribosomes (Cherian et al., 1981) and is under transcriptional control.

MATERIALS AND METHODS

Pregnant Sprague-Dawley rats (Canada Breeding Farm and Laboratories, Saint-Constant, Quebec, Canada) and their newborn pups were used in this study. The experimental details are described in our previous publications (Gallant and Cherian, 1989; Taniguchi and Cherian, 1990). Briefly, rats were housed in individual plastic cages with bedding material in a temperature-controlled room. All diets and water were given ad libitum. In certain experiments, the pregnant rats were fed with zinc deficient or sulfhydryl-deficient diet or control diets (Zeigler Brothers, Gardner, PA) as described previously (Andrews et al., 1987; Gallant and Cherian, 1989) to compare changes in hepatic glutathione or zinc and metallothionein levels in newborn pups. In order to inhibit glutathione synthesis *in utero*, pregnant

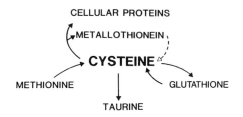

Figure 1. A proposed model of various cysteine pools and its metabolism in newborn rat liver. The arrow showing the release of cysteine from MT is in dotted lines due to lack of supporting experimental data. (Adapted from Gallant and Cherian, 1989.)

rats were given 20 mM buthionine sulfoximine (BSO) in drinking water and newborn pups were killed on day 1 for estimation of glutathione (Tietze, 1969), metals and metallothionein (Scheuhammer and Cherian, 1986). Newborn pups were injected with a single dose of ZnSO$_4$(20 mg/kg s.c.) and were killed on different days (3, 4, 5, 6, 7, 9, 14, 17, and 21) to estimate hepatic zinc and metallothionein. Control pups injected with saline were killed on identical days. In order to study the effect of chelation of zinc or increase in glutathione levels on hepatic metallothionein, rat pups of two different ages (4 and 11 days old) were injected either with 4-MDTC (4-methoxybenzyl-glucamine dithiocarbamate) 1 mmol/kg, s.c. for 3 d or glutathione monopropionyl ester (7 mmol/kg, s.c. for 3 d). Both these compounds were obtained as a gift from Dr. M.M. Jones, Department of Chemistry, Vanderbilt University, Nashville, TN. In certain experiments, cystathionase (Gaull et al., 1972) and γ-glutamyltranspeptidase (Dierickx, 1980) activities were measured in rat liver.

RESULTS

Estimations of hepatic glutathione and metallothionein levels in fetal rat during late gestation (18 to 21 days) and early neonatal period (1, 4, 5, and 11 days of age) showed lower levels of glutathione and higher levels of metallothionein than in adult rats (Table 1). The glutathione levels were below 3 μmol in fetal livers and were above 3 μmol in newborn rat livers. Metallothionein levels gradually increased in fetal livers and were maximum at birth. The levels were maintained high during the first 2 weeks and then declined to adult low levels. However, even in newborn rats metallothionein levels were 160 nmol/g while glutathione levels were 3 to 4 μmol/g.

Injection of zinc sulfate (20 mg/kg) in newborn rats increased both the

TABLE I.
Hepatic Glutathione and
Metallothionein Levels in Rat Liver
During Perinatal Development

| Age (days) | N | Mean ± S.D. | |
		Glutathione (μmol/g)	Metallothionein (nmol/g)
Gestational			
18	3	3.15 ± .71	38 ± 8
19	3	2.92 ± .42	48 ± 6
20	5	2.88 ± .22	69 ± 7
21	4	2.76 ± .44	92 ± 26
Postnatal			
1	9	3.29 ± .68	160 ± 7
4	7	3.57 ± 1.2	142 ± 6
5	3	3.7 ± .53	134 ± 10
11	4	3.9 ± .07	84 ± 5
21	3	4.7 ± .47	5 ± 1

Adapted from Panemangalore et al. (1983), and Taniguchi and Cherian (1990).

hepatic zinc and metallothionein levels to almost double (Figures 2 and 3). These high levels were maintained for ten days, similar to control newborn rats. A similar injection of zinc sulfate in adult rat will increase the hepatic zinc and metallothionein levels but these levels will decrease within 48 h to control values. Therefore in newborn rats there are factors which can retain about 70% of the hepatic zinc as metallothionein during the first two weeks of life (Cherian et al., 1987; Gallant, 1989). There is little information either on these factors or the biological functions of high levels of metallothionein during development.

These results suggest that in newborn rat liver, metallothionein can be a major cysteine storage protein in addition to glutathione (Figure 1). Cysteine can also be synthesized from methionine by transsulfuration pathway. As shown in Figure 4, the synthesis and degradation of hepatic glutathione in newborn rats can be inhibited by BSO or acivicin. The transsulfuration pathway can also be blocked by propargylglycine.

When pregnant rats were fed a zinc-deficient diet from day 12 of gestation, the hepatic levels of metallothionein and zinc of newborn rats were markedly decreased (Table 2.) However this had little effect on hepatic glutathione levels. Feeding of sulphydryl-deficient diet did not alter either metallothionein or glutathione levels in newborn rat liver (Gallant and Cherian, 1989). Treatment of pregnant rats with BSO from day 14 of gestation

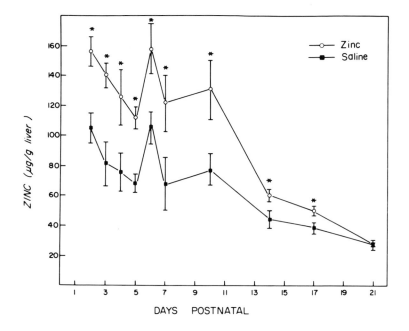

Figure 2. Hepatic zinc levels in newborn rats at different days after a single injection of saline or zinc sulfate (20 mg/kg) on day 1.

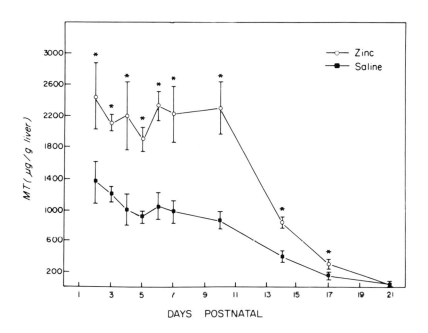

Figure 3. Hepatic metallothionein (MT) levels in newborn rats at different days after a single injection of saline or zinc sulfate (20 mg/kg) on day 1.

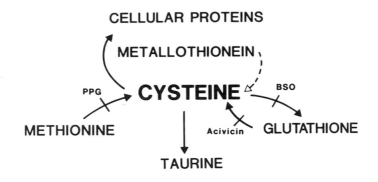

Figure 4. A proposed metabolic model of cysteine in newborn rat liver with various inhibitors to block certain pathways. BSO, buthionine sulfoximine, PPG, propargylglycine.

decreased the glutathione levels without any change in hepatic metallothionein or zinc levels in newborn rats. These results suggest that there is little interaction between the two major sulphydryl pools, glutathione and metallothionein, in newborn rat liver.

Since there is a high activity of γ-glutamyltranspeptidase in newborn rat liver during the first week, glutathione is rapidly degraded and thus may not act as a storage source for cysteine. Therefore, metallothionein with a longer half-time than glutathione may serve to store cysteine during this period. In order to test this hypothesis, the effects of chelation of zinc or increased induced synthesis of glutathione were studied in newborn rats of two age groups — 4 or 11 days old. These age groups were selected because four day old rat pups had high hepatic metallothionein and γ-glutamyltranspeptidase activity with low glutathione levels while eleven day old rat pups had declining levels of hepatic metallothionein and increasing levels of glutathione with low γ-glutamyltranspeptidase activity.

Injection of N-(4-methoxybenzyl)-glucamine dithiocarbamate decreased the hepatic zinc levels in 4-day-old rats. The preliminary studies showed no changes in glutathione, metallothionein, γ-glutamyltranspeptidase or cystathionase activity in newborn rats after chelation of zinc (Table 3). Injections of glutathione mono ester to 4 or 11-day-old rats increased hepatic glutathione levels to adult levels. The increase in hepatic glutathione levels had little effect on the levels of cystathionase or γ-glutamyltranspeptidase activity. However, in 11-day-old rats, injection of glutathione ester resulted in maintaining high levels of metallothionein while in control rat pups, the metallothionein levels decreased (Table 3). These preliminary results suggest that a continuous supply of exogenous cysteine for glutathione synthesis may help to maintain high hepatic levels of metallothionein even at eleven days after birth.

TABLE II.
Effects of Various Treatments of Pregnant Rats on Hepatic MT, Zn, and GSH Levels in Newborn Rats

Treatment[a]	(µg/g tissue ± S.D.)		Glutathione (µmol/g ± S.D.)
	Metallothionein	Zinc	
Control	1247.3 ± 80	104.9 ± 8.8	4.1 ± 0.6
Zn-deficient diet	388.4 ± 29.3	43.4 ± 5.51	4.2 ± 0.8
SH-deficient diet	1158.6 ± 114.6	99.4 ± 12.9	3.8 ± 0.5
BSO	1307 ± 80	91.8 ± 6	1.3 ± 0.2

Adapted from Gallant and Cherian (1989).
[a]Details of treatments are described in "Methods" section. Metallothionein, zinc and glutathione levels were estimated in 1-day-old pups.

TABLE III.
Effects of Injection of GSH Ester or Chelation of Zinc in Newborn Rat Liver

Age (days)	Treatment	GSH (µmol/g)	Cystathionase (µmol cyst/mg P/h)	GGT U/g P	(µg/g)	
					MT	Zn
Four	Control	3.7 ± 0.5	1.7 ± 0.3	6.5 ± 2.2	856	87.8
Four	GSH ester	5.0 ± 1.3	1.6 ± 0.3	6.2 ± 1.5	981	87.8
Four	4-MDTC	3.6 ± 0.5	1.6 ± 0.1	7.8 ± 0.2	912	62
Eleven	Control	3.9 ± 0.7	1.4 ± 0.1	2.3 ± 0.8	680	72
Eleven	GSH ester	6.1 ± 0.5	1.2 ± 0.1	3.1 ± 0.3	1010	84

Newborn pups (4 or 11 d old) were injected with saline (control) or GSH-propionyl ester (7 mmol/ kg, s.c. for 3 d) or 4-MDTC [N-(4-methoxybenzyl) glucamine dithiocarbamate], 1 mmol/kg, s.c. for 3 d. Rats were killed at 24 h later for determinations.

DISCUSSION

A number of biological functions for metallothionein were proposed soon after its isolation and characterization (Kägi and Vallee, 1961). Although the structure of metallothionein has been fully elucidated (Kägi and Kojima, 1987) during the last three decades, there is little direct information on the function of this metalloprotein. The recent reports on the marked changes in metallothionein levels and localization in mammalian livers during development (Webb and Cain, 1982; Panemangalore, et al., 1983; Nartey et al., 1987) and in certain neoplasia (Kontozoglou et al., 1989) suggest a biological function for this protein in cellular differentiation and maturation. The exact role of this protein in mammalian cells during development is not yet understood. The high levels of zinc and copper bound metallothionein in fetal-neonatal livers and the requirement for maternal supply of zinc for its expression in fetal liver suggest a zinc storage function. Thus, the biological role of metallothionein in zinc metabolism is somewhat analogous to that of ferritin in iron metabolism. This conclusion is also supported by the close similarities in the hepatic developmental patterns of these two metal binding proteins: like metallothionein, hepatic ferritin levels are also very high in late gestation and at birth but decline steadily during postnatal development. Moreover, both metallothionein and ferritin are intracellular proteins and have a common site of synthesis on the free polyribosomes in the cytoplasm (Cherian et al., 1981). The nascent polypeptide of metallothionein does not contain any of the signal peptides which are characteristic of secretory proteins.

The significance of the presence of metallothionein in nucleus of hepatocytes during development or partial hepactectomy and also in certain tumour cells is not yet understood but may be related to the interactions of metal ions like zinc with various constituents of the nucleus. The metals which bind to metallothionein may also bind to histones, nucleolar RNA, nuclear acidic proteins and can modify gene expression and phosphorylation of regulatory proteins. They may also cause breakages, excisions, cross-links and transitions on DNA. Presence of metallothionein in the nucleus can effectively chelate and detoxify certain metals and thereby modify various cellular processes.

Most of the proposed functions and metal binding properties of metallothionein are closely related to its high cysteine content (33%). However, little information is available on the biological role of high level of cysteines in metallothionein other than its function on metal binding (Kägi and Kojima, 1987).Although glutathione is a major nonprotein cysteine reservoir in the liver, its hepatic content is at submaximal level in fetal-neonatal rat liver which contains high activity of γ-glutamyltranspeptidase. During this developmental stage, the liver contains high amounts of metallothionein which has a much lower turnover rate than glutathione. Thus cysteine can be retained in the fetal-neonatal liver as metallothionein for a longer period than glutathione. The concentration of glutathione is at about 3 μmol/g tissue and that of metallothionein is about 160 nmol/g liver. Since metallothionein contains about 21 residues of cysteine, the total amount of cysteine in the hepatic metallothionein pool is very similar to that in glutathione in rats at birth (Figure 1). Therefore metallothionein can be considered as a major cysteine storage protein in newborn rat liver.

Much information concerning the functions of a cellular constituent can be derived from experiments in which its metabolism is modified using chemicals which inhibit or stimulate enzymes involved in its synthesis or degradation. Such a study was undertaken in newborn rats to investigate the role of metallothionein in sulphur metabolism by either inhibiting glutathione synthesis with buthionine sulfoximine or stimulating its synthesis by supplying a cysteine source (Figure 4). The results showed little interaction between the two major cysteine pools—glutathione and metallothionein in newborn rat liver (Gallant and Cherian, 1989). The maternal factors which can alter the levels of these two cysteine pools were also studied (Table 2). Although the exact cysteine source for the synthesis of glutathione and metallothionein in newborn rat liver is not yet understood, both these thiol-containing peptides can be effectively synthesized in hepatocytes, even when hepatic glutathione levels in the dams are low and thus limiting the active supply of sulphur amino acids from dams (Gallant and Cherian, 1989; Taniguchi and Cherian, 1990). In contrast to glutathione, the levels of hepatic metallothionein and its mRNA are regulated mainly by maternal factors such as zinc status of the dams. Both metallothionein and its mRNA levels can be markedly decreased when the dams were fed on zinc deficient diet during late gestation (Gallant and Cherian, 1986; Andrews et al., 1987). All these preliminary results suggest that the glutathione concentration in the newborn rat liver can be regulated to some extent by enzymatic activities while metallothionein synthesis is mainly dependent on maternal factors such as transfer of zinc to the fetus. However depletion of glutathione in the dams with BSO injection can also decrease the hepatic glutathione levels in the pups without any change in metallothionein levels. Some of these differences may be due to the two different synthetic pathways for glutathione and metallothionein.

Because of the low activity of cystathionase in human fetal liver, the sulphur metabolism is different from that in rat. Thus methionine cannot be converted into cysteine and the human fetus is entirely dependent on the mother for its supply of cysteine. The developmental pattern of cystathionase enzyme activity and its inverse relationship to metallothionein levels have been demonstrated in the livers of prematurely born children (Zlotkin and Cherian, 1988). In humans, the decrease in hepatic levels of zinc and metallothionein during the first months of life correspond to a period of negative zinc balance and low endogenous cysteine production in the newborn. Therefore metallothionein may play an important role as a storage depot for these two essential nutrients in human fetus during this critical period of active growth. In newborn rats inhibition of cystathionase by repeated injection with propargylglycine can decrease the hepatic levels of both metallothionein and glutathione (Gallant and Cherian, 1989).

Preliminary results showed that injection of glutathione mono ester to eleven day old rats increased the hepatic glutathione levels and it prevented the normal decrease in metallothionein levels (Table 3). There were no changes in metallothionein levels if the glutathione levels were increased in 4-day-old rats. These results thus suggest that the normal fall in hepatic metallothionein in rats after 12 to 14 days of birth may be related to increase in the level of glutathione. Further studies are in progress to investigate the effect of chelation of zinc from metallothionein and inhibition of γ-glutamyltranspeptidase activity in newborn rats on sulphur metabolism.

The present study does not show any direct function of metallothionein in sulphur metabolism in newborn rat liver, although metallothionein can be one of the major sulphur containing pools with a lower turnover rate than glutathione during certain stages in mammalian development.

REFERENCES

Andrews GK, Gallant KR, and Cherian MG (1987): Regulation of the ontogeny of rat liver metallothionein mRNA by zinc. *Eur. J. Biochem.* 166: 527.

Bell JU (1979): Native metallothionein levels in rat hepatic cytosol during perinatal development. *Toxicol. Appl. Pharmacol.* 50: 101.

Cherian MG, Yu S, and Redman CM (1981): Site of synthesis of metallothionein in rat liver. *Can. J. Biochem.* 59: 301.

Cherian MG, Templeton DM, Gallant KR, and Banerjee D (1987): Biosynthesis and metabolism of metallothionein in rat during perinatal development, in *Metallothionein II,* Kägi JHR and Kojima Y, Eds., Birkhäuser-Verlag, Basel, pp. 499–505.

Dierickx PJ (1980): Urinary gamma-glutamyltransferase as a specific marker for mercury after heavy metal treatment of rats. *Toxicol. Lett.* 6: 235.

Gallant KR and Cherian MG (1986): Influence of maternal mineral deficiency on the hepatic metallothionein and zinc in newborn rats. *Biochem. Cell. Biol.* 64: 8.

Gallant KR and Cherian MG (1987): Changes in dietary zinc result in specific alterations of metallothionein concentration in newborn rat liver. *J. Nutr.* 117: 709.

Gallant KR (1989): The metabolism of metallothionein in perinatal rat liver. Ph.D. thesis, University of Western Ontario, London, Ontario, Canada.

Gallant KR and Cherian MG (1989): Metabolic changes in glutathione and metallothionein in newborn rat liver. *J. Pharmacol. Exp. Therap.* 249: 63.

Gaull G, Sturman JA, and Raiha NCR (1972): Development of mammalian sulphur metabolism: absence of cystathionase in human fetal tissues. *Ped. Res.* 6: 538.

Heinonen K (1973): Studies on cystathionase activity in rat liver and brain during development. *Biochem. J.* 136: 1011.

Kägi JHR and Vallee BL (1961): Metallothionein: A cadmium and zinc containing protein from equine renal cortex. *J. Biol. Chem.* 236: 2435.

Kägi JHR and Kojima Y (1987) *Metallothionein II,* Birkhauser-Verlag, Basel.

Kaplowitz N, Aw TY, and Ookhtens M (1985): The regulation of hepatic glutathione. *Ann. Rev. Pharmacol. Toxicol.* 25: 715.

Kontozoglou TE, Banerjee D, and Cherian MG (1989): Immunohistochemical localization of metallothionein in human testicular embryonal carcinoma cells. *Virch. Arch. A. Pathol. Anat.* 415: 545.

Nartey N, Banerjee D, and Cherian MG (1987): Immunohistochemical localization of metallothionein in cell nucleus and cytoplasm of fetal human liver and kidney and its changes during development. *Pathology* 19: 233.

Panemangalore M, Banerjee D, Onosaka S, and Cherian MG (1983): Changes in the intracellular accumulation and distribution of metallothionein in rat liver and kidney during postnatal development. *Dev. Biol.* 97: 95.

States B, Foreman JW, and Segal S (1987): Cysteine and glutathione levels in developing rat kidney and liver. *Ped. Res.* 22: 605.

Taniguchi N, Tsukuda Y, and Nirai H (1974): Acquisition of fetal properties in hepatoma on glutathione metabolism. *Biochem. Biophys. Acta* 351: 161.

Taniguchi M and Inoue M (1986): Ontogenic changes in metabolism and transport of glutathione in the rat. *J. Biochem.* 100: 1457.

Taniguchi M and Cherian MG (1990): Ontogenic changes in hepatic glutathione and metallothionein in rats and the effect of a low-sulphur containing diet. *Brit. J. Nutr.* 63: 97.

Tateishi N, Higashi T, Shinya S, Naruse A, and Sakamoto Y (1974): Studies on the regulation of glutathione level in rat liver. *J. Biochem.* 75: 93.

Tateishi N, Higashi T, Naruse A, Nakashima K, Shiozaki H, and Sakamoto K (1977): Rat liver glutathione: possible role a reservoir of cysteine. *J. Nutr.* 107: 51.

Tateishi N, Higashi T, Nakashina K, and Sakamoto Y (1980): Nutritional significance of increase in γ-glutamyltransferase in mouse liver before birth. *J. Nutr.* 110: 409.

Templeton DM, Banerjee D, and Cherian MG (1985): Metallothionein synthesis and localization in relation to metal storage in rat liver during gestation. *Can. J. Biochem. Cell. Biol.* 63: 16.

Tietze R (1969): Enzymic method for quantitative determination of nanogram amounts of total and oxidized glutathione: application to mammalian blood and other tissues. *Anal. Biochem.* 27: 502.

Webb M and Cain K (1982): Functions of metallothionein. *Biochem. Pharmacol.* 31: 137.

Wirth PJ and Thorgeirsson SS (1978): Glutathione synthesis and degradation in fetal and adult rat liver and Novikoff hepatoma. *Cancer Res.* 38: 2861.

Wong KL and Klaassen CD (1979): Isolation and characterization of metallothionein which is highly concentrated in newborn rat liver. *J. Biol. Chem.* 254: 12399.

Zlotkin SH and Cherian MG (1988): Hepatic metallothionein as a source of zinc and cysteine during the first year of life. *Ped. Res.* 24: 326.

Chapter

11

Cadmium-Binding Proteins in Target Tissues of Cadmium Carcinogenesis

Michael P. Waalkes, Zakaria Z. Wahba,
Toshiaki Koizumi, Alan Perantoni, and Mrinal R. Bhave
Laboratory of Comparative Carcinogenesis
Inorganic Carcinogenesis Section
National Cancer Institute
Frederick Cancer Research and Development Facility
Frederick, Maryland

ABSTRACT

Testes are a well established target site of cadmium (Cd) carcinogenesis in rodents, while the rat prostate was also recently shown to be susceptible to the carcinogenic effects of Cd. Since metallothionein (MT) is thought to be a key factor in tissue resistance to Cd toxicity, the metal binding proteins (BP) in the testes and prostate were analyzed biochemically. Using a combination of reverse-phase high performance liquid chromatography (HPLC) purification and amino acid analysis, both these tissues appeared to be deficient in MT, as indicated by marked differences in amino acid contents of the low molecular weight (M_r) CdBP present. The CdBPs from testes could be readily separated from hepatic MT by gradient SDS-polyacrylamide gel electrophoresis (SDS-PAGE). The CdBPs of the rat and mouse testes and that of the rat prostate were all very low in cysteine (<2%) compared to MT (approximately 30%). In the mouse, the MT-1 gene in the testes was highly methylated in comparison to the same gene in the liver, a condition typically associated with genetic quiescence. Various treatments that make the testes refractory to Cd carcinogenesis, such as high-dose zinc (Zn) and low-dose Cd pretreatments, have no effect on the levels of CdBP in the testes or prostate, when assessed either by Cd binding capacity or by protein concentrations using SDS-PAGE. Thus alternative forms of tolerance were explored. In isolated target cells (interstitial) of the testes, low-dose Cd or high-dose Zn pretreatments *in vivo* prior to isolation made these cells resistant to the cytotoxic effects of Cd *in vitro*. This resistance was associated with an increase in Cd efflux and an increase in glutathione contents. Thus, induced resistance to Cd carcinogenicity in the testes seems not to be due to MT, and alternative mechanisms may be in affect.

INTRODUCTION

There are several target sties of cadmium (Cd) carcinogenesis. In humans Cd is a potent pulmonary carcinogen in occupationally exposed individuals (see Waalkes and Oberdörster, 1990). There are also indications Cd can induce prostatic tumors in humans following occupational (Potts, 1965; Kipling and Waterhouse, 1967) or environmental exposure (Bako et al., 1982). Prostatic cancer is a very important and very deadly form of cancer and its etiology is as yet obscure. Thus a confirmed association with Cd exposure and prostatic cancer would be of great importance. In animal models, Cd has also been shown to be an effective pulmonary carcinogen after chronic inhalation (Takenaka et al., 1983). Like many other metals, Cd is also effective in induction of injection site sarcomas (Gunn et al., 1967; Waalkes et al., 1988a, 1989). Typically fibrosarcomas, such tumors can be induced by Cd at subcutaneous or intramuscular injection sites (Gunn et al., 1967; Waalkes et al., 1988a, 1989). Cd is also a potent testicular tumorigen, inducing interstitial cell tumors in both rats (Gunn et al., 1963, 1964; Waalkes et al., 1988a, 1989) and mice (Gunn et al., 1963) at high incidence. Although these tumors are typically benign, recent data from this laboratory show they can become malignant with repeated Cd exposures (Waalkes et al., 1990). Recent studies have also provided the first definitive experimental evidence that the prostate is a target tissue for Cd carcinogenesis in rodents (Waalkes et al., 1988a, 1989), thus supporting the human data associating Cd with prostate cancer. Tumors of the prostate only occur with Cd doses below those that induce testicular degeneration (Waalkes et al., 1988a) or in cases in which such degeneration is reduced by high dose zinc (Zn) treatment (Waalkes et al., 1989) or low dose Cd pretreatment (Waalkes et al., 1988a). The association of prostatic tumor formation with histologically normal testes indicates the androgen dependency of this tumor type. Lastly, the lymphatic system was recently recognized as a target tissue of Cd carcinogenesis and Cd can increase leukemia incidence in mice (Blakely, 1986) or rats (Waalkes and Rehm, 1990).

Several treatments are effective in reducing or preventing Cd carcinogenesis (Gunn et al., 1963, 1964; Waalkes et al., 1988a, 1989). The ability of Zn to prevent Cd induction of testicular tumors, originally detected by Gunn et al. (Gunn et al., 1963, 1964), was recently shown to be clearly related to Zn dosage (Waalkes et al., 1989). These results would thus indicate that the antagonism of Cd carcinogenesis by Zn is through action at the molecular target sites of Cd. Other treatments that can prevent or reduce Cd carcinogenesis in the testes include pretreatment with Cd at low, subnecrotizing dosage (Waalkes et al., 1988a). This self tolerance is a remarkable aspect of Cd as a metallic toxin and carcinogen.

Metallothionein (MT) is the protein most frequently associated with tolerance to the toxic effects of Cd (see Webb, 1979 for review). With its metal binding ability, high affinity for Cd, and high inducibility, it appears to provide a responsive cellular defense mechanism against the Cd ion (Webb, 1979). Cd and Zn are both potent and efficacious inducers of MT (Onosaka and Cherian, 1981, 1982; Waalkes and Klaassen, 1985), and MT induction is thought to be linked to the ability of Zn or low dose Cd to induce tolerance to normally toxic levels of Cd (Webb, 1979; Goering and Klaassen, 1984).

With regard to tissue specificity in Cd carcinogenesis, several anomalous facts are apparent. In the testes, tumors form despite the fact that less than 1% of a given dose of Cd localizes within this tissue (Gunn et al., 1968; Wong et al., 1980). In contrast, no tumors develop in the liver where the majority of a dose of Cd is typically deposited (Webb, 1979). Thus there appears to be a high tissue specificity in Cd carcinogenesis. Hence our studies have investigated potential tissue susceptibility factors. Since MT is thought to be key in Cd detoxification, we have assessed the nature of Cd binding proteins (CdBP) within target tissues of Cd carcinogenesis. This paper reviews the results of these studies.

MATERIALS AND METHODS

Animals and Sample Preparation

Male BALB/c and NFS mice and Wistar rats were obtained from the Animal Production Area, Frederick Cancer Research and Development Facility (Frederick, MD) and were used at 8 weeks of age or older. Animals were killed by CO_2 asphyxia and the testes or ventral prostate (rats only) were excised, weighed, and homogenized (1:4, w/v) in 20 mM Tris-HCl (pH 8.6 at 4°C) containing 5 mM 2-mercaptoethanol and 250 mM sucrose.

Cytosol was derived by differential centrifugation and used immediately either for gel filtration or further purification by heat treatment and sequential acetone precipitation. Hepatic MT was induced in several groups of mice or rats by injection of Zn. Liver samples were processed as described above.

Partial Purification of Hepatic and Testicular Metal BP

A method for the partial purification of MT from hepatic cytosol (Sobocinski et al., 1978) was applied to testicular, prostatic, and hepatic cytosols. Cytosol was heated to 85°C for 10 min and centrifuged for 15 min at $27,000 \times g$. The heat-stable protein was then subjected to selective acetone precipitation (0 to 40%, 40 to 60%, 60 to 80% acetone by volume) with centrifugation ($27,000 \times g$ for 15 min) between each step. The material precipitating in 80% acetone was stored under argon until reconstitution in either 20 mM Tris-HCl, pH 8.6, containing 5 mM 2-mercaptoethanol and 250 mM sucrose for gel-filtration chromatography or 0.1% trifluoroacetic acid containing 3 M guanidine-HCl for reverse-phase high performance liquid chromatography (HPLC).

Gel Filtration Chromatography

Samples of cytosol were used either directly as prepared or after initial saturation with Cd (containing [109]Cd). Samples partially purified by heat treatment and acetone precipitation were reconstituted in buffer and then saturated with Cd in a similar fashion. Samples were applied to a column (1.5 × 40 cm) of Sephacryl S-200® equilibrated with 20 mM Tris-HCl, pH 8.6, containing 50 mM NaCl, 5 mM 2-mercaptoethanol and 0.02% NaN$_3$, and eluted at a flow rate of 36 ml/h. Forty fractions of 5 min each were collected and assayed for Zn or copper content by atomic absorption spectrophotometry. Cd content was determined by gamma-spectrometry.

Reverse-Phase HPLC

The reverse-phase HPLC method of Klauser et al. (1983), with slight modification (Waalkes and Perantoni, 1986) was used. Partially purified preparations of hepatic, prostatic, and testicular metal BP were used in all cases. Proteins were separated using an Aquapore RP-300® column (Brownlee Labs, Inc. Santa Clara, CA) with a 65-min linear gradient of 25 to 40% acetonitrile in 0.1% trifluoroacetic acid (pH 2.0). Flow rate was 1.0 ml/min, and 60 one-min fractions were collected.

Amino Acid Analysis

Following reverse-phase HPLC, fractions containing the major hepatic, prostatic, or testicular metal BP peaks were combined, divided into two equal parts, and lyophilized to dryness. Samples were then hydrolyzed and amino acid analysis was performed as described (Waalkes and Perantoni, 1986).

Southern Blot Analysis

Southern blot analysis was performed on digests of DNA isolated from testes and liver of mice. After mice were terminated, testes and liver were rapidly removed, trimmed, and homogenized and DNA was isolated using phenol/chloroform and chloroform extractions and ethanol precipitation. DNA was then restricted as described (Bhave et al., 1988; Waalkes et al., 1988b) and Southern blot analysis was carried out with digests (Southern, 1975). Blot hybridization was accomplished by use of the mouse MT-I gene insert in pBX322 (*Stu* I-*Hind* III fragment, 1.99 kb) as the probe (Glanville et al., 1981; Stuart et al., 1984).

Heat-Stable Protein Cd-Capacity

An assay originally designed for assessment of tissue MT concentrations (Onosaka et al., 1978) which takes advantage of the known heat stability of MT (Sobocinski et al., 1978) was applied to cytosol derived from testes, prostate, and liver of control, Cd- and Zn-treated rats or mice. The assay was also applied to cytosol derived from isolated interstitial cells from rat testes. Assay conditions have been previously described (Waalkes et al., 1988b).

Testicular Interstitial Cell Preparation

Testicular interstitial cells were isolated from the pooled (10 to 15 animals per preparation) decapsulated rat testes by the collagenase dispersion method (Waalkes and Poirier, 1985). After isolation, interstitial cells from either untreated control, low dose *in vivo* Cd- or Zn-pretreated rats were suspended in incubation mixture (IM; 131 mM NaCl, 5.2 mM KCl, 0.9 mM MgSO$_4$, 1.0 mM CaCl$_2$, 11.1 mM glucose, Tris-HCl, pH 7.4). Protein was measured by the method of Bradford (1976) and adjusted to a final concentration of 1.0 mg protein per ml. Viability of these preparations, determined by the trypan blue exclusion test consistently exceeded 90%, while contamination with spermatozoa was typically minimal.

Interstitial Cell CdBP Analysis

An aqueous solution of 10.0 mM CdCl$_2$ (0.2 ml) was added to interstitial cell suspensions (1.8 ml) from control and Cd-pretreated rats and were incubated at 32°C for 60 min (final Cd concentration 1.0 mM). Interstitial cell cytosolic fraction was isolated by differential centrifugation. Semiquantitation of low molecular weight (M$_r$) cytosolic testicular CdBP was accomplished by SDS-polyacrylamide gel electrophoresis (SDS-PAGE) using precast gradient gels of 11 to 23% acrylamide, while the amount of metal associated with testicular CdBP was assessed by gel filtration. For SDS-PAGE, samples of cytosol were mixed (9:1) v/v with denaturing solution (Amersham Company, Arlington, IL) and heated for 4 min at 90°C. Samples were prepared from equal wet weights of tissue and then applied to the gel. SDS-PAGE were run at 70 V for the initial 20 min, followed by 140 V for 4 to 5 h. M$_r$ standards were run concurrently. Relative mobilities were determined by use of bromophenol blue, and M$_r$ of unknowns was determined from the relationship between log M$_r$ of standards and relative mobilities. For gel filtration analysis of testicular CdBP metal complement, interstitial cell cytosol (3 ml) was applied to a column of Sephadex G-75® (100 × 2.2 cm I.D.) equilibrated with 20 mM-Tris-HCl, pH 8.6, at 4°C. The cytosol was eluted with the same buffer at a flow rate of 16 ml/h. A 1.0 ml portion of each fraction was used for metal determination.

Cytotoxicity of Cd in Interstitial Cells

Interstitial cells from control, low-dose Cd- and Zn-pretreated rats were suspended in 1.0 mM CdCl$_2$ and incubated at 32°C for 60 min. At the end of incubation, aliquots were removed and intracellular and extracellular fluids were separated by the silicone oil technique as previously described (Waalkes and Poirier, 1985). Extracellular GOT was assayed with a commercially available kit (Sigma Chemical Company, St. Louis, MO) and intracellular K was determined by atomic absorption spectrometry.

Interstitial Cell Influx and Efflux of Cd

For influx determination, cells isolated from control, low-dose Cd-, or Zn-pretreated animals were suspended in 70.0 μM CdCl$_2$ (containing [109]Cd) in IM and were incubated at 32°C. Three aliquots were removed from the reaction mixture after 0.5, 1.0, 6.0, 15.0, and 60 min and intracellular and extracellular fluid were separated. Intracellular Cd was then measured by gamma spectrometry. For efflux determination, cells isolated from control and Zn-pretreated animals were suspended in 70.0 μM CdCl$_2$ and incubated at 32°C for 60 min. After incubation, the cells were centrifuged at 120 × g

for 10 min. The cells were gently resuspended in 10 ml of IM and centrifuged at $120 \times g$ for 10 min, a total of three times. Then the cells were resuspended in 6.0 ml of IM and aliquots of 100 µl were immediately removed (time 0) and intracellular and extracellular fluids were separated. The remaining cell suspension was incubated for a further 30 min in Cd-free media prior to removal of aliquots and separation of intra- and extracellular fluids. Intracellular Cd was then measured by gamma spectrometry.

Interstitial Cell Subnuclear Distribution of Cd

For assessment of the subnuclear distribution of Cd in intact cells, ICs isolated from either control or Zn-pretreated rats were suspended in buffer containing ^{109}Cd and incubated for 1 h at 32°C. Nuclei were then purified according to the method of Windel and Tata (1964) and DNA was purified by extraction with chloroform-isoamyl alcohol mixture (Ciccarelli and Wetterhahn, 1984).

Influence of CdBP on Interstitial Cell Nuclear Uptake

The testicular CdBP and MT were labeled with ^{109}Cd *in vitro* and isolated and concentrated by use of heat treatment and acetone precipitation (Waalkes and Perantoni, 1986). A 500-µl aliquot containing either 0.2 µCi ^{109}Cd or 1.5 mg MT (labeled with 0.10 µCi ^{109}Cd) or 1.4 mg testicular CdBP (labeled with 0.09 µCi ^{109}Cd) was added to 2.5 ml isolated nuclei at a concentration of 2.0×10^6 cellular equivalents per ml. The reaction mixture was incubated at 32°C and aliquots were removed at 0.5, 2.5, 5.0, 7.5, and 10 min and centrifuged for 15 s to assess the amount of free or protein-bound Cd taken up into nuclei.

Glutathione Determination

Cytosolic, mitochondrial, microsomal, and nuclear fractions of interstitial cells derived from control animals or animals pretreated with low dose Cd or Zn were isolated by differential centrifugation. For determination of glutathione levels all the samples were adjusted to a consistent volume based on an equal amount of source tissue in ice-cold 50 mM Tris-HCl buffer, pH 7.4. Glutathione content was measured according to the method of Baars and Breimer (1983), using 1-chloro-2,4-dinitrobenzene derivatives and analyzing the product by reverse-phase HPLC. Glutathione derivatives were identified by elution times based on commercially available standards. Levels of glutathione were assessed in interstitial cells after *in vitro* exposure to Cd (1.0 mM, for 60 min).

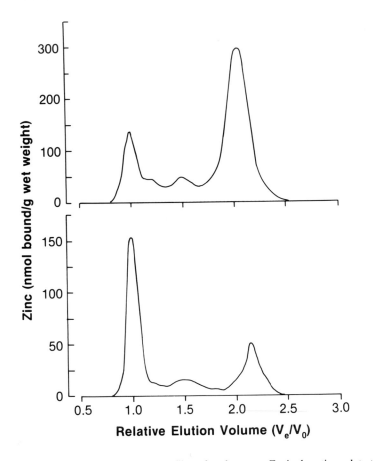

Figure 1. Representative gel filtration profiles of endogenous Zn in hepatic and testicular cytosol. Testicular cytosol (bottom panel) was derived from control rats, whereas hepatic cytosol (top panel) was isolated 24 h after treatment with Zn acetate. The Sephacryl S-200® column was eluted with 20 mM Tris-HCl (pH 8.6) containing 50 mM NaCl, 5 mM 2-mercaptoethanol, and 0.02% NaN$_3$ at a flow rate of 48 ml/h. Fractions (5 min) were collected and assayed for Zn by atomic absorption. (From Waalkes and Perantoni [1986]: *J. Biol. Chem.* 261: 13097.)

RESULTS AND DISCUSSION

Figure 1 shows the elution profile of ZnBP in cytosol from rat testes and liver after gel filtration. A prominent low M_r ZnBP was detected in the testes. This protein eluted at a relative elution volume similar to that of authentic MT from the liver of Zn-treated rats. This testicular protein also binds Cd after *in vitro* saturation with Cd or after Cd treatment (Deagen and Whanger, 1985). This testicular protein can also be extracted by a series of heat treatment and acetone precipitations (Waalkes and Perantoni, 1986) developed for isolation of MT (Sobocinski et al., 1978).

Such preparations were further purified with reverse-phase HPLC using the method developed for isolation of isoforms of MT (Klauser et al., 1983). The rat testicular CdBP was separated into two distinct isoforms eluting at 50 and 57 min (Figure 2). This method elutes the 2 forms of rat hepatic MT at between 50 and 55 min (Waalkes and Perantoni, 1986). Thus the testicular forms and the forms of authentic MT have similar retention times within this system.

Marked differences become evident, however, when these proteins isolated by HPLC are subjected to amino acid analysis (Table I). The results for the rat testicular forms as compared to the forms of hepatic MT indicate that the testicular protein clearly can not be classified as a MT. This is particularly true when differences in cysteine content are considered. The

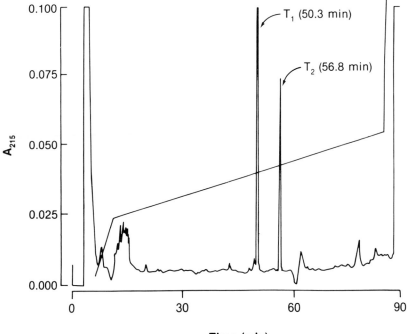

Figure 2. Further purification of partially purified low M_r testicular Cd/Zn BP by HPLC. Samples partially purified by heat treatment and acetone precipitation were reconstituted in 1.0 ml of 0.1% trifluoroacetic acid/g wet weight equivalent containing 3 M guanidine HCl, and 250 μl of this solution was injected. Chromatography was performed at 1 ml/min with a linear gradient of 25 to 40% acetonitrile (linear plot) in 0.1% trifluoroacetic acid. Two major peaks were detected, termed T_1 and T_2 by order of elution. Peaks eluting prior to 20 min were found to be due to traces of constituents of the isolation buffer (Tris, 2-mercaptoethanol). (From Waalkes and Perantoni [1986].)

TABLE I.
Amino Acid Composition of Rat Hepatic Metallothionein and Cd Binding Protein from the Rat Testes and Ventral Prostate[a]

| | Liver | | Testes | | Prostate |
Amino acid	MT-Form 1	MT-Form 2	T_1	T_2	VP_1
Asp	4.5 (5)	5.0 (5)	5.6 (6)	5.1 (5)	4.3 (4)
Thr	2.1 (2)	2.6 (3)	3.7 (4)	5.3 (5)	4.4 (4)
Ser	7.5 (8)	10.3 (10)	4.9 (5)	3.4 (3)	5.8 (6)
Glu	3.7 (4)	4.0 (4)	12.1 (12)	11.3 (11)	12.6 (13)
Pro	2.2 (2)	1.9 (2)	2.9 (3)	2.5 (3)	6.2 (6)
Gly	4.5 (5)	5.6 (6)	1.7 (2)	1.7 (2)	2.6 (3)
Ala	5.5 (6)	5.2 (5)	2.9 (3)	3.7 (4)	3.1 (3)
Val	1.1 (1)	1.5 (2)	0.0 (0)	0.0 (0)	3.0 (3)
1/2 Cys	19.4 (19)	16.9 (17)	0.8 (1)	0.6 (1)	0.4 (0)
Met	1.0 (1)	1.0 (1)	0.9 (1)	0.8 (1)	1.0 (1)
Ile	0.9 (2)	0.9 (1)	2.4 (2)	3.0 (3)	2.2 (2)
Leu	0.0 (0)	0.0 (0)	2.5 (3)	2.4 (2)	3.7 (4)
Tyr	0.0 (0)	0.0 (0)	0.0 (0)	0.0 (0)	0.9 (1)
Phe	0.0 (0)	0.0 (0)	1.3 (1)	1.2 (1)	1.4 (1)
His	0.0 (0)	0.0 (0)	0.0 (0)	0.0 (0)	1.1 (1)
Lys	8.7 (9)	8.3 (8)	10.0 (10)	9.0 (9)	7.4 (7)
Arg	0.0 (0)	0.0 (0)	0.0 (0)	0.0 (0)	0.7 (1)
Total residues	64	64	53	47	61

[a]Data are expressed as residues/molecule (nearest whole number). Forms are defined by order of elution following reverse-phase HPLC. Half-cysteine determined as cysteic acid after performic acid oxidation. From Waalkes and Perantoni (1986) and Waalkes et al. (1989).

low levels of cysteine in the testicular protein most likely would result in a lower affinity for Cd (Waalkes and Perantoni, 1986), as this amino acid is a preferred bioligand of Cd. In this protein, glutamate replaces cysteine as the prominent amino acid and probably accounts for the binding of Cd. Leucine and aromatic amino acids are also contained within the testicular protein but does not occur in MT.

When the HPLC method was also applied to CdBP from ventral prostate, only a single form was eluted at 47 min (Waalkes et al., 1989). Marked differences from MT were also evident when this prostatic CdBP isolated by HPLC was subjected to amino acid analysis (Table I). Results indicate that this prostatic protein also can not be classified as a MT, especially based on differences in cysteine content. Again in this protein glutamate replaces cysteine as the prominent amino acid. Leucine and aromatic amino acids are also present. It is noteworthy that the prostatic protein was quite similar to the proteins isolated from the testes.

Marked differences between the testicular CdBP of the mouse testes and MT are also quite apparent (Waalkes et al., 1988b). These proteins are again deficient in cysteine, and instead contain glutamate as the predominant amino acid (Waalkes et al., 1988b). Thus it appears that the remarkable testopathic effects of Cd may be related to a MT deficiency at least with regard to the protein purified from whole testes.

The second forms of the testicular protein and MT can be physically separated by several methods, including reverse-phase HPLC (Waalkes and Perantoni, 1986) and SDS-PAGE (Waalkes et al., 1984).

This glutamate-rich protein in the rodent testes and prostate was also found to be uninducible by treatments such as Cd or Zn that result in a marked induction of MT in tissues able to synthesize this protein, such as liver (Table II). These data are derived from whole tissues, measuring heat-stable CdBP by the method of Onosaka et al. (1978). The testicular and prostatic MT-like protein is heat stable and is detected by this method. The dosage levels of Zn and low-dose Cd used here make the testes refractory to the carcinogenic effects of higher dose Cd.

Likewise the testicular protein was also found to be uninducible within specific target cells of Cd carcinogenesis (Table III). Shown here are heat-stable CdBP levels in isolated interstitial cells of the testes after treatment *in vivo* with Zn. Again there was no effect, despite the fact that Zn makes the testes resistant to Cd carcinogenesis (Gunn et al., 1963; Waalkes et al.,

TABLE II.
Effect of Zn or Cd Treatments on the Levels of
Heat-Stable Metal BP in Rat Liver, Testes, and Prostate[a]

Treatment	Liver	Testes	Prostate
Control	5.5 ± 1.3	80.1 ± 3.1	2.40 ± 0.29
Cd (3 μmol/kg, s.c.)	55.8 ± 7.2	79.8 ± 1.2	2.81 ± 0.32
Zn (1.0 mmol/kg, s.c.)	58.2 ± 3.5	82.1 ± 5.5	2.68 ± 0.40

[a]Determined by the Cd-hemoglobin assay (Onosaka, 1978). Data are the mean $\pm$ S.E.M. in nmol Cd/g tissue for three separate determinations. Levels were measured 24 h after treatment. (From Waalkes and Perantoni [1988].)

TABLE III.
Concentrations of Testicular Metal
BP in Isolated Interstitial Cells
After Zn Treatment[a]

Treatment	Interstitial Cells
Control	27.0 ± 5.0
Zn (1.0 mmol/kg, s.c.)	29.5 ± 5.6

[a]Data expressed as mean $\pm$ S.E.M. in nmol Cd/g equivalent of tissue and was determined 24 h after treatment. (From Waalkes and Perantoni [1988].)

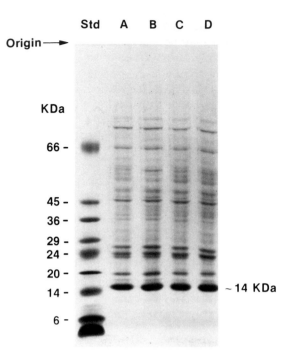

Figure 3. SDS-PAGE of interstitial cell cytosol derived from control or low dose *in vivo* Cd-pretreated rats with or without *in vitro* exposure to Cd. Lanes: A, control; B, low dose *in vivo* Cd-pretreatment; C, control with *in vitro* exposure to Cd; D, low dose *in vivo* Cd-pretreatment with *in vitro* Cd exposure. Neither low dose *in vivo* Cd-pretreatment or *in vitro* Cd exposure appeared to greatly alter levels of the low M_r (approximately 14 kDa) testicular CdBP. (From Wahba et al. [1990].)

1989) and these particular cells refractory to the cytotoxic effects of Cd (Koizumi and Waalkes, 1989a).

SDS-PAGE analysis of interstitial cell cytosolic proteins indicated that no marked increases in levels occurred with low-dose Cd treatment (Figure 3). No apparent differences in cytosolic proteins occurred. This includes both the low M_r proteins and higher M_r proteins. Again this low-dose Cd pretreatment makes the testes resistant to the carcinogenic effects of Cd (Waalkes et al., 1988a) and the interstitial cells themselves resistant to the effects of Cd (Wahba and Waalkes, 1989).

Furthermore, the MT gene within the mouse testes was found to be highly methylated (Bhave et al., 1988; Waalkes et al., 1988b), a condition typically associated with quiescence (Compere and Palmiter, 1981). Southern blot analysis of the methylation status of the mouse MT-1 gene in testes and liver of mice resistant (BALB/c) and susceptible (NFS) to the testopathic effects of Cd clearly indicated hypermethylation of the testicular gene (Bhave et al., 1988). Zn pretreatments at levels making the testes of susceptible mice refractory to the testopathic effects of Cd also had no effect on methylation (Waalkes et al., 1988b). Methylation is thought to control, at least in part, the expressibility of the MT gene and hypermethylation is associated with quiescence (Compere and Palmiter, 1981). Thus it appears there may be a genetic basis for the lack of responsiveness of the MT gene within the testes.

Thus, there appears to be a deficiency of MT in every target tissue of Cd carcinogenesis thus far studied. This includes the rat and mouse testes, and the rat prostate. However, it should be noted that the present results do not completely eliminate the possibility that MT may be present in a few specific cells within these heterogenous tissues in relatively small amounts overall. In any event, in view of the apparent deficiency of MT or of an inducible MT system, alternative mechanisms of tolerance must be considered. To study such tolerance, we have used an isolated cell system, namely isolated interstitial cells of the rat testes (Waalkes and Poirier, 1985; Koizumi and Waalkes, 1989a,b, 1990; Wahba and Waalkes, 1989; Wahba et al., 1990). The effects of *in vivo* treatments that make the testes refractory to Cd carcinogenesis, such as Zn or low-dose Cd, on the *in vitro* effects of Cd were thus assessed in interstitial cells isolated from rats given such treatments (Koizumi and Waalkes, 1989a,b, 1990; Wahba and Waalkes, 1989; Wahba et al., 1990). Figure 4 shows the effect of low dose *in vivo* Cd pretreatment on the cytotoxic effects of Cd *in vitro* in isolated interstitial cells as assessed by GOT loss. Low dose Cd pretreatment markedly reduced Cd cytotoxicity. The same was true for other indices of Cd toxicity in these cells such as K loss or lipid peroxidation (Wahba and Waalkes, 1989). Likewise *in vivo* Zn pretreatment will reduce the cytotoxicity of Cd in these cells (Koizumi and Waalkes, 1989a).

The Cd content of the low M_r testicular protein was assessed to determine if this tolerance to Cd within these target cells of Cd carcinogenesis might be linked to a greater disposition of the metal within this protein in a fashion analogous to that which occurs with MT. Figure 5 shows the effects of low dose *in vivo* Cd pretreatment with and without an *in vitro* Cd exposure. In marked contrast to what occurs with MT-based tolerance to Cd, low-dose Cd pretreatment at levels making the testes and these cells, in particular, resistant to Cd actually resulted in a large reduction in the Cd content of the testicular metal binding protein. Although not immediately apparent, this may in fact be important for the development of tolerance to Cd carcinogenesis. Since, when Cd is associated with this testicular protein there is dramatic increase in the nuclear disposition of Cd (Koizumi and Waalkes, 1989b), reductions here could reduce the amount of Cd that becomes associated with genetic material. Reduced levels of Cd in the nucleus could reduce interaction with nuclear material and thus possibly prevent Cd-induced tumor formation. This assumes of course that DNA is a target molecule of Cd carcinogenesis, an assumption as yet not proven.

Thus, alternative mechanisms for Cd tolerance were considered. In this regard, glutathione is thought to constitute a first line of defense against toxic metal ions (Singhal et al., 1987; Suzuki and Cherian, 1989). Glutathione levels in interstitial cells were significantly increased by low dose *in vivo* Cd pretreatment by approximately 20% (Wahba et al., 1990). This was true overall in whole cells and appeared to be a specific effect in the cytosol. Glutathione is known to bind metals and glutathione deficiency enhances Cd toxicity (Singhal et al., 1987). Thus glutathione increases may account, at least in part, for the reduction in Cd toxicity to these cells.

Likewise Zn pretreatment, which can make animals resistant to Cd-induced testicular carcinogenicity, prevents Cd cytotoxicity in isolated interstitial cells (Koizumi and Waalkes, 1989a) in a fashion similar to low dose Cd. This is despite the fact that *in vivo* Zn pretreatment actually in-

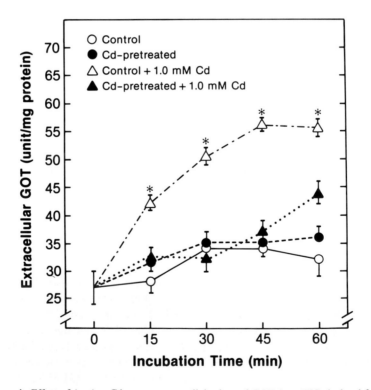

Figure 4. Effect of *in vitro* Cd exposure on cellular loss of GOT from TICs isolated from rat with or without *in vivo* Cd pretreatment. Results are the mean ± S.E.M. of 5–6 preparations and asterisks indicate a significant difference from appropriate control. Note broken X-axis. (From Wahba and Waalkes [1989].)

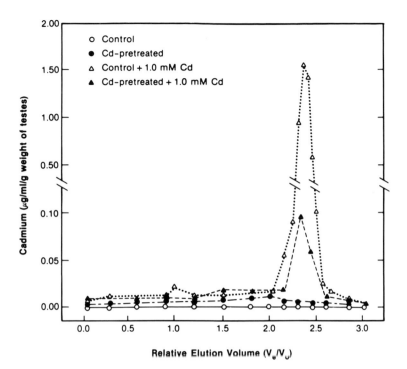

Figure 5. Gel-filtration chromatography elution profile of cytosolic Cd prepared from ICs isolated from control or low dose *in vivo* Cd-pretreated rats with and without exposure to *in vitro* Cd. Gel-filtration was carried out as specified in the Materials and Methods section. A prominent testicular CdBP eluted in the low M_r range with relative elution volume (V_e/V_o) approximately 2.0 to 2.5. *In vivo* Cd-pretreatment markedly reduced the amount of Cd associated with this protein. Note broken Y-axis. (From Wahba et al. [1990].)

creased *in vitro* Cd uptake into interstitial cells (Koizumi and Waalkes, 1989a). The increases in Cd influx were small, however, when compared to the increases in the efflux of Cd that were induced by Zn pretreatment (Table IV). *In vivo* Zn pretreatment increased Cd efflux by a factor of at least 4.5-fold. Given the very small amount of Cd that actually reaches the testes (Gunn et al., 1968; Wong et al., 1980), this increased loss of Cd from specific target cells could have potentially dramatic effects. Indeed, this appears to be the case when the nuclear content of Cd is considered. Overall, *in vivo* Zn pretreatment resulted in a marked reduction in the nuclear content of Cd within interstitial cells (Koizumi and Waalkes, 1989a). There was also a reduction in the Cd content of DNA isolated from interstitial cells from Zn pretreated animals and exposure *in vitro* to Cd (Koizumi and Waalkes, 1990). This indicates that Zn interactions with DNA may also directly reduce Cd interactions with genetic material.

TABLE IV.
Efflux of Cd from Rat Testicular Interstitial Cells
With or Without *In Vivo* Zn Pretreatment[a]

Experimental	Cd Content in Cells (%)		Efflux Rate
	0 min	30 min	
Control cells	5300 ± 200 (100%)	4500 ± 100 (85%)	1600
Zn-pretreated cells	$6700 \pm 100^*$ (100%)	$3000 \pm 150^*$ (44%)	7400

[a]Data represents the mean $\pm$ S.E. (percent time 0) of 4 independent cell preparations and are expressed as [109]Cd cpm/mg protein (content) or [109]Cd cpm/mg protein/h (efflux rate). Time 0 equals the point at which the cells were transferred to a Cd-free medium. Asterisks indicate a significant difference ($p \leq 0.05$) from control cells.

In summary, tolerance to Cd carcinogenicity within the testes does not seem to be due to MT. This is true of induced tolerance, such as that seen with Zn or low dose Cd pretreatments, or genetically based tolerance, as seen in resistant strains of mice. Furthermore it does not seem to be due to the available low M_r proteins, at least not entirely. Alternative mechanisms therefore must be explored. Such mechanisms could be due to multiple factors including possibly a combination of increased glutathione levels and increased Cd efflux. The glutathione could possibly sequester the Cd molecule until it can be extruded by a more active transport system. Alternatively the ability of Zn and low dose Cd to prevent Cd carcinogenesis may be through entirely distinct mechanisms. Further research is required to resolve this question.

REFERENCES

Baars AJ and Breimer DD (1983): Determination of glutathione in biological material by high pressure liquid chromatography. *Pharm. Weekbl. [Sci.]* 5: 145.

Bako G, Smith ESO, Hanson J, and Dewar R (1982): The geographical distribution of high cadmium concentrations in the environment and prostate cancer in Alberta. *Can. J. Public Health* 73: 92.

Bhave MR, Wilson MJ, and Waalkes MP (1988): Methylation status and organization of the metallothionein-I gene in livers and testes of strains of mice resistant and susceptible to cadmium. *Toxicology* 50: 231.

Blakley BR (1986): The effect of cadmium- and viral-induced tumor production in mice. *J. Appl. Toxicol.* 6: 425.

Bradford MM (1976): A rapid and sensitive method for the quantitation of microgram quantities of protein utilizing the principle of protein-dye binding. *Anal. Biochem.* 72: 248.

Ciccarelli RB and Wetterhahn KE (1984): Nickel-bound chromatin, nucleic acids, and nuclear proteins from kidney and liver of rats treated with nickel carbonate *in vivo. Cancer Res.* 44: 3892.

Compere SJ and Palmiter RD (1981): DNA methylation controls the inducibility of the mouse metallothionein-I gene in lymphoid cells. *Cell* 25: 233.

Deagen JT and Whanger PD (1985): Properties of cadmium-binding proteins in rat testes: characteristics unlike metallothionein. *Biochem. J.* 231: 279.

Glanville N, Durnam DM, and Palmiter RD (1981): Structure of mouse metallothionein-I gene and its mRNA. *Nature* 292: 267.

Goering PL and Klaassen CD (1984): Zinc-induced tolerance to cadmium hepatotoxicity. *Toxicol. Appl. Pharmacol.* 74: 299.

Gunn SA, Gould TC, and Anderson WAD (1963): Cadmium-induced interstitial cell tumors in rats and mice and their prevention by zinc. *J.N.C.I.* 31: 745.

Gunn SA, Gould TC, and Anderson WAD (1964): Effects of zinc on cancerogenesis by cadmium. *Proc. Soc. Exp. Biol. Med.* 115: 653.

Gunn SA, Gould TC, and Anderson WAD (1967): Specific response of mesenchymal tissue to cancerigenesis by cadmium. *Arch. Pathol. Lab. Med.* 83: 493.

Gunn SA, Gould TC, and Anderson WAD (1968): Failure of ^{109}Cd to traverse spermatogenic pathway. *J. Reprod. Fertil.* 16: 125.

Kipling MD and Waterhouse JAH (1967): Cadmium and prostatic carcinoma. *Lancet* 1: 730.

Klauser S, Kagi JHR, and Wilson KJ (1983): Characterization of isoprotein patterns in tissue extracts and isolated samples of metallothionein by reverse-phase high-pressure liquid chromatography. *Biochem. J.* 209: 71.

Koizumi T and Waalkes MP (1989a): Effects of zinc on the distribution and toxicity of cadmium in isolated interstitial cells in the rat testes. *Toxicology* 56: 137.

Koizumi T and Waalkes MP (1989b): Interactions of cadmium with rat testicular interstitial cell nuclei: alterations induced by zinc pretreatment and cadmium binding proteins. *Toxicology In Vitro* 3: 215.

Koizumi T and Waalkes MP (1990): Effects of zinc on the binding of cadmium to DNA: assessment with testicular interstitial cell and calf thymus DNAs. *Toxicology In Vitro.* In press.

Onosaka S, Tanaka K, Doi M, and Okahara K (1978): A simplified procedure for determination of metallothionein in animal tissues. *Eisei Kagaku* 24: 128.

Onosaka S and Cherian MG (1981): The induced synthesis of metallothionein in various tissues of rat in response to metals. I. Effect of repeated injection of cadmium salts. *Toxicology* 22: 91.

Onosaka S and Cherian MG (1982): The induced synthesis of metallothionein in various tissues of rat in response to metals. II. Influence of zinc status and specific effect on pancreatic metallothionein. *Toxicology* 23: 11.

Potts CL (1965): Cadmium proteinuria—the health of battery workers exposed to cadmium oxide dust. *Ann. Occup. Hyg.* 8: 55.

Singhal RK, Anderson ME, and Meister A (1987): Glutathione, a first line of defense against cadmium toxicity. *FASEB J.* 1: 220.

Sobocinski PZ, Canterbury WJ, Mapes CA, and Dinterman RE (1978): Involvement of hepatic metallothionein in hypozincemia associated with bacterial infection. *Am. J. Physiol.* 234: E399.

Southern EM (1975): Detection of specific sequences among DNA fragments separated by gel electrophoresis. *J. Mol. Biol.* 118: 503.

Stuart GW, Searle PF, Chen HY, Brinster RL, and Palmiter RD (1984): A 12-base-pair DNA motif that is repeated several times in metallothionein gene promoters confers metal regulations to a heterologous gene. *Proc. Natl. Acad. Sci. U.S.A.* 81: 7318.

Suzuki CA and Cherian MG (1989): Renal glutathione depletion and nephrotoxicity of cadmium-metallothionein in rats. *Toxicol. Appl. Pharmacol.* 98: 544.

Takenaka S, Oldiges H, König H, Hochrainer D, and Oberdörster G (1983): Carcinogenicity of cadmium chloride aerosols in Wistar rats. *J.N.C.I.* 70: 367.

Waalkes MP, Chernoff SB, and Klaassen CD (1984): Cadmium-binding proteins of rat testes: characterization of a low molecular mass protein which lacks identity with metallothionein. *Biochem. J.* 220: 811.

Waalkes MP and Klaassen CD (1985): Concentration of metallothionein in major organs of rats after administration of various metals. *Fundam. Appl. Toxicol.* 5: 473.

Waalkes MP and Poirier LA (1985): Interactions of cadmium with interstitial tissue of the rat testes: uptake of cadmium by isolated interstitial cells. *Biochem. Pharmacol.* 34: 2513.

Waalkes MP and Perantoni A (1986): Isolation of a novel metal-binding protein from rat testes: characterization and distinction from metallothionein. *J. Biol. Chem.* 261: 13097.

Waalkes MP and Perantoni A (1988): *In vitro* assessment of target cell specificity in cadmium carcinogenesis: interactions of cadmium and zinc with isolated interstitial cells of the rat testes. *In Vitro Cell Dev. Biol.* 24: 558.

Waalkes MP, Rehm S, Riggs CW, Bare RM, Devor DE, Poirier LA, Wenk ML, Henneman JR, and Balaschak MS (1988a): Cadmium carcinogenesis in the male Wistar [Crl:(WI)BR)] rat: Dose-response analysis of tumor induction in the prostate, the testes and at the injection site. *Cancer Res.* 48: 4656.

Waalkes MP, Perantoni A, Bhave MR, and Rehm S (1988b): Strain dependence in mice of resistance and susceptibility to the testicular effects of cadmium: assessment of the role of testicular cadmium-binding proteins. *Toxicol. Appl. Pharmacol.* 93: 47.

Waalkes MP and Perantoni A (1989): Apparent deficiency of metallothionein in the Wistar rat prostate. *Toxicol. Appl. Pharmacol.* 101: 83.

Waalkes MP, Rehm S, Riggs CW, Bare RM, Devor DE, Poirier LA, Wenk ML, and Henneman JR (1989): Cadmium carcinogenesis in Wistar [Crl:(WI)BR] rats: Dose-response effects of zinc on tumor induction in the prostate, in the testes, and at the injection site. *Cancer Res.* 49: 4282.

Waalkes MP, Konishi N, Rehm S, Bare RM, and Ward JM (1990): Carcinogenic effects of repeated injections of cadmium in Wistar and Fischer rats. *The Toxicologist.* 10: 2.

Waalkes MP and Oberdörster G (1990): In *Biological Effects of Heavy Metals, Vol. II, Mechanisms of Metal Carcinogenesis.* Foulkes EC, Ed., CRC Press, Boca Raton, pp. 129–158.

Waalkes MP and Rehm S (1990): Effects of dietary zinc deficiency on cadmium carcinogenesis in rats. *Proc. Am. Assoc. Cancer Res.* 31: 140.

Wahba ZZ and Waalkes MP (1989): Effect of *in vivo* low-dose cadmium pretreatment on the *in vitro* interactions of cadmium with isolated interstitial cells of the rat testes. *The Toxicologist* 9: 131.

Wahba ZZ, Hernandez L, Issaq H, and Waalkes MP (1990): Involvement of sulf-hydryl metabolism in tolerance to cadmium in testicular interstitial cells. *The Toxicologist.* 10: 159.

Webb M, Ed., In *The Chemistry, Biochemistry and Biology of Cadmium,* Elsevier/ North-Holland, Amsterdam, 1979.

Wong KL, Cachia R, Klaassen CD (1980): Comparison of the toxicity and tissue distribution of cadmium in newborn and adult rats after repeated administration. *Toxicol. Appl. Pharmacol.* 56: 317.

Chapter 12

Absorption of Cadmium-Metallothionein from the Gastrointestinal Tract

N. Sugawara and C. Sugawara
Department of Public Health
Sapporo Medical College
Sapporo, Japan

INTRODUCTION

When Cd is given orally, it normally induces metallothionein (MT) synthesis in the intestine as well as in the liver and kidney. To understand the Cd absorption from the gastrointestine, the role of MT cannot be excluded. Previous reports (Foulkes and McMullen, 1986; Sugawara and Sugawara, 1987) showed that Cd-MT is directly related to the mucosal uptake of Cd absorbed from the intestine, but is inversely related to its transfer to the blood circulation. It is of interest that Cd-MT itself hardly crosses through the basolateral membrane (Foulkes and McMullen, 1986). In the blood, almost all of Cd is associated with albumin.

If exogenous Cd-MT exists in the duodenum lumen, the protein is absorbed in a different manner from other Cd salts (Cherian et al., 1978). However, its mechanism is still under discussion. We have studied absorption of exogenous Cd-MT from the intestine of the mouse *in vivo*. This may provide a better understanding of the physiological role of MT in Cd absorption.

RESULTS AND DISCUSSION

Absorption of ^{109}Cd-MT and ^{109}CdCl$_2$ from the Intestine

Cadmium chloride or Cd-MT [MT(II) isolated from rat liver] was given orally to the upper part of duodenum of mice. Mice were sacrificed 30 min and 2 h after the oral intubation. The sum radioactivity in the liver and kidney was markedly lower in the MT group than in the CdCl$_2$ group at 30 min and 2 h (Table I). The ratio of deposited-^{109}Cd in the liver to deposited-^{109}Cd in the liver and kidney was decreased in the MT group. These ratios show that there was a difference of metabolism in the two compounds (Tanaka et al., 1975). The absorption of the two compounds was estimated from the deposited-^{109}Cd in the liver and kidney. MT-bound Cd was absorbed more poorly than Cd as CdCl$_2$ (Table I).

Table II shows the ^{109}Cd uptake of the two compounds *in vivo,* and the excretion of ^{109}Cd into the urine. The experiment was carried out under the same conditions in Table I. A 20-cm length of small intestine was removed from the pylorus. In comparison with Cd in CdCl$_2$, the uptake of MT-bound Cd decreased significantly at 30 min and 2 h. Consequently, the poor absorption of Cd-MT (Table I) is due to the decrease of Cd-MT uptake into the intestine (Table II).

Cherian and Shaikh (1975) demonstrated that Cd-MT given i.v. was excreted rapidly to the urine. However, the observation has not been previously found in the case of the MT-bound Cd given orally. Table II indicates that even when MT was given perorally, it was excreted rapidly into the urine. It is not likely that the rapid excretion is due to the acute renal dysfunction, because of the small dose of Cd administered. The metabolism of Cd may therefore be different between the two Cd compounds.

When the total excretion of ^{109}Cd into the urine for 30 min was calculated, it was estimated to be roughly between 100 to 200 cpm. The rough estimation is clearly less than the difference of about 1,400 cpm between the CdCl$_2$ (2,600 cpm in the liver and kidney) and MT (1,200 cpm in the liver and kidney) group. The result therefore confirms that MT-bound Cd was absorbed less than Cd in CdCl$_2$.

Cd Absorption from the Intestinal Tract Pretreated with Zn

To identify the form of Cd passing through the brush border membrane (BBM), we studied the effect of pretreatment with Zn. 50 μg Cd as CdCl$_2$ was given orally to mice pretreated with Zn (900 μg) or only deionized water. In the pretreated-group, the uptake of Cd into the intestine and intestinal MT concentration were increased significantly (Table III). However,

TABLE I. Deposition of ^{109}Cd in the Liver and Kidney

		Liver (cpm/organ)	Kidney (cpm/organs)	Liver and Kidney (cpm/organs)	Absorption (%)	Ratio
CdCl$_2$	30 min (5)	2420 ± 660**	220 ± 50	2640 ± 710*	0.12 ± 0.03**	0.91 ± 0.0**
	2 h (3)	4400 ± 2820	530 ± 260*	4950 ± 3070	0.23 ± 0.14	0.87 ± 0.0**
MT	30 min (5)	900 ± 530	280 ± 70	1190 ± 530	0.05 ± 0.02	0.71 ± 0.1
	2 h (5)	1710 ± 450	1290 ± 360	3000 ± 530	0.13 ± 0.02	0.56 ± 0.0

CdCl$_2$ or ^{109}Cd-Mt (5.7 μg Cd with 2.25 μCi/mouse) was given with a capillary tube to the upper part of the duodenum of mice (ICR male, 6-week-old). Mice were sacrificed 30 min and 2 h after the dosing. Data are expressed as mean ± S.D. Ratio is expressed as hepatic ^{109}Cd/hepatic and renal ^{109}Cd. Absorption was estimated by the deposited ^{109}Cd in the liver and kidney. The significance of the difference between the groups was calculated by Student's t-test (*p <0.05, **p <0.01).

TABLE II.
^{109}Cd Activity in Intestine and Urine

		Intestine ($100 \times$ cpm/g tissue)	Urine (cpm/Cr)
CdCl$_2$	30 min	$351 \pm 175^*$ (5)	— (0)
	2 h	$241 \pm 98^*$ (4)	60 ± 120 (2)
MT	30 min	104 ± 77 (5)	310 ± 10 (4)
	2 h	62 ± 38 (5)	460 ± 200 (5)

The experimental procedures are as for in Table I. Urine was collected from the bladder with a capillary. Data are expressed as mean $\pm$ S.D. Creatinine (Cr) concentration was determined by the method of Jaffé, using a commercially available kit (Wako Pure Chemical Industries, Ltd., Osaka, Japan). $^*p < 0.05$.

TABLE III.
CdCl$_2$ Absorption from the Intestine of Mouse Pretreated with Zn

	Intestinal Uptake (Cd μg/g tissue)	Intestinal MT (Cd μg/mg protein)	Absorption (%)	Ratio
Water CdCl$_2$ (6)	3.1 ± 0.7	0.07 ± 0.01	2.3 ± 1.1	0.8 ± 0.0
Zn CdCl$_2$ (6)	$6.5 \pm 3.1^*$	$0.18 \pm 0.04^{**}$	1.6 ± 0.6	0.8 ± 0.0

Mice (male ICR, 6-week-old) were given orally Zn (900 μg/mouse) as ZnSO$_4$ or deionized water (control). One hour later, Cd (50 μg/mouse) was given orally. Mice were killed 6 h after the Cd dosing. Cd was measured with flame or flameless AAS. MT was determined by the modified method of Cd/hemoglobin affinity (Sugawara and Sugawara, 1987). The absorption was estimated by the deposited Cd in the liver and kidney. Ratio is expressed as the hepatic Cd/hepatic and renal Cd. Data are expressed as means $\pm$ S.D. $^*p < 0.05$, $^{**}p < 0.01$.

Cd absorption decreased considerably (Table III). The ratio of hepatic Cd/ hepatic and renal Cd was the same in both groups.

When Cd-MT instead of CdCl$_2$ was introduced into the same experimental system, the intestinal ^{109}Cd uptake and MT concentration were not increased by Zn pretreatment (Table IV). Interestingly, the absorption of ^{109}Cd-MT was increased by the pretreatment with Zn. The results in these two tables (Tables III and IV) suggest that lumenal Cd-MT (given perorally) was internalized in the cells in the form which cannot bind to the preinduced MT.

Mode of Cd-MT Uptake into the Mucosa

When CdCl$_2$ is given orally, Cd ($+2$) may cross cell membranes by the following mechanism: (1) a non-specific binding step to the outside of the membrane; (2) an internalization process to carry the Cd through the membrane (Foulkes, 1988). However, the mode of MT entry into the mucosa cells is still being debated. Pinocytosis is one possible mechanism. Pinocytosis is only active in suckling animals (Keller and Doherty, 1980). We therefore focused on MT uptake by a receptor mediated endocytosis. Monodancyl cadaverine (MDC) is known to be an inhibitor of endocytosis. As shown in Table V, the drug did not inhibit the uptake of Cd-MT or deposition of Cd in the liver and kidney. The endocytosis may therefore not be related to the Cd-MT absorption from the gastrointestine. Mugitani et al. (1987) reported that transferrin was internalized through the transferrin receptor mediated system. Furthermore, they suggested that ferric and ferrous form of Fe salts also utilized the system. Further study needs to clarify the internalization of lumenal Cd compounds.

TABLE IV.
^{109}Cd-MT Absorption from the Intestine of Mouse Pretreated with Zn

	Intestinal Uptake (cpm/mg tissue)	Intestinal MT (cpm/mg protein)	Absorption (%)	Ratio
Water ^{109}Cd-MT (6)	170 ± 110	1500 ± 1100	0.57 ± 0.3	0.6 ± 0.1
Zn ^{109}Cd-MT (6)	190 ± 100	2300 ± 1100	1.35 ± 0.9	0.7 ± 0.0

Zn (900 µg/mouse) or deionized water was given orally to mice (male ICR, 6-week-old). One hour later, Cd-MT (13.7 µg Cd with 2 µCi/mouse) was given orally. They were killed 6 h after the Cd dosing. Intestinal MT is expressed as ^{109}Cd activity in the supernatant heated at 85°C for 5 min. Absorption was estimated by the deposited-^{109}Cd in the liver and kidney. Ratio is expressed as hepatic ^{109}Cd/hepatic and renal ^{109}Cd. Data are expressed as mean ± S.D.

TABLE V.
Effect of Cadaverine on ^{109}Cd-MT Absorption

MDC (µmol)	Intestine (100 × cpm/g tissue)	Liver and Kidney (100 × cpm/organs)	Absorption (%)
0 (4)	76 ± 55	92 ± 30	0.32 ± 0.1
0.5 (5)	75 ± 70	101 ± 61	0.35 ± 0.2

MDC (monodancylcadaverine) was given orally 30 min before the oral intubation of ^{109}Cd-MT (12 µg Cd with 2.5 µCi/mouse). Mice (ICR male, 6-week-old) were killed 6 h after the MT intubation. Absorption was estimated by the deposited-^{109}Cd in the liver and kidney. Data are expressed as mean ± S.D.

CONCLUSION

When Cd-MT entered into the intestinal lumen, its absorption was clearly less than that of $CdCl_2$. This decrease may be due to the reduction of MT uptake into the intestinal mucosa. Although MT crossed through the membrane in the metalloprotein form, our experiment did not support the hypothesis that it is moved by endocytosis. An intracellular MT originating from lumenal MT may transfer through the basolateral membrane in an intact form. This hypothesis was also supported by the rapid excretion of [109]Cd into the urine.

REFERENCES

Cherian MG and Shaikh ZA (1975): Metabolism of intravenously injected cadmium-binding protein. *Biochem. Biophys. Res. Commun.* 65: 863–869.

Cherian MG, Goyer RA, and Valberg LS (1978): Gastrointestinal absorption and organ distribution of oral cadmium chloride and cadmium-metallothionein in mice. *J. Toxicol. Environ. Health* 4: 861–868.

Foulkes EC and McMullen DM (1986): Endogenous metallothionein as a determinant of intestinal cadmium absorption: a reevaluation. *Toxicology* 38: 285–291.

Foulkes EC (1988): On the mechanism of transfer of heavy metals across cell membranes. *Toxicology* 52: 263–272.

Keller CA and Doherty RA (1980): Correlation between lead retention and intestinal pinocytosis in the suckling mouse. *Am. J. Physiol.* 239: G1114–G112.

Mugitani K, Hisayasu S, and Yoshino Y (1987): Detection of transferrin in digestive juices and its possible role in iron absorption in rats (in Japanese). *Diges. Absorp.* 10: 68–71.

Sugawara N and Sugawara C (1987): Role of mucosal metallothionein preinduced by oral Cd or Zn on the intestinal absorption of a subsequent Cd dose. *Bull. Environ. Contam. Toxicol.* 38: 295–299.

Tanaka K, Sueda K, Onosaka S, and Okahara K (1975): Fate of 109Cd-labeled metallothionein in rats. *Toxicol. Appl. Pharmacol.* 33: 258–266.

Chapter

13

Role of Metallothionein in Epithelial Transport and Sequestration of Cadmium

E.C. Foulkes
Departments of Environmental Health
and Physiology/Biophysics
University of Cincinnati
College of Medicine
Cincinnati, Ohio

ABSTRACT

The likely contribution of MT to transport of Cd from liver to kidney and to renal Cd uptake is well supported by results from many laboratories and is further characterized in the present paper. Much of the available information is based on results obtained with exogenous CdMT and this protein may not behave exactly as does endogenous MT. The additional suggestion that endogenous MT traps Cd in epithelial cells and thus reduces transepithelial passage of the metal is also reviewed, both in the light of newer results on Cd absorption in the intestine, and by a comparison of Zn and Cd fluxes into and out of the rabbit kidney *in vivo*. Cd is taken up by the kidney as CdMT from the lumen, and as Cd or certain low-molecular weight complexes both from lumen and blood; this Cd does not return to blood at a significant rate. In contrast, Zn taken up from blood or urine can be recovered in the renal vein within 2 to 3 min of uptake. In the rat jejunum *in vivo*, Cd absorption follows a transcellular pathway, and this process is specifically reduced by endogenous MT. As a result, only small amounts of Cd appear in portal venous blood within 20 min of the metal being placed into the intestinal lumen, unless endogenous MT becomes saturated; Ni and Zn, in contrast, normally reach blood after a time delay of only a few minutes. The concept that Cd trapped in this manner by endogenous MT is toxicologically inert, even though supported by considerable evidence, does not fully explain the toxicokinetics of the metal.

INTRODUCTION

Among the various biological functions proposed for metallothionein (MT), a role in cadmium transport has found considerable experimental support. Soon after the discovery of the protein, Piscator (1964) suggested that Cd is released from the liver as CdMT, and in this form is carried to the kidney where it accumulates. Direct evidence for renal uptake of CdMT was furnished by Vostal and Cherian (1974) and subsequently by Nomiyama and Foulkes (1977). The attractive hypothesis of the mediation of Cd movement from liver to kidney by MT has been repeatedly reviewed (see, for instance, Foulkes, 1974). It is strengthened by the confirmation of the ready renal uptake of circulating CdMT (Foulkes, 1978), and by repeated observation of the release of CdMT from the damaged liver with consequent accumulation in the kidney (see e.g. Cain and Griffiths, 1980). Other and more recent experiments bearing on the uptake of CdMT by epithelial cells are reviewed in the present paper. An important and unresolved question here is whether injected CdMT adequately mimics the behavior of endogenous MT circulating in plasma.

In addition to the proposed involvement of extracellular MT in Cd transport across epithelial cell membranes, it has also been suggested that endogenous MT may be important in sequestering and thus trapping heavy metals in epithelial cells (Richards and Cousins, 1975); indeed, the long biological half life of Cd in renal cortex may well be related to such a reaction. Cadmium sequestered as CdMT is generally considered to be toxicologically relatively inert (Nomiyama and Nomiyama, 1982). However, even though considerable evidence supports the trapping function of MT, inactivation of Cd as CdMT cannot fully explain the toxicokinetics of the metal following its acute or subchronic administration. These problems were also further explored in the present work.

METHODS

Unpublished experiments reported in this paper were carried out with male New Zealand white rabbits as described elsewhere (Foulkes and Blanck, 1990a). In short, the animals (average weight 2.6 kg) were anesthetized with pentobarbital sodium (Nembutal) and catheters inserted as required; renal venous blood after arterial bolus injections was continuously collected through an indwelling catheter connected to a withdrawal pump. The bolus could be trapped in the kidney, as previously described, by transiently occluding the aorta (Foulkes and Blanck, 1990b). During the resulting prolonged artery-to-vein transit time, barrier-limited solute uptake from blood into tubular epithelium can thus more closely approach completion than is possible during free flow. Transient anoxia during a 40 s occlusion does not interfere with continued capacity of the kidney normally to transport PAH and amino acids (Foulkes and Blanck, 1990a,b).

RESULTS AND DISCUSSION

Renal Uptake of CdMT

Filtration and reabsorption of CdMT in the kidney forms the basis of its suggested role in Cd transport from liver to kidney (Piscator, 1964). The apical membranes of the proximal tubule readily reabsorb filtered CdMT, a process mediated by a mechanism specific for anionic proteins (Foulkes, 1978). No appreciable fraction of the Cd filtered and reabsorbed as exogenous CdMT reappeared in renal venous blood during the first 4 min after injection and filtration (Foulkes, 1982).

Non-filtering (stop-flow) kidneys, unlike normal kidneys, accumulate little Cd following intra-arterial injection of CdMT (Foulkes, 1978). This finding suggests that basolateral cell membranes, in contrast to the brush-border, do not react with CdMT. To test the possibility that non-filtered CdMT might be extracted from blood, but only at a slow rate, advantage was taken of a recently developed technique in which an aortic bolus is trapped in the kidney (Foulkes and Blanck, 1990b) by transiently interrupting the circulation with a balloon catheter in the aorta. The resultant prolonged contact time between injected solute and basolateral membranes permits relatively slow (barrier-limited) uptake processes to approach steady state.

Application of this technique for the study of barrier-limited basolateral solute uptake may be illustrated as in Figure 1 for the renal extraction of non-filtered Cd in the rabbit kidney in presence of mercaptoethanol (ME). Under control conditions (on the left), no removal of Cd from venous blood was observed; recovery of Cd was here compared to that of 3H-methoxy-inulin which served as extracellular marker. Actually, more Cd was recovered in this experiment than inulin, due presumably to a small amount of protein binding. In some other similar experiments (Foulkes and Blanck, 1990a), a small uptake of Cd occurred under these conditions. It is clear

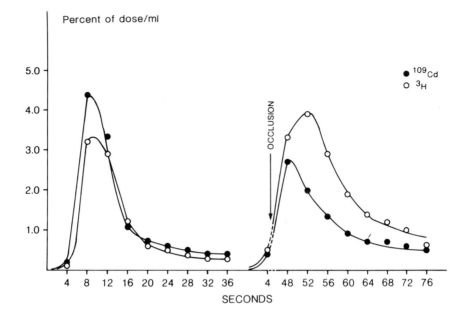

Figure 1. Diffusion-limitation of renal uptake of non-filtered Cd in presence of ME. (From EC Foulkes [1987], *Biol. Trace Elem. Res.* 21: 195–200. With permission)

that the short contact time between CdME and basolateral cell membranes during a single non-restricted passage through the kidney, of the order of only a few seconds (Foulkes, 1974), does not permit extensive extraction of Cd.

In contrast, when a second Cd bolus was injected into the same animal, and the bolus was allowed to remain in contact with the basolateral cell membranes during a 40 s occlusion of the aorta, fractional uptake of Cd increased greatly (Figure 1, right). The fact that this uptake could be inhibited by Zn (Foulkes and Blanck, 1990a) indicates that Cd did not move across the cell membrane by diffusion of the lipid-soluble CdME complex, whose uptake should not be affected by other metals. Presumably the CdME complex dissociates in competition with the high affinity binding sites on the basolateral cell membrane; it is the binding to such sites which is known to be sensitive to inhibition by Zn and other metals, at least in jejunal epithelium (Foulkes, 1989). None of the Cd accumulated during the transient occlusion could subsequently be extracted from the kidney with EDTA, so that the Cd cleared from postglomerular blood appears to become internalized. Internalized Cd is here operationally distinguished from Cd externally bound to cell membranes by the fact that EDTA does not readily penetrate cells and thus does not rapidly remove cellular Cd (Foulkes, 1988).

The requirement for low-molecular weight thiol compounds in such studies arises from the need to prevent sequestration of the metal by high-molecular weight plasma protein (Foulkes, 1974). When basolateral Cd uptake by kidney cortex slices was measured in protein-free Ringer solution, ME actually depressed Cd uptake (unpublished results). This finding further supports the conclusion that under conditions illustrated in Figure 1 it is not the Cd-thiol complex which is taken up. In contrast, when Cd is tightly bound in a lipid-soluble complex as for instance with diethyldithiocarbamate, its renal uptake is as rapid and flow-dependent as that of paraaminohippurate (Foulkes and Blanck, 1990a). In the form of Cd-EDTA, a tight and water-soluble complex, Cd remains restricted to the extracellular fluid (Foulkes, 1974).

In the absence of a specific mechanism for transport of anionic protein such as is involved in reabsorption of filtered CdMT from tubular urine, it may be predicted on the basis of these results that non-filtered Cd circulating as CdMT, a water-soluble and very stable complex, will not react with basolateral membranes. In accord with this prediction, a previous report described the finding that the artery-to-vein transit of CdMT across a normal kidney closely resembles that of inulin (Foulkes, 1978). As further shown in Figure 2, no appreciable fraction of non-filtered CdMT is retained by the

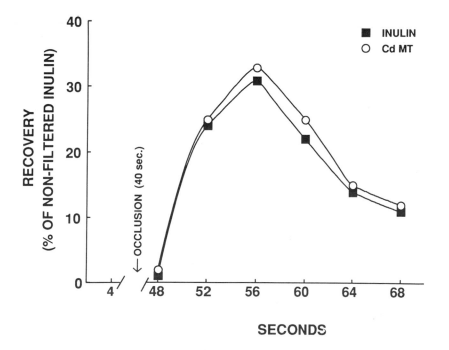

Figure 2. Absence of renal uptake of nonfiltered CdMT during aortic occlusion.

kidney, even during 40 s aortic occlusion: in contrast to CdME (see Figure 1), venous recovery of CdMT after such occlusion is still very similar to that of inulin. It is this finding which led to the conclusion cited above that basolateral cell membranes of tubular epithelium, unlike apical membranes, do not react with CdMT. Basolateral Cd uptake may nevertheless be toxicologically significant to the extent that plasma Cd circulates as complexes other than CdMT, especially after acute Cd exposure.

It is important to emphasize that, as in the studies just cited, much of what is known about CdMT transport and distribution is based on experiments with exogenous CdMT. The implicit assumption is therefore made that injected CdMT is identical with that circulating in plasma. There are some discordant observations, however, which may bring this assumption into question. Thus, Nomiyama and Foulkes (1977) reported that the (rabbit) kidney effectively reabsorbs filtered radioactive CdMT, so that none of the filtered load is excreted in the urine of normal animals below plasma levels of approximately 0.5 nmol Cd as CdMT/ml plasma. In contrast, immunologically identified endogenous MT is excreted in the urine of normal rats at plasma levels as low as 0.0005 nmol/ml (Sato et al., 1989). Shaikh and Tohyama (1984) had previously observed the excretion of immunologically characterized MT in humans. Unless urinary MT were assumed to be all derived from the kidney, its ready excretion at low plasma levels would not have been predicted on the results of Nomiyama and Foulkes (1977). Care clearly needs to be taken in extrapolating the results obtained with exogenous MT to the behavior of low concentrations of endogenous compounds. It is not known whether this problem refers to differences in the metal composition of exogenous and endogenous MT, or whether other differences exist between the two classes of molecules.

Apical Uptake of CdMT in Intestine

Cherian (1979) described the occurrence of transepithelial transport of CdMT, or at least of some of its partial breakdown products, from the lumen of the mouse intestine into the kidney. In the rat, the rate of apical CdMT uptake by intestinal epithelium is no faster than that of $CdCl_2$ (Foulkes and McMullen, 1986). There is thus no evidence to suggest that apical MT transport mechanisms similar to those described in the renal tubule are active in the intestine. A specific role of extracellular MT in mediating intestinal absorption of heavy metals thus seems unlikely.

Trapping Function of Intracellular MT in the Intestine

Such a function was suggested by Richards and Cousins (1975) in relation to control of Zn absorption in the rat, and discussed specifically for

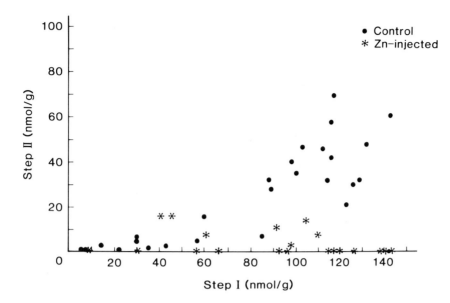

Figure 3. Effect of Zn pretreatment on mucosal trapping of Cd in rat jejunum. (From EC Foulkes and DM McMullen, [1986], *Toxicology* 38: 285–291. With permission.)

Cd by Squibb et al. (1976). Evidence for trapping of Cd by endogenous MT has been described in rat jejunum perfused *in situ* (Foulkes and McMullen). Figure 3 illustrates the finding that, as uptake of Cd from the lumen (step 1 of Cd absorption) is increased by raising the Cd concentration in the perfusate, the basolateral extrusion of the metal from the mucosa (step 2) remains low in control animals until the cumulative load transferred by step 1 reaches values of 60 to 80 nmol/g. At that stage, the capacity of cells to retain Cd is exceeded, and step 2 begins to rise steeply and proportionately to further increases in step 1. In contrast, animals pretreated with Zn in order specifically to increase their mucosal MT content can retain all Cd taken up to values of step 1 as high as 140 nmol/g; it is worth emphasizing that the Zn treatment in these experiments stimulated protein synthesis only in the MT fraction. Under the conditions where retention of Cd is increased, that of Ni, a metal with low affinity for MT, remains at control levels. Further evidence in support of the suggestion by Squibb et al. (1976) that endogenous MT may sequester significant amounts of Cd taken up from the lumen was presented by Goon and Klaassen (1989) with an elegant perfusion technique *in vivo,* and more indirectly by Ohta et al. (1989) *in vitro* using everted sacs of small intestine.

In a different study, in which the kinetics of metal transport from in testinal lumen into the portal vein were analyzed in the intact rat (Foulkes and McMullen, 1987), the time required for different metals (Ni, Zn and

TABLE I.
Transepithelial Transit
Time (TET) of Heavy Metals
in Rat Jejunum

Metal	n	TET (min)	EC_{50} (μM)
Ni	10	5 ± 2	473
Zn	8	9 ± 2	8
Cd	3	>20	1

TET measures the time required for transcellular transfer of the metal from lumen into
the portal vein. EC_{50} is the concentration of
the metal required to displace 50% of ^{65}Zn
from MT (Waalkes et al., 1984). (Modified
from Foulkes and McMullen, 1987.)

Cd) to cross the epithelial barrier from lumen into the portal vein was found
to vary inversely with their affinity for MT. This is illustrated in Table I,
and provides additional support for the trapping role of MT in the intestinal
mucosa.

Trapping Function of MT in the Renal Tubule

The remarkably long biological half life of Cd in the kidney is commonly attributed to its binding as CdMT. Given the fact that Zn is bound
to MT much less tightly than is Cd, such an interpretation leads to the
prediction that Zn taken up by the kidney should return to blood much faster
than Cd. This prediction was tested in the series of experiments shown in
Table II (Foulkes and Blanck, 1990a). A bolus containing per kg body
weight 1 to 15 μmol of labeled $ZnCl_2$ or $CdCl_2$ (^{65}Zn, ^{109}Cd), in addition
to inulin as glomerular marker and 300 μmol mercaptoethanol, was injected
into the aorta. Four seconds later, circulation was transiently interrupted, as
described above, to trap the bolus in the kidney and permit uptake of the
metal to proceed. Given the high fractional reabsorption of filtered metals
($>90\%$) under these conditions (Foulkes, 1974), and assuming an average
filtration fraction of 0.2, apical uptake is calculated as approximately 20%
of the renal load; total uptake therefore equalled 20% plus the fraction
directly removed from the peritubular circulation. Essentially none of that
Cd returned to venous blood over a period of almost 3 min from the end
of occlusion. In contrast, the major portion of Zn which had been taken up
during occlusion could subsequently be recovered in renal venous blood
during that same time period.

Results like those in Table II confirm the well-documented fact that the
renal cortex effectively retains Cd, and are fully compatible with the hypothesis that CdMT is involved in this process. Attempts were made to

obtain more direct support for this likely role of endogenous CdMT by measuring Cd retention after the kidneys had been induced to synthesize MT by prior treatment with Zn, as described above for the intestinal mucosa. However, even in control animals the renal cortex contains sufficient endogenous Cd-binding compounds to retain most of the Cd taken up following injection of as much as 15 μmol/kg in presence of ME (see Table II); no further stimulation of Cd retention could therefore be demonstrated following Zn pretreatment. Of course, Zn administration is well known to increase the ability of the kidney to accumulate Cd over longer time periods than studied here (Webb, 1986). In any case, the results described here, contrasting the instantaneous trapping of Cd with the rapid release of freshly accumulated Zn, are fully compatible with a role of MT in the renal trapping of Cd.

Role of Endogenous MT as Modulator of Cytotoxic Actions of Cd

It has repeatedly been suggested that intrarenal Cd bound to endogenous MT is toxicologically inert (see, for instance, Nomiyama and Nomiyama, 1982). Such compartmentation can, however, not explain the initiation period before overt malfunction appears following acute loading of the renal cortex with Cd, as described in rats (Maitani et al., 1986) and rabbits (Foulkes and Blanck, 1990a). Even after more chronic exposure, renal functional

TABLE II. Renal Retention of Cd and Zn

			Percent of Renal Load	
Experiment No.	Dose[a] (μmol/kg)	Basolateral Uptake	Total Uptake[b]	Return to Blood[c]
Cadmium 1	1	16	36	0
2	1	6	26	0
3	12	16	36	0
4	12	8	28	5
5	14	24	44	0
6	15	3	23	6
Zinc 1	2	19	39	14
2	2	20	40	27
3	5	26	46	30
4	12	25	45	44

(Modified from Foulkes and Blanck, 1990a.)

[a]Administered in arterial bolus.
[b]The sum of basolateral uptake, and load reabsorbed from filtrate (average filtration fraction 20%, see text).
[c]Over 3 min from injection.

damage only occurred considerably later than the achievement of maximal steady-state levels of both metallothionein Cd and non-MT Cd in rabbit kidney cortex (Nomiyama and Nomiyama, 1982).

Acute injection of Cd-cysteine into rats did not lead to malfunction for at least 12 hours (Maitani et al., 1986), even though the maximum renal Cd concentration was achieved within 4 h; similarly, between 6 and 16 hours were required in rabbits to cause renal malfunction after administration of CdME (Foulkes and Blanck, 1990a). Obviously, renal MT concentrations in untreated animals are likely to be significantly lower than 12 hours or longer following administration of Cd in doses known to induce synthesis of MT. If malfunction was caused by Cd through direct inhibition of various solute transport systems, then the early effect of the metal should therefore be more pronounced than after a prolonged delay. On the other hand, if one argued that initial binding of Cd to endogenous MT suffices to abolish an early toxic effect, then the initiation delay should be much longer than the observed 6–16 hours, given the relatively long half life of endogenous MT in rabbit kidney cells (Kobayashi et al., 1982).

All these facts suggest (1) that endogenous MT in the kidney under present conditions is not the only factor determining toxicity of a given renal Cd load, and (2) that Cd does not exert its toxic action directly on epithelial solute transport.

CONCLUSIONS

Evidence from many sources has shown that MT may play a variety of essential roles. The findings described here emphasize especially the functions of MT in Cd transport to the kidney, and in the trapping of the metal in renal and intestinal epithelium; there is strong support for both of these functions. However, the concept of endogenous CdMT as a toxicologically relatively inert Cd pool cannot account for the toxicokinetics of Cd after acute or subchronic exposure.

ACKNOWLEDGMENTS

Original work described here was supported by NIH Grants ES-02416, ES-02453 and ES-00159.

REFERENCES

Cain K and Griffiths B (1980): Transfer of liver cadmium to the kidney after aflatoxin induced liver damage. *Biochem. Pharmacol.* 29: 1852–1855.

Cherian MG (1979): Metabolism of orally administered Cd-metallothionein in mice. *Env. Health Perspectives* 28: 127–130.

Foulkes EC (1974): Excretion and retention of Cd, Zn and Hg by the rabbit kidney. *Am. J. Physiol.* 227: 1356–1360.

Foulkes EC (1978): Renal tubular transport of CdMT. *Tox. Appl. Pharmacol.* 45: 505–512.

Foulkes EC (1982): Role of metallothionein in transport of heavy metals. In: *Biological Roles of Metallothionein*. Foulkes EC, Ed., Elsevier/North Holland, Amsterdam, pp. 131–140.

Foulkes EC and McMullen DM (1986): Endogenous metallothionein as determinant of intestinal cadmium absorption: A reevaluation. *Toxicology* 38: 285–291.

Foulkes EC and McMullen DM (1987): Kinetics of transepithelial movement of heavy metals in rat jejunum. *Am. J. Physiol.* 253: G134–G138.

Foulkes EC (1988): On the mechanism of transfer of heavy metals across cell membranes. *Toxicol.* 52: 263–272.

Foulkes EC (1989): On the mechanism of cellular cadmium uptake. *Biol. Trace Elem. Res.* 21: 195–200.

Foulkes EC and Blanck S (1990a): Acute cadmium uptake by rabbit kidneys: mechanisms and effects. *Tox. Appl. Pharmacol.* 102: 464–473.

Foulkes EC and Blanck S (1990b): Site of uptake of nonfiltered amino acid in the rabbit kidney. *Proc. Soc. Exp. Biol. Med.* 193: 56–59.

Goon G and Klaassen CD (1989): Dosage-dependent absorption of cadmium in the rat intestine measured *in situ*. *Toxicol. Appl. Pharmacol.* 100: 41–50.

Kobayashi S, Imano M, and Kimura M (1982): Turnover of metallothionein in mammalian cells. In: *Biological Roles of Metallothionein,* Foulkes EC, Ed., Elsevier/North Holland, Amsterdam, pp. 305–322.

Maitani T, Watahiki A, and Suzuki KT (1986): Acute renal dysfunction by cadmium injected with cysteine in relation to renal critical concentration of cadmium. *Arch. Toxicol.* 58: 36–140.

Nomiyama K and Foulkes EC (1977): Reabsorption of filtered cadmium metallothionein in the rabbit kidney. *Proc. Soc. Exp. Biol. Med.* 156: 97–99.

Nomiyama K and Nomiyama H (1982): Tissue metallothionein in rabbits chronically exposed to cadmium, with special reference to the critical concentration of cadmium in the renal cortex. In: *Biological Roles of Metallothionein,* Elsevier/North Holland, New York, 1981, pp. 47–67.

Ohta H, DeAngelis MV, and Cherian MG (1989): Uptake of cadmium and metallothionein by rat everted intestinal sacs. *Toxicol. Appl. Pharmacol.* 101: 62–69.

Piscator M (1964): Cadmium in the kidneys of normal human beings and the isolation of metallothionein from liver of rabbits exposed to cadmium. *Nord. Hyg. Tidskr.* 45: 76–82.

Richards MP and Cousins RJ (1975): Mammalian Zn homeostasis: requirement for RNA and metallothionein synthesis. *Biochem. Biophys. Res. Comm.* 64: 1215–1223.

Sato M, Nagai Y, and Bremner I (1989): Urinary excretion of metallothionein-I and its degradation products in rats treated with cadmium, copper, zinc or mercury. *Toxicol.* 56: 23–33.

Shaikh ZA and Tohyama C (1984): Urinary metallothionein as an indicator of cadmium body burden and of cadmium-induced nephrotoxicity. *Environ. Health Perspec.* 54: 171–174.

Squibb KS, Cousins RJ, Silbon BL, and Levin S (1976): Liver and intestinal metallothionein: Function in acute cadmium toxicity. *Exp. Mol. Pathol.* 25: 163–171.

Vostal JJ and Cherian MG (1974): Effects of cadmium metallothionein on the renal tubular transport of sodium. *Fed. Proc.* 33: 519 (abstract).

Waalkes MP, Harvey MJ, and Klaassen CD (1984): Relative *in vitro* affinity of hepatic metallothionein for metals. *Toxicol. Lett.* 20: 33–39.

Webb M (1986): Role of metallothionein in cadmium metabolism. In: Cadmium, Foulkes EC, Ed., *Handbook of Experimental Pharmacology,* 80, Springer-Verlag, Berlin, pp. 281–337.

Chapter 14

Hepatic Calcium Level and Induction of Zinc-Thionein

Tamio Maitani, Yukio Saito, and Kunitoshi Yoshihira
National Institute of Hygienic Sciences
Setagaya, Tokyo, Japan

Kazuo T. Suzuki
National Institute for Environmental Studies
Tsukuba, Ibaraki, Japan

SUMMARY

Hepatic zinc-thionein (Zn-MT) was induced after administration of carrageenan, dextran sulfate, endotoxin, and other toxic compounds. At the same time, the increase of hepatic calcium (Ca) concentration was observed. A good correlation between the increase of hepatic Ca level and the induction of Zn-MT was apparent in several cases. The time-courses of hepatic Ca concentration after administration of the above compounds were quite different from that after Ca loading. The possible mechanisms through which hepatic Zn-MT is induced in our systems are discussed.

INTRODUCTION

Although metallothionein (MT) was first isolated as a cadmium (Cd) and zinc (Zn)-binding protein (Margoshes and Vallee, 1957), MT also plays an important role in Zn homeostasis (Bremner and Davies, 1975). The protein is induced as Zn-thionein (Zn-MT) not only by Zn administration (Suzuki and Yamamura, 1979) but also by a variety of physiological stresses

(Oh et al., 1978) and dexamethasone (Etzel et al., 1979). Since it has been reported that the induction of Zn-MT may be associated with inflammatory reactions (Sobocinski et al., 1978), we have been very interested in the induction of Zn-MT after administration of inflammatory drugs. Inflammatory reactions are fundamental to disease states and could be the key to the elucidation of the role of Zn-MT in the living body.

When our studies on MT were undertaken, a new analytical method for metals, inductively coupled plasma-atomic emission spectroscopy (ICP-AES), had been only recently developed and had become commercially available. With this spectrometer, a simultaneous multi-elemental analysis of samples is possible. Therefore, we started research to investigate the induction of MT and the changes of essential metal levels in organs after administration of inflammatory drugs. In the course of the studies, we found that the increase of hepatic Ca concentration was correlated with the hepatic Zn-MT induction. The details will be described below.

Determination of MT and Analysis of Chemical Forms of Metals

Several analytical methods for MT determination have been reported so far. Those are divided into two categories. One is those which are based on the determination of the metals in MT and the other on the protein. The Cd-hemoglobin method (Onosaka et al., 1978) and radioimmunoassay (Vander Mallie and Garvey, 1978; Tohyama and Shaikh, 1978) are the representatives of the former and the latter, respectively. The HPLC-AAS method, which consists of a combination of a high performance liquid chromatograph (HPLC) equipped with, for example, a gel-filtration column (G3000SW, Tosoh) and an atomic absorption spectrometer (AAS), is a method in the former category and has been used for MT determination in this study and is especially practical, because isometallothioneins can be detected separately when the column is eluted with a slightly alkaline buffer (Suzuki, 1980). Zn-MT was determined as Cd-MT because of the higher stability of Cd-MT and the higher sensitivity of Cd by AAS. A representative chromatogram for MT determination is given in Figure 1.

Chemical forms of metals in tissues were analysed by HPLC-ICP, a method analogous but more sophisticated than HPLC-AAS. With our system in NIHS, 20 elements selected out of 45 measurable elements can be monitored simultaneously and continuously. After a measurement is completed, HPLC chromatograms for the respective elements can be monitored on the display of a computer by using a new program developed specifically for the HPLC-ICP method.

Essential metal concentrations in organs were determined with the ICP-AES after wet-digestion with a mixed acid (HNO_3:$HClO_4$, 5:1, v/v).

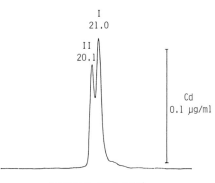

Retention Time (min)

Figure 1. A typical MT determination by HPLC-AAS chromatogram of liver supernatant. Mice were injected intraperitoneally with lambda-carrageenan at a dose of 2.5 mg per animal and killed at 1 day. Livers from each mouse were pooled and homogenized in 3 vol. of buffer solution. The homogenate was centrifuged. Cd solution was added to the supernatant and the excess Cd was removed by heat-treatment and centrifugation. A 100-μl portion of heat-treated supernatant was applied to HPLC-AAS system with a gel-filtration column. The detector level of AAS was set as indicated by a vertical bar. I and II indicate MT-I and -II, respectively.

The Induction of Zn-MT and the Increase of Hepatic Ca Level After Administration of Lambda-Carrageenan

Initially, we studied carrageenan as an inflammatory drug. Carrageenans are a group of sulfated polygalactans extracted from various red seaweeds. They are widely used in foods and cosmetics. As a food additive, it is a GRAS (generally recognized as safe) compound according to the classification of the FDA in the U.S. and is also used widely in Japan as so-called natural (not synthetic) food additive. However, it is also well-known as an inflammatory drug when injected parenterally (Winter et al., 1962).

When lambda-carrageenan was injected intraperitoneally into mice at a dose of 2.5 mg per animal, hepatic Zn concentrations showed a transitory increase with a maximum at 2 days as shown in Figure 2 (Maitani and Suzuki, 1981). The transitory increase of Zn concentration could be ascribed to the induction of Zn-MT.

At the same time, hepatic Ca concentrations also showed a transitory increase with a time-course change similar to that of Zn concentration (Figure 2). In the liver, the influx of extracellular Ca (namely the increase of Ca concentration) is regarded as the final step of the hepatic cell death (El-Mofty et al., 1975; Smith et al., 1981). Therefore, the magnitude of increase in hepatic Ca concentration may suggest the hepatotoxicity of the injected compound.

Essential metal concentrations in the spleen also changed after the administration. Splenic Ca levels increased while iron (Fe) levels decreased with a splenomegaly. The splenomegaly is considered to be closely related in its effects to the immunosuppressive character of carrageenan (Aschheim and Raffel, 1972).

The Induction of Zn-MT and the Changes of Essential Metal Levels After Administration of Three Kinds of Dextran Sulfate with Different Molecular Weights

Dextran sulfate (DS) is a synthetic sulfated polyglucan and bears a structural resemblance to carrageenan (polygalactan). When DS of 500,000 molecular weight (MW) was injected intraperitoneally, Zn-MT was induced and the induced amount showed a linear dose-dependency up to 60 mg/kg body weight (Maitani and Suzuki, 1982a). The increase of hepatic Ca con-

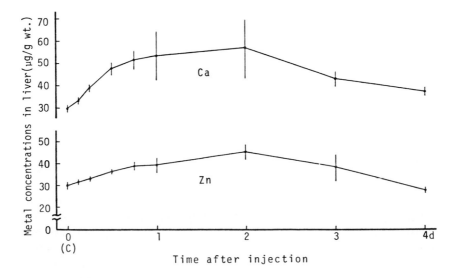

Figure 2. Changes of Ca and Zn concentrations in liver after injection of lambda-carrageenan. The animals were killed after 3, 6, 12, and 18 h, and 1, 2, 3, and 4 d. Vertical bars indicate S.D. of the mean (6 mice per group).

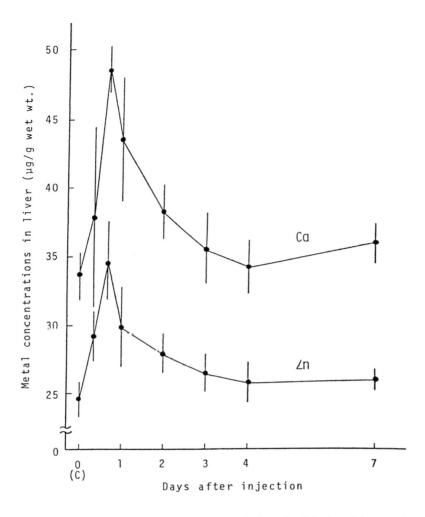

Figure 3. Changes of Ca and Zn concentrations in liver after injection of dextran sulfate. Mice were injected intraperitoneally with DS at a dose of 40 mg/kg body weight. The animals were killed after 8 and 16 h, and 1, 2, 3, 4, and 7 d. Vertical bars indicate S.D. of the mean (6 mice per group).

centration was also observed in the DS treatment. Time-courses of hepatic Zn and Ca concentrations were followed at a dose of 40 mg/kg body weight. Similar time-courses of Zn and Ca were observed as shown in Figure 3. The splenomegaly with the increase of Ca and the decrease of Fe concentration was also observed (Figure 4). Thus, the injection of DS of 500,000 MW effectively induced hepatic Zn-MT. In the subcellular distribution study, the increase of Zn level was observed in the supernatant fraction, while the increase of hepatic and splenic Ca levels was ascribed to that in the precipitated fractions. However, both fractions contributed to the decrease of Fe level in the spleen (Maitani and Suzuki, 1983).

Hirono et al. (1983) reported that DS of 54,000 MW exhibited a carcinogenic activity in the colon and rectum when it was given to rats orally as 2.5% diet, whereas those of 520,000 and 9500 MW showed no significant

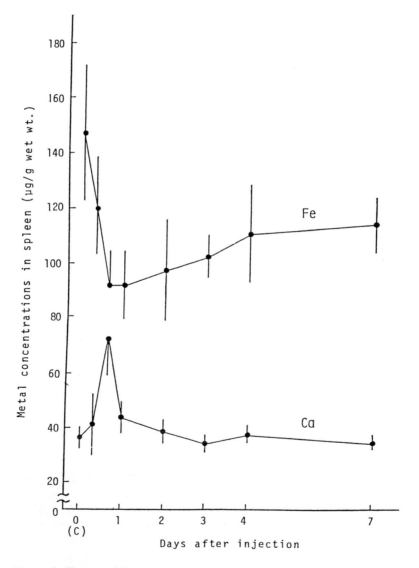

Figure 4. Changes of Ca and Fe concentrations in spleen after injection of dextran sulfate (see caption to Figure 3).

carcinogenicity. The carcinogenicity of DS of 54,000 MW has also been confirmed by Ishioka et al. (1987). At the present time, DS of 8,000 MW is attracting keen interest because of its anti-HIV (human immunodeficiency virus) activity (Nakashima et al., 1987; Mitsuya et al., 1988). Thus, the activities of DS seem much dependent on MW. Therefore, the ability of DS to induce hepatic Zn-MT was compared among the three kinds of DS with different MWs.

Three molecular weight fractions of DS (500,000, 54,000, and 8,000 MW) were injected intraperitoneally or subcutaneously into mice. The intraperitoneal (i.p.) injection of DS of 500,000 MW induced 8 times more hepatic Zn-MT than the subcutaneous (s.c.) injection. DS of lower MWs did not induce so much Zn-MT as DS of 500,000 MW in ip injection. The different abilities of DS to induce Zn-MT are not explained from the differences in the sulfate content of DS, because sulfur concentrations (namely sulfate contents) of three kinds of DS determined by ICP-AES were in the range of 17.6 to 18.8 weight %.

The hepatic Ca concentration exhibited a significant increase only after the ip injection of DS of 500,000 MW, which was in accord with an effective induction of Zn-MT. This fact also suggests a correlation between the hepatotoxicity of DS and the ability to induce hepatic Zn-MT.

Administration of Endotoxin into Endotoxin-sensitive and Endotoxin-resistant Strains of Mice

In our preliminary study, bacterial endotoxin was found to induce hepatic Zn-MT with the augmentation of hepatic Ca level (Maitani et al., 1981). The induction was not so much dependent on the injection routes as in DS (0.56 and 0.45 μg Cd/100 μl supernatant fraction for ip and sc injections, respectively, at a dose of 1 mg/kg body weight). It is known that C3H/HeJ mouse shows a lower sensitivity to bacterial endotoxin than the corresponding responder C3H/HeN mouse (Sultzer, 1968; Glode et al., 1976).

To investigate the correlation between the induction of hepatic Zn-MT and the increase of hepatic Ca level further, bacterial endotoxin (lipopolysaccharide *Escherichia coli* 0111:B4 Westphal method) was injected intraperitoneally into the endotoxin-sensitive C3H/HeN strain and the endotoxin-resistant C3H/HeJ strain at two different doses. Figure 5 shows the induced hepatic Zn-MT level at 24 h after the injection of endotoxin (Maitani et al., 1986). At a lower dose (0.25 mg/kg body weight), endotoxin-sensitive mice induced much more hepatic Zn-MT than endotoxin-resistant mice. However, comparable amounts of Zn-MT were observed in both strains at a higher dose (10 mg/kg body weight).

The changes of hepatic Ca concentrations are given in Table I. At the

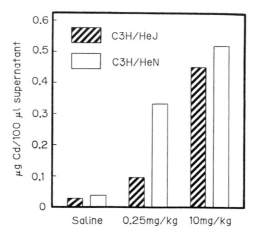

Figure 5. The induced hepatic Zn-MT level in endotoxin-resistant C3H/HeJ and endotoxin-sensitive C3H/
HeN mice at 24 h after injection of endotoxin at two
different doses. A portion of the liver from each mouse
was pooled in each group and Zn-MT was determined
for the groups (see caption to Figure 1).

lower dose, the significant increase of hepatic Ca level was observed only
in endotoxin-sensitive mice. At the higher dose, however, hepatic Ca level
was significantly higher in both strains as compared to the respective controls. A significant increase of splenic Ca level was observed only in the
endotoxin-sensitive mice at the higher dose. Thus, the increase in hepatic
Ca level was parallel to the induced amount of hepatic Zn-MT again. These
results also suggest that the induction of hepatic Zn-MT after bacterial endotoxin treatment is correlated to the hepatotoxic action of endotoxin.

Thus, the dose-related differences in response to bacterial endotoxin
were observed between two strains of C3H mice. The mechanism through

TABLE I.
Calcium Concentration (μg/g) in Various
Tissues of Mice After Endotoxin Treatment[a]

Endotoxin	Liver		Spleen	
dose (mg/kg)	HeJ	HeN	HeJ	HeN
Control	35.9 ± 0.9	37.4 ± 2.2	36.5 ± 1.9	35.2 ± 1.7
0.25	37.1 ± 2.0	43.5 ± 2.5^b	38.7 ± 2.1	37.4 ± 3.5
10	40.6 ± 1.1^b	49.5 ± 5.3^b	34.9 ± 1.5	41.6 ± 5.3^b

[a]Expressed as mean ± S.D. for 5 mice.
[b]Significantly different from the control value ($p < 0.05$).

which hepatic Zn-MT is induced by bacterial endotoxin is not clear yet. However, it has been previously reported that the induction is not mediated by glucocorticoid hormones (Durnam et al., 1984). Even so, it is true that the toxicity of endotoxin is highly related to glucocorticoid, since the adrenalectomized mouse shows 6,000 times higher sensitivity to endotoxin (Chedid et al., 1963). C3H/HeJ and C3H/HeN mice may be a useful tool to study the mechanism through which Zn-MT is induced by endotoxin.

Other Substances which Induce Hepatic Zn-MT with the Augmentation of Hepatic Ca Level

Zn is a primary inducer of MT and the coding of metal responsive elements in MT gene has been already clarified (Karin et al., 1987). However, when Zn was injected intraperitoneally at a high dose (10 mg Zn/kg and more), the increase of hepatic Ca level was observed (Maitani et al., 1981). The increase of Ca level may suggest that, when a high dose is injected intraperitoneally, Zn induces Zn-MT probably through two mechanisms, namely the mechanism as a primary inducer and that as a hepatotoxin mentioned in this study.

Cd is also a primary inducer of MT. The intravenous (i.v.) injection of Cd solution at a dose of 0.9 mg Cd/kg body weight did not produce the increase of hepatic Ca level. However, the i.v. injection of $CdCO_3$ suspension resulted in an increase of hepatic Ca level and, at the same time, the induction of Zn-MT as well as (Cd,Zn)-MT was also observed (Maitani and Suzuki, 1982b).

Indomethacin (Maitani et al., 1981) and turpentine oil also induced hepatic Zn-MT with the augmentation of hepatic Ca level.

Induction of Hepatic Zn-MT After Administration of Ca and Sr

It has been reported that the administration of Ca itself (Onosaka et al., 1983) or Ca-related vitamin D_3 (Karasawa et al., 1987) and catecholamine (Brady and Helvig, 1984) also induce Zn-MT. This led us to investigate the relation between hepatic Ca level and induction of Zn-MT after Ca loading. Sr, which belongs to the same group as Ca in the periodic table, was also administered to assess the specificity of Ca in the Zn-MT induction.

The s.c. injection of Ca at a dose of 2 mmol/kg body weight induced hepatic Zn-MT when observed at 24 h (about 0.4 μg/100 μl supernatant). Moreover, Sr injection also induced Zn-MT to half the amount of Ca administration. Thus, both Ca and Sr induced hepatic Zn-MT effectively.

The time-course of hepatic Ca concentration after Ca loading was followed. The Ca concentration showed a transitory increase with a maximum at 0.5 h. Ca concentration after DS (500,000 MW) treatment showed a

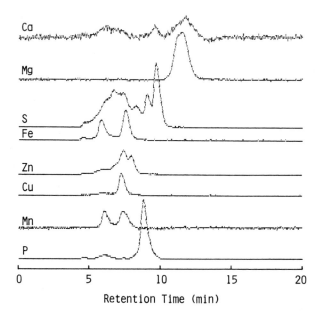

Figure 6. HPLC-ICP chromatograms of liver supernatant from Ca-injected mice. Mice were injected subcutaneously with Ca at a dose of 2 mmol/kg body weight and killed at 1 h. Livers from two mice were combined and homogenized in 3 vol. of buffer solution. The homogenate was centrifuged. A 100 μl portion of the supernatant was applied to HPLC-ICP system with a gel-filtration column (Asahipak GFA-50F®). The scales of enlargement in the ordinate for the respective elements are: Ca, ×50; Mg, ×10; S, ×3; Fe, ×5; Zn, ×20; Cu, ×20; Mn, ×200; P, ×1.

maximum at 16 h as mentioned above (Figure 3) (Maitani and Suzuki, 1982a). Thus, the time-courses of hepatic Ca level were markedly different between Ca and DS administrations.

Figure 6 represents HPLC-ICP chromatograms of liver supernatant fractions obtained from mice administered with Ca and killed at 1 h. Ca was detected at the retention times of 7, 10, and 12 min. Compared to the control, most of the additive Ca ions were detected at the retention time of free Ca ions (12 min) under the experimental conditions used. However, in HPLC-ICP analysis of plasma obtained from control mice, most of Ca ions were also detected as free ions. Therefore, the result suggests that, in HPLC analysis with a gel-filtration column, the roles of high-molecular-weight proteins may be underestimated with respect to the binding with Ca. This is attributable to the fact that a gel-filtration column for HPLC is liable to adsorb metals bound weakly to high-molecular-weight proteins (Suzuki, 1980).

What is the Primary Inducer of Zn-MT Induction in Our Systems?

As described above, Zn-MT induction by several compounds was observed with a concomitant increase of hepatic Ca level. This leads us to ask the fundamental question, what is the primary inducer? Zn and glucocorticoid hormones are primary inducers of Zn-MT and metal responsive elements and glucocorticoid responsive elements in MT genes have been clarified (Karin et al., 1984). Therefore, an explanation such that glucocorticoid hormones participate in the Zn-MT induction by inflammatory drugs is very attractive, because glucocorticoid hormones have an anti-inflammatory action. However, Sobocinski et al. (1981) had reported that adrenalectomized and normal rats induced comparable amounts of Zn-MT after administration of turpentine oil. Therefore, glucocorticoid hormones which are secreted from adrenal cortex were ruled out as the primary inducer in turpentine treatment. Thereafter, Durnam et al. (1984) also found with transgenic mice that the Zn-MT induction by bacterial endotoxin is not mediated by glucocorticoid hormones. Consequently, it is most unlikely that glucocorticoid hormones may be the primary inducer in our systems. In fact, our preliminary experiments showed that dexamethasone treatment produces the decrease of hepatic Ca level.

Interleukin-1 (IL-1) is a polypeptide (about 15 kDa) and is an endogenous inflammation mediator. Recently, it has been found that IL-1 also induces MT (Karin et al., 1985). IL-1 is produced in acute inflammation reactions such as bacterial infection or endotoxin treatment (Dinarello, 1984). Carrageenan treatment also results in a release of IL-1 from human monocytes (Sugawara et al., 1982). Therefore, it could be considered that IL-1 might be commonly involved in the Zn-MT induction in our systems. As for the release of IL-1, moreover, Auron et al. (1984) presented the attractive explanation that the extracellular appearance of IL-1 is the result of leakage upon cellular injury rather than active transport. This seems true at least for IL-1B (Bakouche et al., 1987). Consequently, if IL-1 is the primary inducer in our systems, both increases of hepatic Ca concentration and Zn-MT induction through IL-1 may be explained from the viewpoint of cellular injury. However, Iijima et al. (1987) have recently reported that the Zn-MT induction by, at least, bacterial endotoxin is mediated by a macrophage factor other than IL-1. The factor may be transforming growth factor-α (Iijima et al., 1989). It is not clear whether the factor is also involved in the Zn-MT induction by other compounds studied in this study.

Thornalley and Vašák (1985) have reported with a spin trapping technique of ESR that MT is an effective hydroxyl radical scavenger. Since MT is also induced after X-irradiation (Shiraishi et al., 1989), the protective effect of Zn-MT against free radicals appears to be a logical conclusion.

We have just started an *in vitro* study to investigate whether hydroxyl radicals or superoxide radicals are produced by macrophages or neutrophils when treated with inflammatory drugs. By using the spin trapping method with DMPO (5,5-dimethyl-1-pyrroline-1-oxide) as a spin-trapping agent, we could detect hydroxyl radicals produced by neutrophils when treated with some inflammatory drugs. Although carrageenan and endotoxin mainly act on macrophages, the detection of free radicals produced by macrophages has not been performed yet. Further studies are required to investigate whether oxygen radicals participate in the Zn-MT induction observed in our systems.

REFERENCES

Aschheim L and Raffel S (1972): The immunodepressant effect of carrageenin. *J. Reticuloendothel. Soc.* 11: 253.

Auron PE, Webb AC, Rosenwasser LJ, Mucci SF, Rich A, Wolff SM, and Dinarello CA (1984): Nucleotide sequence of human monocyte interleukin 1 precursor cDNA. *Proc. Natl. Acad. Sci. U.S.A.* 81: 7907.

Bakouche O, Brown DC, Lachman LB (1987): Liposomes expressing IL-1 biological activity. *J. Immunol.* 138: 4256.

Brady FO and Helvig B (1984): Effect of epinephrine and norepinephrine on zinc thionein levels and induction in rat liver. *Am. J. Physiol.* 247: E318.

Bremner I and Davies NT (1975): The induction of metallothionein in rat liver by zinc injection and restriction of food intake. *Biochem. J.* 149: 733.

Chedid L, Skarnes RC, and Parant M (1963): Characterization of Cr^{51}-labeled endotoxin and its identification in plasma and urine after parenteral administration. *J. Exp. Med.* 117: 561.

Dinarello CA (1984): Interleukin-1. *Rev. Infect. Dis.* 6: 51.

Durnam DM, Hoffman JS, Quaife CJ, Benditt EP, Chen HY, Brinster RL, and Palmiter RD (1984): Induction of mouse metallothionein-I mRNA by bacterial endotoxin is independent of metals and glucocorticoid hormones. *Proc. Natl. Acad. Sci. U.S.A.* 81: 1053.

El-Mofty SK, Scrutton MC, Serroni A, Nicolini C, and Farber JL (1975): Early, responsible plasma membrane injury in galactosamine-induced liver cell death. *Am. J. Pathol.* 79: 579.

Etzel KR, Shapiro SG, and Cousins RJ (1979): Regulation of liver metallothionein and plasma zinc by the glucocorticoid dexamethasone. *Biochem. Biophys. Res. Commun.* 89: 1120.

Glode LM, Scher I, Osborne B, and Rosenstreich DL (1976): Cellular mechanism of endotoxin unresponsiveness in C3H/HeJ Mice. *J. Immunol.* 116: 454.

Hirono I, Kuhara K, Yamaji T, Hosaka S, and Golberg L (1983): Carcinogenicity of dextran sulfate sodium in relation to its molecular weight. *Cancer Lett.* 18: 29.

Iijima Y, Takahashi T, Fukushima T, Abe S, Itano Y, and Kosaka F (1987): Induction of metallothionein by a macrophage factor and the partial characterization of the factor. *Toxicol. Appl. Pharmacol.* 89: 135.

Iijima Y, Fukushima T, and Kosaka F (1989): Involvement of transforming growth factor-α secreted by macrophages in metallothionein induction by endotoxin. *Biochem. Biophys. Res. Commun.* 164: 114.

Ishioka T, Kuwabara N, Oohashi Y, and Wakabayashi K (1987): Induction of colorectal tumors in rats by sulfated polysaccharides. *CRC Crit. Rev. Toxicol.* 17: 215.

Karasawa M, Hosoi J, Hashiba H, Nose K, Tohyama C, Abe E, Suda T, and Kuroki T (1987): Regulation of metallothionein gene expression by 1,25-dihydroxyvitamin D_3 in cultured cells and in mice. *Proc. Natl. Acad. Sci. U.S.A.* 84: 8810.

Karin M, Haslinger A, Holtgreve H, Richards RI, Krauter P, Westphal H, and Beato M (1984): Characterization of DNA sequences through which cadmium and glucocorticoid hormones induce human metallothionein-II_A gene. *Nature (London)* 308: 513.

Karin M, Imbra RJ, Heguy A, and Wong G (1985): Interleukin 1 regulates human metallothionein gene expression. *Mol. Cell. Biol.* 5: 2866.

Karin M, Haslinger A, Heguy A, Dietlin T, and Cooke T (1987): Metal—responsive elements act as positive modulators of human metallothionein-II_A enhancer activity. *Mol. Cell. Biol.* 7: 606.

Maitani T and Suzuki KT (1981): Alterations of essential metal levels and induction of metallothionein by carrageenan injection. *Biochem. Pharmacol.* 30: 2353.

Maitani T, Suzuki KT, and Kubota K (1981): Increase of hepatic calcium level on metallothionein induction. *Ipn. J. Hyg.* 36: 366.

Maitani T and Suzuki KT (1982a): Induction of metallothionein in liver and changes of essential metal levels in selected tissues by three dextran derivatives. *Biochem. Pharmacol.* 31: 3051.

Maitani T and Suzuki KT (1982b): Changes of essential metal levels in selected tissue and splenomegaly induced by the injection of suspending cadmium salt into mice. *Toxicol. Appl. Pharmacol.* 62: 219.

Maitani T and Suzuki KT (1983): Age- and sex-dependent variations of essential metal levels in tissues and responses to dextran sulfate treatment which induces zinc-thionein. *Chem. Pharm. Bull.* 31: 4456.

Maitani T, Saito Y, Fujimaki H, and Suzuki KT (1986): Comparative induction of hepatic zinc-thionein and increase in tissue calcium by bacterial endotoxin in endotoxin-sensitive (C3H/HeN) and endotoxin-resistant (C3H/HeJ) mice. *Toxicol. Lett.* 30: 181.

Margoshes M and Vallee BL (1957): A cadmium protein from equine kidney cortex. *J. Am. Chem. Soc.* 79: 4813.

Mitsuya H, Looney DJ, Kuno S, Ueno R, Wong-Staal F, and Broder S (1988): Dextran sulfate suppression of viruses in the HIV family: inhibition of virion binding to $CD4^+$ cells. *Science* 240: 646.

Nakashima H, Yoshida O, Tochikura TS, Yoshida T, Mimura T, Kido Y, Motoki Y, Kaneko Y, Uryu T, and Yamamoto N (1987): Sulfation of polysaccharides generates potent and selective inhibitors of human immunodeficiency virus infection and replication *in vitro*. *Jpn. J. Cancer Res. (Gann)* 78: 1164.

Oh SH, Deagen JT, Whanger PD, and Weswig PH (1978): Biological function of metallothionein V. Its induction in rats by various stresses. *Am. J. Physiol.* 234: E282.

Onosaka S, Tanaka K, Doi M, and Okahara K (1978): A simplified procedure for determination of metallothionein in animal tissues. *Eisei Kagaku* 24: 128.

Onosaka S, Yoshiya S, Min K-S, Fukuhara T, and Tanaka K (1983): The induced synthesis of metallothionein in various tissues of rat after injection of various metals. *Eisei Kagaku* 29: 221.

Shiraishi N, Hayashi H, Hiraki Y, Aono K, Itano Y, Kosaka F, Noji S, and Taniguchi S (1989): Elevation in metallothionein messenger RNA in rat tissues after exposure to X-irradiation. *Toxicol. Appl. Pharmacol.* 98: 501.

Smith MT, Thor H, and Orrenius S (1981): Toxic injury to isolated hepatocytes is not dependent on extracellular calcium. *Science* 213: 1257.

Sobocinski PZ, Canterbury Jr., WJ, Mapes CA, Dinterman RE, Hauer, EC and Abeles FB (1978): Hypozincemia of inflammation: sequestration of zinc by hepatic metallothioneins. *Fed. Proc.* 37: 890.

Sobocinski PZ, Canterbury Jr., WJ, Knutsen GI, and Hauer EC (1981): Effect of adrenalectomy on cadmium- and turpentine-induced hepatic synthesis of metallothionein and α_2-macrofetoprotein in the rat. *Inflammation* 5: 153.

Sugawara I, Ishizaka S, and Moeller G (1982): Carrageenans highly sulfated polysaccharides and macrophage toxic agents newly found human T-lymphocyte mitogens. *Immunobiology* 163: 527.

Sultzer BM (1968): Genetic control of leucocyte responses to endotoxin. *Nature* 219: 1253.

Suzuki KT and Yamamura M (1979): Dose dependent formation of zinc-thionein in livers and kidneys of rats and mice by zinc injection. *Biochem. Pharmacol.* 28: 2852.

Suzuki KT (1980): Direct connection of high-speed liquid chromatograph (equipped with gel permeation column) to atomic absorption spectrophotometer for metalloprotein analysis: Metallothionein. *Anal. Biochem.* 102: 31.

Thornalley PJ and Vašák M (1985): Possible role for metallothionein in protection against radiation-induced oxidative stress. Kinetics and mechanism of its reaction with superoxide and hydroxyl radicals. *Biochim. Biophys. Acta* 827: 36.

Tohyama C and Shaikh ZA (1978): Cross-reactivity of metallothioneins from different origins with rabbit anti-rat hepatic metallothionein antibody. *Biochem. Biophys. Res. Commun.* 84: 907.

Vander Mallie RJ and Garvey JS (1978): Production and study of antibody produced against rat cadmium thionein. *Immunochemistry* 15: 857.

Winter CA, Risley EA, and Nuss GW (1962): Carrageenin-induced edema in hind paw of the rat as an assay for antiinflammatory drugs. *Proc. Soc. Exp. Biol. Med.* 111: 544.

Chapter

15

Discriminative Uptake of Cadmium, Copper and Zinc by the Liver

Kazuo T. Suzuki, Sanae Kawahara, Hiroyuki Sunaga,
and Etsuko Kobayashi
National Institute for Environmental Studies
Ibaraki, Japan

SUMMARY

Discriminatory regulation between essential and nonessential heavy metals was studied using a combination of essential (copper and zinc) and nonessential metals (cadmium) during the uptake process of the three metals by the liver from the bloodstream. Each heavy metal injected intravenously into rats disappeared from the bloodstream and accumulated in the liver with different time course curves; cadmium disappeared rapidly from the bloodstream and accumulated concomitantly, while copper and zinc disappeared slowly from the bloodstream and started to accumulated after 2 h postinjection. Pretreatment with a small dose of cadmium before 24 h did not affect the disappearance and accumulation curves of the three metals. However, pretreatment with cadmium before 6 h enhanced the disappearance and accumulation of copper (and possibly zinc) but not of cadmium. Two possibilities were raised to explain the discriminatory uptake mechanisms. One is the discriminatory influx and assumes a regulatory process for the influx of an essential metal. The other is the discriminatory efflux which requires a specific efflux channel for an essential metal but not for a nonessential metal. Endogenous zinc was effluxed by injection of cadmium, whereby zinc bound to metallothionein and alcohol dehydrogenase were replaced with cadmium. The results suggest that excess zinc ions but not cadmium ions are effluxed from the liver cells. Therefore, the discriminatory uptake between essential and nonessential heavy metals was explained by the discriminative efflux between essential (copper and zinc) and nonessential heavy metals (cadmium).

INTRODUCTION

Discrimination between essential and nonessential heavy metals together with the homeostatic regulation of the former metals by the body are considered to be fundamental biological processes. Many places at which biological discriminatory processes occur can be defined such as uptake and absorption at the gastrointestinal tract, binding to plasma components followed by site-specific distribution, and excretion and reabsorption by the kidney (Suzuki et al., 1990a).

Elements belonging to the same column of the periodic table resemble each other in their chemical properties. Zinc (Zn) and cadmium (Cd) are transition metals both belonging to group IIb. Zn is known as one of the most important essential heavy metals while Cd is one of the representative toxic heavy metals. The two metals are therefore likely to be a good combination to examine the biological discrimination mechanism between essential and nonessential heavy metals.

Zn and Cd are both known to induce metallothionein (MT) in various organisms and bind to the protein by sharing the same ligands (Kägi and Kojima, 1987). Further, the two metals bind preferentially to albumin in the bloodstream (Scott and Bradwell, 1983; Suzuki et al., 1986). These facts indicate that Zn and Cd are present in the same chemical forms before the uptake by the liver (i.e., bound to albumin) and after the accumulation in the liver (i.e., bound to MT). However, the uptake process for each metal into the liver may be different.

Copper (Cu) is also bound preferentially to albumin in the bloodstream and to MT in the liver when the metal is administered intravenously into rats (Suzuki et al., 1989). Cu induces MT efficiently in the liver and kidney (Kägi and Kojima, 1987). Further, Cu and Zn both 1st row transition metals, are always bound to MT as co-existing metals even if the protein is induced by Cd (Suzuki, 1982).

These facts suggest that the three heavy metals, two essential (Cu and Zn) and one nonessential (Cd) heavy metals are a good combination of elements to elucidate metal uptake processes by the liver. They also represent excellent candidates to study as one of the principal biological discriminatory processes of the living body. The present study was initiated to clarify the uptake process for the three metals by the liver from the standpoint of the discrimination in the body.

Disappearance from plasma and accumulation in the liver were compared among the three metals after a single intravenous injection of each metal with or without pretreatment. The results are discussed from the viewpoint of the discrimination mechanism for the uptake of essential and nonessential heavy metals by the liver, and a new working hypothesis is presented for the discriminative uptake process.

DISAPPEARANCE FROM PLASMA AND ACCUMULATION IN THE LIVER OF Cd, Cu AND Zn AFTER A SINGLE INTRAVENOUS INJECTION INTO RATS

Time-courses of the disappearance from plasma (Figure 1) and accumulation in the liver (Figure 2) were compared among the three metals after injecting each metal into rats. Cd disappeared rapidly from plasma and Cd concentration in plasma was decreased to approximately 20% of the estimated initial concentration by 5 min after the injection. Compared to Cd, Cu and Zn disappeared slowly from plasma and they took more than 3 h to return to the respective control levels (Figure 1).

In accordance with the rapid disappearance of Cd from plasma, the metal was taken up (and concurrently accumulated) in the liver (Figure 2).

Plasma Cu concentration decreased to about a half of the estimated initial level by 20 min and more than 80% of the metal disappeared from plasma within 1 h. However, concentration of Cu in the liver stayed almost at the control level during this period and started to increase only after 3 h post-injection. This result indicates that most of Cu administered into the bloodstream is not taken up by the liver or does not accumulate in the liver during the initial disappearance process from plasma. The amount of Cu excreted into bile and urine during this period was too low to explain the metal disappeared from plasma (Suzuki et al., 1990a) and its distribution is presently unexplained.

Although Zn concentration in the liver showed a transitory increase shortly after the injection, it returned to the control level and remained nearly at this level up to 3 h post-injection. The transitory increase of Zn concentration in the liver may correlate to the faster disappearance of Zn from plasma than that of Cu.

The disappearance curves from plasma (Figure 1) and accumulation curves in the liver (Figure 2) for the three metals suggest that the three metals are discriminated during the uptake process by the liver from plasma despite that the three metals are all bound to albumin before the uptake process.

Although Cd accumulated much faster than Cu and Zn in the liver, MT

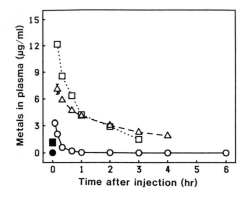

Figure 1. Disappearance curves of Cd (○), Cu (□) and Zn (△) from plasma with time after a single intravenous injection of each metal into rats (Suzuki et al., 1990a). Cd, Cu, or Zn was injected singly into female Wistar rats (8-week-old; mean body weight, 160 g) at a dose of 0.8 mg/kg body weight (in 0.1 ml saline per rat) and the animals (3 rats per group) were killed after 5, 10, 20, 40 min, 1, 2, 3, 4, and 6 h for the Cd group; after 10, 20, 40 min, 1, 2, and 3 h for the Cu group; and after 10, 20, 40 min, 1, 2, 3, and 4 h for the Zn group. Control animals (5 rats per group; Cd (●), Cu (■), and Zn (▲) groups) were killed without any treatment by exsanguination under pentobarbital anesthesia. Symbols without vertical bars indicate that S.D. are within the symbols. Plasma concentrations of the injected metals were estimated to be 17 μg/ml at the time of injection by assuming even distribution of each metal. Concentrations of Cu and Zn in control plasma were 1.9 and 1.7 μg/ml, respectively.

synthesis was induced after the same lag time of 2 h for the three metals (Figure 3). This result suggests that the nonessential metal Cd is taken up by the liver without any regulation and the metal accumulated in the liver induces MT synthesis, while the essential metals Cu and Zn are taken up by the liver only in a small quantity until MT synthesis is induced. It is also suggested that the uptake by the liver or accumulation in the liver of the essential metals Cu and Zn may be regulated by the available amount of MT for sequestration of those metals, while the nonessential metal Cd is related to MT synthesis only after the accumulation of the metal in the liver.

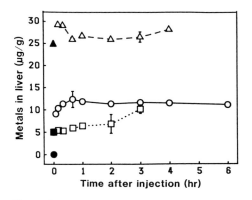

Figure 2. Accumulation curves of Cd, Cu and Zn in the liver with time after a single intravenous injection of each metal into rats (Suzuki et al., 1990a). Livers were excised from the corresponding rats in Figure 1. See the legend to Figure 1. Cd (○), Cu (□) and Zn (△).

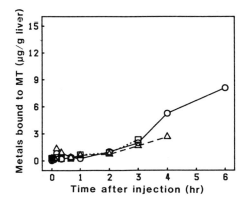

Figure 3. Changes in concentrations of Cd, Cu, and Zn bound to MT in the liver with time after a single intravenous injection of each metal into rats (Suzuki et al., 1990a). The corresponding livers in Figure 2 were homogenized in 3 volumes of 0.1 *M* Tris-HCl buffer (pH 7.4, containing 0.25 *M* glucose) and the homogenates were centrifuged at 170,000 × *g* for 60 min. A 1.0 ml portion of the supernatants from each rat was pooled in each group and a 0.1 ml aliquot of the pooled supernatants was applied to an Asahipak GST-520® column (Asahi Chemical Co., Ltd., Tokyo; 7.6 × 500 mm) and the column was eluted with 10 m*M* Tris-HCl buffer (pH 7.4, containing 0.9% NaCl and 0.05% NaN$_3$). Concentrations of each metal bound to MT were estimated from peak area by HPLC-ICP (Sunaga et al., 1987). Cd (○), Cu (□) and Zn (△).

EFFECTS OF PRETREATMENT WITH Cd ON THE DISAPPEARANCE FROM PLASMA AND ACCUMULATION IN THE LIVER OF Cd, Cu AND Zn INJECTED SUBSEQUENTLY INTO RATS

The disappearance curves in Figure 1 and the accumulation curves in Figure 2 indicated that the uptake process by the liver for the essential heavy metals may be related to the induction of MT synthesis or the capacity to sequester excess metal ions as MT.

When MT is induced in the liver by injection of Cd, Cu or Zn, a lag time of several hours is known to be required for the synthesis of the protein as also observed in Figure 2 (Cempel and Webb, 1976). Pretreatment with a nontoxic dose of heavy metals reduces the harmful effects of the subsequent toxic doses of heavy metals by synthesizing MT without lag and/or by sequestering the toxic metals by replacing Zn bound to MT (Cempel and Webb, 1976; Lever and Miya, 1976; Suzuki and Yoshikawa, 1974). These facts indicate that pretreatment with a small dose of metals may facilitate the uptake of the subsequent high dose of metals by inducing MT synthesis promptly without lag when uptake by the liver is assumed to be regulated by the availability of MT for sequestration of excess metal ions.

Pretreatment effects on the discriminative uptake among the three metals were examined for the disappearance curves (Figure 4) and the accumulation curves (Figure 5). Cd was administered in a small quantity as pretreatment because the metal remains in the liver for a long time bound to MT. Although Cd is bound to MT at a steady state, the protein is always degraded and resynthesized (Suzuki, 1982; Webb, 1979), indicating that mRNA for MT (MTmRNA) is maintained at an elevated level even at a steady state.

Cd, Cu, or Zn was injected after 24 h post-pretreatment with Cd and the disappearance curve (solid symbols) of each metal was compared with the corresponding curve without pretreatment (small solid symbols with a solid line) as shown in Figure 4. The three metals disappeared from plasma exactly with the same time-course curves as those without pretreatment (Figure 4). The three metals accumulated in the liver also with the same time-course curves as those without pretreatment when the elevated levels of Cd (Figure 5a) and Zn (Figure 5c) by the pretreatment are taken into consideration (Figure 5). These results indicate that the pretreatment was not effective on the disappearance and accumulation of not only Cd but also Cu and Zn. However, MTmRNA level might be lowered after 24 h post-injection.

Pretreatment effects were then examined by injected Cd 6 h before the subsequent high doses of Cd and Cu (open symbols in Figures 4 and 5). Although Cd disappeared from plasma with the same time-course curve as the other two, disappearance of Cu was enhanced by a shorter time interval between pretreatment and subsequent dose (Figure 4). Accumulation of Cd

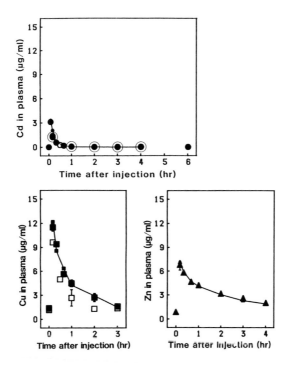

Figure 4. Disappearance curves of Cd (a), Cu (b), and Zn (c) from plasma after a single intravenous injection of each metal with different time intervals after pretreatment with Cd (Suzuki et al., 1990b). Cd was injected subcutaneously into rats at a dose of 0.3 mg/kg body weight as pretreatment. Cd, Cu, or Zn was subsequently injected after 6 (open symbols) or 24 h (solid symbols) post-treatment. Small solid symbols with a solid line indicate the corresponding curve without pretreatment shown in Figure 1 (shown without S.D.). Symbols without vertical bars indicate that S.D. are within the symbols.

in the liver was also not enhanced by pretreatment with the shorter time interval (Figure 5). In accordance with the enhanced disappearance of Cu from plasma in Figure 4b, Cu accumulated in the liver with an enhanced rate as shown in Figure 5b.

The pretreatment experiments mentioned above suggest that the essential metals Cu and possibly Zn, too, but not the nonessential metal Cd are taken up by the liver in connection with induction of MT synthesis (Suzuki et al., 1990b). Uptake processes of Cu and Zn by the liver have been studied in relation to the induction of MT synthesis (Cousins, 1982, 1985; Dunn and Cousins, 1989; Ettinger et al., 1986; Mehra and Bremner, 1987; Pattison and Cousins, 1986). These processes have also been studied from the viewpoint of a disturbance of metal metabolism such as Menkes' disease (Herd et al., 1987; Kimelberg and Norenberg, 1989). Accumulation of metals in the liver is a result of higher uptake rate or slower efflux rate as pointed out in these studies.

Rapid uptake and accumulation of Cd are certainly caused by high uptake and slow efflux rates of Cd. On the other hand, slow accumulation of the essential metals Cu and Zn and its relation to induction of MT synthesis may be explained by either one of the following two possibilities (Suzuki et al., 1990a). One is that the liver does not take up the essential metals until MT synthesis is induced and can sequester excess Cu and Zn ions in the cell. The other is that the liver excretes Cu and Zn at the same rate as it takes up the two metals. The former explanation assumes a discriminative uptake process at the membrane, while the latter explanation assumes a different efflux mechanism between essential and nonessential metals.

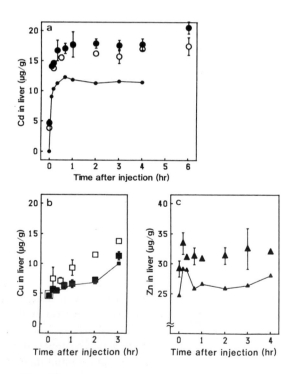

Figure 5. Accumulation curves of Cd (a), Cu (b), and Zn (c) in the liver after a single intravenous injection of each metal with different time intervals after pretreatment with Cd (Suzuki et al., 1990b). Livers were obtained from the corresponding rats in Figure 4. Symbols also correspond to those in Figure 4.

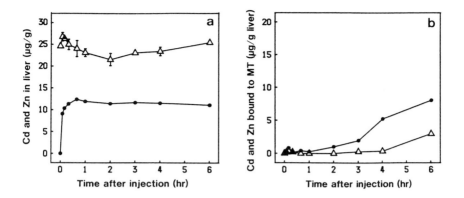

Figure 6. Changes in concentrations of Zn (a) and Zn bound to MT (b) in the liver with time after a single intravenous injection of Cd into rats (Suzuki et al., 1990c). Concentrations of Zn ($\triangle$) were determined together with Cd for the livers shown in Figure 2 and for the metal bound to MT shown in Figure 3. Concentrations of Cd ($-\bullet-$) correspond to those in Figures 2 and 3 (shown without S.D.).

EFFLUX OF ENDOGENOUS Zn BY REPLACEMENT WITH Cd

From the time-course curves of the disappearance from plasma and the accumulation in the liver for the essential and non-essential metals, two possibilities were raised to explain the discriminative uptake. Pretreatment effects have been explained by induction of MT synthesis without lag and/ or by replacement of Zn bound to MT with Cd as mentioned above. The latter mechanism for the pretreatment effects indicates that Zn ions are liberated within the cell and the fate of the endogenous Zn may give a clue to clarify the mechanism for the discriminative uptake process.

Figure 6 shows the changes of Zn concentrations in the liver and the metal bound to MT with time after Cd injection without pretreatment. Concentration of Zn in the liver showed a transitory increase immediately after Cd injection as also observed in Figures 2 and 3 when Zn was injected without and with pretreatment, respectively. After the transitory increase, the concentration of Zn decreased to a lower level than the initial control level (Figure 6a). The decrease of Zn concentration in the liver was due to that in the supernatant fraction (data not shown) but not due to the metal bound to MT (Figure 6b). In a separate study in our laboratory, Cd was shown to bind to alcohol dehydrogenase (ADH) in the liver by replacing Zn in ADH before induction of MT synthesis (Sunaga et al., 1989). The decrease of Zn in Figure 6a was due to the decrease in the supernatant fraction but not due to MT (Figure 6b), suggesting that Zn liberated from ADH is excreted by the uptake of Cd. In fact, Zn bound to ADH was decreased on an HPLC-ICP profile (data not shown).

Pretreatment with Cd induced MT containing Cd and Zn and concentration of Zn in the liver was increased (compare Zn concentrations at time 0 in Figures 6a and 7a). The concentration of Zn in the liver decreased without a transitory increase when Cd was injected into the rats that had been pretreated with Cd before 24 h (Figure 7a). The extent of the decrease was more than that in Figure 6a and it was due to that in the supernatant (data not shown). Further, it was shown that Zn bound to MT in the pretreated rat liver was decreased by the subsequent injection of Cd (Figure 7b). The HPLC-ICP profiles of the supernatants indicated that Zn bound to MT and ADH were replaced by Cd, suggesting that the Zn liberated from both proteins were excreted (data not shown).

The excretion of the endogenous Zn shown in Figures 6 and 7 indicates that excess Zn ions are excreted when the metal is not sequestered by MT owing to the shortage of the available protein. This result also indicates that excess Zn but not Cd ions in the cell are excreted, thereby suggesting that the influx of the essential metal is balanced by the efflux. However, the non-essential metal is not effluxed.

CONCLUSION

The uptake processes by the liver of essential and nonessential heavy metals were studied because it is one of the representative examples of biological discriminatory processes among heavy metals.

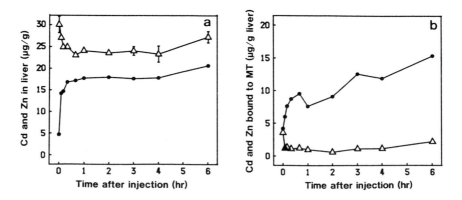

Figure 7. Changes in concentrations of Zn (a) and Zn bound to MT (b) in the liver with time after a single intravenous injection of Cd into the rats that were pretreated with Cd before 24 h. Concentrations of Zn (△) and the metal bound to MT were determined for the corresponding livers with a 24 h interval shown by solid symbols in Figure 5a. Concentrations of Cd (–●–) correspond to those in Figure 5a (shown without S.D.).

From the time-course curves for the disappearance from plasma and accumulation in the liver of Cd, Cu, and Zn injected with and without pretreatment, it was suggested that the essential and non-essential metals are taken up discriminatively by the liver. Cd is taken up by the liver without any regulation and then induces MT synthesis. On the other hand, Cu (and Zn) is taken up only to a limited extent by the liver until MT synthesis is induced to sequester the excess essential metals in the cell.

Efflux of endogenous Zn occurred when Cd was taken up by the liver and the origin of the endogenous Zn was suggested to be ADH and MT.

From these results, the discriminative uptake process by the liver between essential and non-essential heavy metals was explained as follows; the influx of the essential heavy metals Cu and Zn is balanced by the efflux of the same metals, while the efflux of the non-essential heavy metal Cd does not occur as its ionic form.

The present results also suggest that induction of MT synthesis is not the cause for the uptake and accumulation of both the essential (Cu and Zn) and non-essential heavy metals (Cd), but is the result of influx or accumulation in the cell. This conclusion implies that MT is induced to sequester excess heavy metal ions in the cell, thereby MT removes or reduces the toxicity of nonessential harmful heavy metals as well as with that of excess essential heavy metals.

REFERENCES

Cempel M and Webb M (1976): The time-course of cadmium-thionein synthesis in the rat. *Biochem. Pharmacol.* 25: 2067.

Cousins RJ (1982): Relationship of metallothionein synthesis and degradation to intracellular zinc metabolism. In Foulkes EC, Ed., *Biological Roles of Metallothionein,* Elsevier/North-Holland, New York, pp 251–260.

Cousins RJ (1985): Absorption, transport, and hepatic metabolism of copper and zinc: special reference to metallothionein and ceruloplasmin. *Physiol. Rev.* 65: 238.

Dunn MA and Cousins RJ (1989): Kinetics of zinc metabolism in the rat: effect of dibutyl cAMP. *Am. J. Physiol.* 256: E420.

Ettinger MJ, Darwish HM, and Schmitt RC (1986): Mechanism of copper transport from plasma to hepatocytes. *Fed. Proc.* 45: 2800.

Feldman SL, Squibb KS, and Cousins RJ (1978): Degradation of cadmium-thionein in rat liver and kidney. *J. Toxicol. Environ. Health* 4: 805.

Herd MD, Camakaris J, Christofferson R, Wookey P, and Danks DM (1987): Uptake and efflux of copper-64 in Menkes' disease and normal continuous lymphoid cell lines. *Biochem. J.* 247: 341.

Kägi JHR and Kojima Y (1987): Chemistry and biochemistry of metallothionein. In, Kägi JHR and Kojima Y, Eds., *Metallothionein II,* Birkhäuser-Verlag, Basel, pp 25–61.

Kimelberg HK and Norenberg MD (1989): Astrocytes. *Sci. Am.,* April, Vol. 44.

Lever AP and Miya TS (1976): A mechanism for cadmium- and zinc-induced tolerance to cadmium toxicity: involvement of metallothionein. *Toxicol. Appl. Pharmacol.* 37: 403.

Mehra RK and Bremner I (1987): Induction of synthesis and degradation of metallothionein-I in the tissues of rats injected with zinc. In, Kägi JHR and Kojima Y, Eds., *Metallothionein II,* Birkhäuser-Verlag, Basel, pp 565–572.

Pattison SE and Cousins RJ (1986): Zinc uptake and metabolism by hepatocytes. *Fed. Proc.* 45: 2805.

Scott BJ and Bradwell AR (1983): Identification of the serum-binding proteins for iron, zinc, cadmium, nickel, and calcium. *Clin. Chem.* 29: 629.

Sunaga H, Kobayashi E, Shimojo N, and Suzuki KT (1987): Detection of sulfur-containing compounds in control and cadmium-exposed rat organs by high performance liquid chromatography-vacuum-ultraviolet inductively coupled plasma-atoic emission spectrometry (HPLC-ICP). *Analyt. Biochem.* 160: 160.

Sunaga H, Yamane Y, Aoki Y, and Suzuki KT (1989): The major cadmium-binding protein before induction of metallothionein in the rat liver is alcohol dehydrogenase. *Eisei Kagaku,* 35: p-21.

Suzuki Y and Yoshikawa H (1974): Role of metallothionein in the liver in protection against cadmium toxicity. *Ind. Health* 12: 141.

Suzuki KT, Sunaga H, Kobayashi E, and Shimojo N (1986): Mercaptalbumin as a selective cadmium-binding protein in rat serum. *Toxicol. Appl. Pharmacol.* 86: 466.

Suzuki KT (1982): Induction and degradation of metallothionein and their relation to the toxicity of cadmium. In, Foulkes EC, Ed., *Biological Roles of Metallothionein,* Elsevier/North-Holland, New York, pp 215–235.

Suzuki KT, Karasawa A, and Yamanaka K (1989): Binding of copper to albumin and participation of cysteine *in vivo* and *in vitro. Arch. Biochem. Biophys.* 273: 572.

Suzuki KT, Kawahara S, Sunaga H, Kobayashi E, and Shimojo N (1990a): Discriminative uptake of metals by the liver and its relation to induction of metallothionein by cadmium, copper and zinc. *Comp. Biochem. Physiol.* 95C: 279.

Suzuki KT, Kawahara S, Sunaga H, and Shimojo N (1990b): Effects of pretreatment with cadmium on the discriminative uptake of subsequent cadmium, copper or zinc by the liver. *Comp. Biochem. Physiol.* 95C: 285.

Suzuki KT, Kawahara S, Sunaga H, and Shimojo N (1990c): Efflux of endogenous zinc liberated from metallothionein and alcohol dehydrogenase in the liver by replacement with cadmium. *Toxicol. Appl. Pharmacol.* 105: 413.

Webb M (1979): Functions of hepatic and renal metallothioneins in the control of the metabolism of cadmium and certain other bivalent cations. In, Kägi JHR and Nordberg N, Eds., *Metallothionein,* Birkhäuser-Verlag, Basel, pp 313–320.

Chapter 16

Tissue-Specific Metallothionein Induction by Non-Binding Metals: Evidence of an Associated Inflammatory Response

Charles C. McCormick and Rodney R. Dietert
Cornell University, Ithaca, New York

INTRODUCTION

It has been over three decades since the discovery of the unique metal-binding protein, metallothionein (MT). Since then and through the advent of techniques in molecular biology, the MT gene has been examined in detail in several species and has emerged as a eukaryotic model for inducible gene expression. In fact, it is thought that the control of MT gene expression is due exclusively to transcriptional regulation (Searle, 1987). Although the list is probably not complete, the various inducers of MT gene transcription appear to fall into at least three general categories: (1) metals—cadmium, zinc, and copper, (2) glucocorticoids and (3) cytokines—interleukin-1 and interferon. While the specific promoter sequences for the first two of these have been identified in various species, the latter (cytokine) awaits more definitive study. Nonetheless, there seems to be little doubt that each of the factors listed above directly stimulates the initiation of MT mRNA transcription and thus the induction of MT in various tissues. At present, there is increasing evidence that DNA binding proteins are an integral part of this process (Seguin and Hamer, 1987; Seguin and Prevost, 1988; Westin and Schaffner, 1988; Garg et al., 1989).

In addition to the above factors, other agents (conditions) have been recognized to stimulate the synthesis of MT *in vivo* by mechanisms which are not understood. In fact, Bracken and Klaassen (1987) have suggested that the nature of induction of MT by some compounds *in vivo* must be "indirect" since no induction can be demonstrated *in vitro*. Earlier, Durnam and Palmiter (1984) had indicated that some compounds must be "gratuitous" inducers since MT has no apparent relationship to their metabolism. The question that has intrigued us over the past several years concerns the mechanism by which MT is induced indirectly. Some investigators have suggested that indirect induction of MT may involve changes in zinc homeostasis and/or secretion of glucocorticoids as might occur during general stress (Bracken and Klaassen, 1987). Thus, this would explain why certain substances are effective *in vivo* but not *in vitro*. Over the past several years, we have investigated the nature of MT induction by various metals. We have consistently observed an effect which appears to be: (1) dependent on the route of metal administration, and (2) related to the indirect induction of MT. Our results indicate that it is independent of either zinc homeostasis or stress and that inflammation is an associated event.

MT INDUCTION BY ZINC: SECONDARY EFFECTS

The induction of hepatic MT by zinc is thought to result from the interaction of zinc ions and nuclear factors leading to the synthesis of MT mRNA (Hamer, 1986). This implies that the zinc ion directly effects the induction of tissue MT. Since there are data to support this suggestion, zinc as well as cadmium are presently considered to directly stimulate the synthesis of MT mRNA, requiring only sufficient nuclear-binding factors for normal expression. Much of the initial work concerning the regulation of MT induction has been conducted *in vivo*. Since this experimental model is confounded by influences which cannot be controlled, the results of these studies may be difficult (if not impossible) to interpret. For example, the induction of MT by glucocorticoids was originally thought to represent an indirect action of the hormone on zinc flux into the cell. Glucocorticoids stimulated the uptake of zinc by cells and consequently the induction of MT. Therefore, MT induction by glucocorticoids was considered to be a secondary response resulting from changes in the concentration of intracellular zinc. It is now clear that glucocorticoids directly affect the synthesis of MT independent of changes in cellular zinc (Karin et al., 1980). This example serves to illustrate difficulties in separating the "cause and effect" of related events.

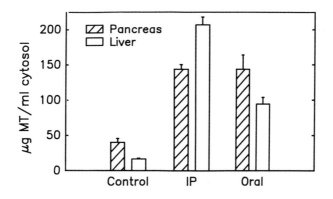

Figure 1. The accumulation of metallothionein in liver and pancreas of chicks as influenced by the route of zinc administration. Young chicks were given zinc by intraperitoneal (i.p.) injection (i.p., 5 mg Zn/kg) or by oral (p.o.) gavage (p.o., 32 mg Zn). Controls received normal saline i.p. Twenty-four hours following treatments, liver tissue was obtained for MT analysis (Cd-radio-assay). The results indicated that MT accumulation in the pancreas was similar in both groups (i.p. and oral) suggesting that exposure to zinc was comparable. In contrast, the accumulation of MT in liver was nearly twice as great when zinc was given IP (vs. Oral). The data suggest that zinc given IP causes an additional direct (tissue-specific) induction of MT which is not related to zinc exposure.

We have examined the induction of MT in various tissues following the administration of zinc. We (as many others) have found that MT accumulates in several tissues following the administration of zinc. While this was not surprising, we believed that, under certain conditions, the response to parenteral zinc is confounded by physiological (secondary) processes initiated by the mere injection of the metal. Our first observation in this regard is evidence shown in Figure 1 (Fleet et al., 1988). The data illustrate that if zinc were given intraperitoneally (versus orally) the tissue response is considerably different. For example, the accumulation of MT in the pancreas of chicks given zinc either i.p. or orally was essentially the same. This implied that exposure of chicks in both groups to zinc at the cellular level was approximately equal. Assuming that this were the condition, the hepatic response then reflects a marked deviation from the expected response. The accumulation of MT in the liver was nearly twice as great in chicks given zinc i.p. when compared to that of chicks given zinc orally. These results strongly suggest that the i.p. administration of zinc causes an additional (liver-specific) effect unrelated to the level of zinc exposure. Although the quantitative nature of zinc exposure at the cellular level could not be proven, we have obtained additional data with copper which support such a suggestion, and thus, the indirect effects of the intraperitoneally administration of metal.

MT INDUCTION BY COPPER: SECONDARY EFFECTS

The induction of MT by the administration of copper has historically been a controversial area of investigation (see Bremner, 1987 for review). Originally, many considered MT induction by copper to be an indirect consequence of changes in zinc metabolism. Specifically, the parenteral administration of copper was thought to initiate changes in the hepatic content of zinc which then stimulated the synthesis of hepatic MT. However, it now seems that copper can directly effect the induction of hepatic MT independent of changes in liver zinc. Mercer and Grimes (1986) clearly showed that the intraperitoneal injection of copper caused increased hepatic MT mRNA prior to detectable changes in hepatic zinc. As a result of this and other studies (Kobayashi et al., 1985) copper is now considered to be a direct effector of MT synthesis. In the course of our studies on the induction of hepatic MT in the chick, we have observed markedly different results depending on the route of copper administration (McCormick and Fleet, 1988). If copper were administered intravenously, there was virtually no change in the concentration of hepatic total zinc. On the other hand, if copper were given intraperitoneally, hepatic zinc increased approximately two-fold. Most notably, the accumulation of total hepatic copper under these conditions was equal, strongly suggesting that the exposure of both groups to copper was also comparable. As might be expected, the changes observed in hepatic total metal were a direct reflection of the concentration of hepatic MT (unpublished data). Thus, the additional accumulation of hepatic zinc in chicks given copper i.p. corresponded directly to changes in the concentration of hepatic MT. These results are consistent with a secondary (additional) effect of copper when it is given intraperitoneally. In other words, when copper is given by intraperitoneal injection, an additional effect is manifested in changes in the accumulation of hepatic zinc and MT. We have focused on this additional or secondary effect and have attempted to discern a mechanism by which the induction of MT occurs under these conditions (only). Perhaps the clearest evidence of secondary effects has been obtained in studies of the induction of MT by a metal which does bind to MT, i.e., iron.

MT INDUCTION BY IRON

Several years ago, we reported that the parenteral administration of iron caused the accumulation of MT in liver of chicks (McCormick, 1984). Since we observed no effect of iron in either the kidney or pancreas, we considered the response to be tissue-specific. In addition, data from a feeding trial within that same study suggested that the effect was clearly indirect. Feeding iron (which accomplished similar changes in hepatic iron) had no effect on hepatic MT. Recently, we have focused on further characterizing the effect parenteral iron and have concluded that, analogous to results presented above for zinc and copper, the effect of iron is strongly dependent on the route of iron administration. This conclusion is based on results obtained in an experiment where chicks received an equal amount of iron as ferrous gluconate either by intravenous (i.v.), subcutaneous (s.c.), or intraperitoneal (i.p.) injection. Twenty-four hours later, the concentration of hepatic MT was 25.5 ± 5.0, 23.4 ± 8.4 and 135.7 ± 17.9 μg MT per ml cytosol, respectively (control = 15.5 ± 3.1 μg MT/ml, mean ± SEM). The data clearly showed that only in those chicks given iron by i.p. injection was hepatic MT elevated significantly. From these and other results, we began to suspect that the introduction of a reactive metal (iron or others) into the peritoneal cavity initiated events which led to the induction specifically of hepatic MT. Over the past few years, we have attempted to determine the mechanism of this effect.

The first question that we addressed focused on the chemical nature of the metal. That is, was iron unique or were other chemically similar metals as effective? Our approach was simply to assess the potency of other metals which were chemically similar to iron. We chose two metals considered part of the iron triad, nickel and cobalt, and two others closely positioned in the periodic table, chromium and manganese. Young chicks received (i.p.) equimolar amounts of these metals and iron. After 24 h, liver was obtained and analyzed (by cadmium radioassay) for hepatic MT. The results were quite surprising in that nickel and cobalt were much less effective (28%, $p < .05$) than iron (100%) whereas chromium and manganese were significantly more effective (125%, $p < .05$). These results indicated that the chemical nature of the metal was an important part of the effect and that this may provide a clue for a potential mechanism.

The results obtained with chromium provided a unique opportunity to further investigate the importance of metal chemistry. This metal can exist in several valence states of which two are biologically relevant ($Cr + 3$ and $Cr + 6$). Chromium as $Cr + 6$ is considered carcinogenic and the form which easily crosses cell membranes. On the other hand, $Cr + 3$ lacks genotoxicity and cannot normally penetrate cell membranes (Hansen and Stern, 1986). We initiated an experiment to assess the effects of either form of chromium on the induction of hepatic MT. Young chicks received (i.p.) equal molar injections of either sodium dichromate ($Cr + 6$) or two $Cr + 3$ compounds, potassium dichromate or chromium chloride. At 24 h following the injection, liver was obtained for MT analysis. The results of the experiment (Fleet et al., 1990) were particularly surprising and again indicated that the nature of the metal was an important aspect of the effect. Chromium as $Cr + 6$ was virtually ineffective in causing the accumulation (induction) of hepatic MT.

In contrast, both compounds of chromium as Cr + 3 caused a marked increase in hepatic MT (Figure 2). These data suggest that the valence may be an important factor in the effect of metals on the induction of hepatic MT. In addition and perhaps more importantly, the results may indicate that reactive (reducing) metals which are not well absorbed from the peritoneal cavity (Cr + 3 vs. Cr + 6) are those which are most potent. By incorporating this latter possibility, we have developed a hypothesis to account for the indirect effects of some reactive substances on the induction of hepatic MT. This hypothesis arose only after extensive study of other more obvious possibilities such as have been indicated previously, i.e. changes in zinc metabolism or stress (glucocorticoids).

The parenteral administration of iron (or chromium) causes a marked depression in the concentration of plasma zinc shortly following injection. Originally this observation suggested that perhaps changes in zinc metabolism may directly effect the induction of MT and thus represent the signal by which parenteral iron initiated induction. Several lines of evidence indicate that this is probably not the case. For example, dietary zinc depletion, a condition which reduces plasma zinc markedly, has no effect on the induction of hepatic MT by iron injection (unpublished data). Moreover, and

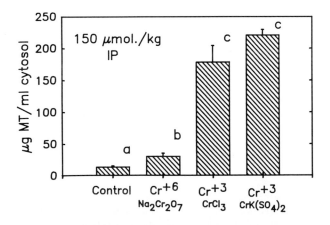

Figure 2. The effect of different parenterally administered chromium compounds on the induction of hepatic MT in the chick. Young chicks were given (i.p.) 150 μmol Cr/kg either as Cr + 6 (disodium chromate), Cr + 3 (CrCl₃) or Cr + 3 (CrK(SO₄)₂) or an equivalent volume of saline (control). Twenty-four hours later, tissues were obtained for MT analysis. Only chromium as Cr + 3 was effective in causing the induction (accumulation) of hepatic MT. These results indicate that Cr valence may be an important factor in the mechanism of MT induction. On the other hand, the results may reflect the inability of Cr + 3 to cross cell membranes.

perhaps more importantly, if one examines the temporal nature of hepatic MT induction following iron injection (by analysis of MT mRNA), changes in plasma zinc are preceded considerably by changes in hepatic MT mRNA. At 3 or 6 h following iron administration, hepatic MT mRNA is increased three to six-fold despite no significant change in the concentration of plasma zinc (unpublished results). Finally, the lack of MT induction due to parenteral iron in other tissues such as the pancreas and kidney seems to indicate that general systemic changes in zinc metabolism cannot account for the observed tissue-specific effect of iron (McCormick, 1984). This latter characteristic has always been considered to be an important clue concerning the mechanism of the iron effect. In this context, we have considered that glucocorticoids may mediate directly the induction of MT during the potentially stressful condition of i.p. Iron administration.

Several years ago, Hager and Palmiter (1981) indicated that the relative induction of MT by glucocorticoids in different tissues was related to the abundance of glucocorticoid receptors in the various tissues. They demonstrated that MT mRNA was highest in liver following dexamethasone treatment and that this coincided with the considerably higher concentration of glucocorticoid receptors in this tissue. We surmised from this and other information that glucocorticoids may represent the effectors of MT induction following iron administration. This clearly was consistent with not only the known effects of glucocorticoids on MT induction but also the observed tissue-specific effects of the iron. We then initiated studies to investigate glucocorticoids as a potential mediator of the iron effect. The results of several studies indicated that circulating glucocorticoids (corticosterone), although elevated moderately following iron injection, were not related to the induction of hepatic MT. Moreover, we showed that parenteral iron caused comparable accumulation of hepatic MT in both intact and adrenalectomized rats (McCormick, 1987). Finally, Petro and Hill (1987) found no relationship in their studies with chicks using glucocorticoid synthesis inhibitors. Therefore, the conclusion from these studies must be that while circulating adrenal hormones may be part of the overall response to iron, hepatic MT induction does not appear to be directly related. In summary then, neither changes in zinc homeostasis nor circulating glucocorticoids represent the principal mechanism accounting for the indirect induction of hepatic MT by nonbinding metals. What then is the mechanism?

INDIRECT MT INDUCTION: THE INFLAMMATORY RESPONSE

One of the well-known characteristics of iron (as well as other trace elements) is its ability to catalyze the formation of hydroxyl radicals from superoxides. This product is thought to be the reactive oxygen radical responsible for the biological toxicity of oxygen (Halliwell, 1987). Since iron can catalyze the formation of damaging free radicals, we began to consider processes which involve production of superoxides. The respiratory burst of phagocytes is the initial stage of inflammation and represents clearly a process which involves the production of superoxides. We began to consider the possibility that parenteral iron might initiate inflammation especially since the route of administration seemed so critical, i.e., only i.p. injections were effective. We initiated studies to assess the infiltration of phagocytic cells into the peritoneal cavity of chicks receiving iron or other substances. Our hypothesis was that i.p. injected iron stimulated the infiltration of phagocytic cells which upon activation produced the signal for hepatic MT induction. The chicken is perhaps an ideal model for this kind of experimental work since this species, in contrast to mammals, does not possess a significant population of "resident" peritoneal macrophages (Rose and Hesketh, 1974). Therefore, a significant change in the number of peritoneal phagocytic cells represents a condition under which cells have been recruited. Our first study focused on assessing whether iron injections caused an increase in the infiltration of cells into the peritoneal cavity. Preliminary results suggested that there was little or no change in the number of macrophages present in the peritoneal cavity at 24 h following the administration of iron (Fleet et al., 1988). However, after further study at earlier time points (3 hours), we have found that iron injection causes a significant increase in the number (and activation state) of heterophils in the peritoneal cavity (Fleet et al., 1990). At this early time point, hepatic MT induction was occurring as evidenced by the increased concentration of hepatic MT mRNA. It appeared then that the infiltration of heterophils into the peritoneal cavity might be an event which is related to the induction of hepatic MT. Interesting, macrophage infiltration was not evident in this experiment suggesting that these cells were not important. The former cells, avian heterophils, are equivalent to mammalian neutrophils and represent in both species the first cells to be recruited during the inflammatory response (Movat et al., 1987). The lack of infiltration of macrophages may be important in considering a mechanism by which hepatic MT induction occurs under these conditions.

Our final study focused on the induction of hepatic MT (or lack of) following the administration of various forms of chromium. If infiltration of phagocytic cells (namely heterophils) were an important and related response in metal-induced hepatic MT accumulation, then we would predict that $Cr+6$ would not cause the infiltration of peritoneal cells. This hypothesis is predicated on our previous observation that this form of chromium (in contrast to $Cr+3$) was not effective in stimulating the accumulation of hepatic MT. The results of our study suggested that indeed our predictions

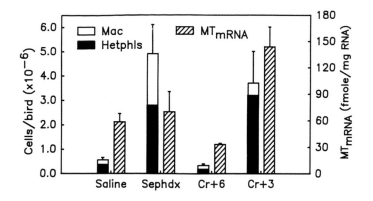

Figure 3. The infiltration of phagocytic cells and the accumulation of hepatic MT mRNA at 3 h following the administration of chromium or Sephadex® (Sephdx). Young chicks were given (i.p.) either Cr + 6 (disodium chromate) or Cr + 3 (chromium chloride) at 150 μmol Cr/kg. Other chicks received 1 ml/kg of a suspension (3%) of cross-linked dextran (G50 Sephadex®, Pharmacia Co.) or an equivalent volume of saline (Saline). At 3 h following treatments, total peritoneal exudate cells were collected and analyzed for macrophages (Mac) and heterophils (Hetphls). Liver was also obtained for MT mRNA analysis. The administration of Cr + 6 did not result in inflammation, i.e., the infiltration of phagocytic cells into the peritoneal cavity, nor did it cause MT induction. In contrast, Cr + 3 administration caused significant infiltration primarily of heterophils and extensive MT induction. The Sephadex® treatment resulted in significant infiltration of both macrophages and heterophils but no significant MT induction. These latter results suggest that MT induction during inflammation may be more closely related to heterophil (vs. macrophage) infiltration or recruitment.

were justified. Equimolar injection of Cr + 6 neither induced hepatic MT nor caused a significant change in the number of either heterophils or macrophages when compared to controls (Figure 3). In contrast, Cr + 3 caused a significant increase in heterophils (but not macrophages) and extensive MT induction. Interestingly, Sephadex® injections which are known to cause the infiltration of phagocytic cells, (Sabet et al., 1977; Trembicki et al., 1984; Qureshi et al., 1986) caused the infiltration of considerably greater numbers of macrophages and a variable response in hepatic MT induction. After several experiments, we have concluded that there appears to be a relationship between the inflammatory response and hepatic MT induction. The correlation is greatest with heterophils both in absolute numbers and in terms of percent of total peritoneal exudate cells. Thus the variable response with Sephadex® may be due to the relatively fewer number (percent) of heterophils elicited by this treatment. Overall, our results suggest that iron (metal) injections cause an inflammatory response and that these events somehow lead to the induction of hepatic MT. Precisely how this may be accomplished is not clear.

In future research, we will consider two principal possibilities. The first of these is that during inflammation phagocytes such as macrophages secrete cytokines which effect (as discussed earlier) the induction of MT. We have indicated, however, that the metal-induced response appears to be more closely related to the infiltration of heterophils, cells not thought to secrete cytokines (Hanson et al., 1980; Dinarello, 1984). Alternatively, the respiratory burst of heterophils in the early stages of the inflammatory response may provide the substrates for iron-catalyzed production of inflammatory metabolites, elements necessary in the events leading to MT induction. Specifically what factor(s) may mediate the induction is not clear. It may be that a serum component(s) is transformed by superoxides (free radicals) during inflammation and that this product represents directly or indirectly the effector of MT synthesis. Precedence for such a suggestion may be indicated in a report by Petrone et al. (1980). These workers demonstrated that inflammation initiated by carrageenan administration causes the formation of a serum factor which was chemotactic to neutrophils. The direct role of superoxides was evidenced by their results showing that the inflammatory response was inhibitable by superoxide dismutase (SOD). In other words, the formation of the chemotactic factor during carrageenan-induced inflammation was completely blocked by prior treatment *(in vivo)* with stabilized SOD. These workers went on to show that albumin (or fatty acids bound to albumin) may represent the chemotactic factor. Thus, we speculate that the respiratory burst of heterophils, initiated by parenteral iron or other substances, results in the formation of a serum factor which leads to the induction of MT. This factor would then represent the signal by which hepatic MT induction is initiated under these conditions. Future work in our laboratory will be aimed at identifying/isolating the factor(s) responsible in this transduction pathway.

REFERENCES

Bracken WM and Klaassen CD (1987): Induction of metallothionein in rat primary hepatocyte cultures: evidence for direct and indirect induction. *J. Toxicol. Environ. Health.* 22: 163.

Bremner I (1987): Involvement of metallothionein in the hepatic metabolism of copper. *J. Nutr.* 117: 19.

Dinarello CA (1984): Interleukin-1. *Rev. Infect. Dis.* 6: 51.

Durnam DM and Palmiter RD (1984): Induction of metallothionein-I mRNA in cultured cells by heavy metals and iodoacetate: evidence for gratuitous inducers. *Mol. Cell. Biol.* 4: 484.

Fleet JC, Qureshi MA, Dietert RR, and McCormick CC (1988): Tissue-specific accumulation of metallothionein in chickens as influenced by the route of zinc administration. *J. Nutr.* 118: 176.

Fleet JC, Golemboski KA, Andrews GK, Dietert RR, and McCormick CC (1990): Induction of hepatic metallothionein by intraperitoneal metal injection in chicks: an associated inflammatory response. *Am. J. Physiol.* 258: G926.

Garg LC, Dixit A, Webb ML, and Jacob ST (1989): Interaction of a positive regulatory factor(s) with a 106-base pair upstream region controls transcription of metallothionein-I gene in the liver. *J. Biol. Chem.* 264: 2134.

Hager LJ and Palmiter RD (1981): Transcriptional regulation of mouse liver metallothionein-I gene by glucocorticoids. *Nature* 291: 340.

Halliwell, B (1987): Oxidants and human disease: some new concepts. *FASEB J.* 1: 358.

Hamer DH (1986): Metallothionein. *Ann. Rev. Biochem.* 55: 913.

Hansen K and Stern RM, Eds. (1986): *Carcinogenic and Mutagenic Metal Compounds: Environmental and Analytical and Biological Effects*, Gordon and Breach, New York, pp. 207–212.

Hanson DF, Murphy PA, and Windle BE (1980): Failure of rabbit neutrophils to secrete endogenous pyrogen when stimulated with staphylococci. *J. Exp. Med.* 151: 1360.

Karin M, Andersen RD, Slater E, Smith K, and Herschman HR (1980): Metallothionein mRNA induction in HeLa cells in response to zinc or dexamethasone is a primary induction response. *Nature* 286: 295.

Kobayashi S, Imano M, and Kimura M (1985): Induction and degradation of Zn-, Cu- and Cd-thionein in Chang liver cells. *Chem. Biol. Interact.* 52: 319.

McCormick CC (1984): The tissue-specific accumulation of hepatic zinc metallothionein following parenteral iron loading. *Proc. Soc. Exp. Biol. Med.* 176: 392.

McCormick CC (1987): Iron-induced accumulation of hepatic metallothionein: the lack of glucocorticoid involvement. *Proc. Soc. Exp. Biol. Med.* 185: 413.

McCormick CC and Fleet JC (1988): The toxicity of parenteral copper in the chick: dependence on route of administration. *J. Nutr.* 118: 1398.

Mercer JFB and Grimes A (1986): Variation in the amounts of hepatic copper, zinc and metallothionein mRNA during development in the rat. *Biochem. J.* 238: 23.

Movat HZ, Cybulsky MI, Colditz IG, Chan MKW, and Dinarello CA (1987): Acute inflammation in Gram-negative infection: endotoxin, interleukin-1, tumor necrosis factor, and neutrophils. *Fed. Proc.* 46: 97.

Petro A and Hill CH (1987): Response of hepatic metallothionein to iron administration. *Biol. Trace Elem. Res.* 14: 255.

Petrone WF, English DK, Wong K, and McCord JM (1980): Free radicals and inflammation: superoxide-dependent activation of a neutrophil chemotactic factor in plasma. *Proc. Natl. Acad. Sci. U.S.A.* 77: 1159.

Qureshi MA, Dietert RR, and Bacon LD (1986): Genetic variation in the recruitment and activation of chicken peritoneal macrophages. *Proc. Soc. Exp. Biol. Med.* 181: 560.

Rose ME and Hesketh P (1974): Fowl peritoneal exudate cell: collection and use for macrophage migration inhibition test. *Avian Pathol.* 3: 297.

Sabet T, Hsia WC, Stanisz W, El-Domeiri A, and VanAlten PA (1977): Simple method for obtaining peritoneal macrophages from chickens. *J. Immunol. Methods* 14: 103.

Searle PF (1987): Metallothionein gene regulation. *Biochem. Soc. Trans.* 15: 584.

Seguin C and Hamer DH (1987): Regulation *in vitro* of metallothionein gene binding factors. *Science* 235: 1383.

Seguin C and Prevost J (1988): Detection of a nuclear protein that interacts with a metal regulatory element of the mouse metallothionein 1 gene. *Nucleic Acids Res.* 16: 10547.

Trembicki KA, Qureshi MA, and Dietert RR (1984): Avian peritoneal exudate cells: a comparison of stimulation protocols. *Dev. Comp. Immunol.* 8: 395.

Westin G and Schaffner W (1988): A zinc-responsive factor interacts with a metal-regulated enhancer element (MRE) of the mouse metallothionein-I gene. *Embo. J.* 7: 3763.

Metallothionein Synthesis in Rats Exposed to Radical Generating Agents

Masao Sato
*Division of Environmental
Pollution Research
Fukushima Medical College
Fukushima, Japan*

ABSTRACT

The induction of metallothionein (MT) synthesis by radical generating agents has been investigated. The administration of paraquat (PQ), a superoxide radical generating agent, to rats increased the pulmonary concentrations of metallothionein-I (MT-I) on day 1 but concentrations returned to the control level by day 5. Synthesis of MT-I was dose-dependent and tissue specific, insofar as the induction occurred in the lung and liver but not in the kidney. The MT synthesized in the liver contained zinc as the bound metal. Induction of MT-I by PQ may reflect *de novo* synthesis since the response in the liver was decreased by pretreatment with actinomycin D. The administration of PQ or carbon tetrachloride (CCl_4) increased the hepatic concentrations not only of MT-I but also of thiobarbituric acid-reactive substances, indicating the occurrence of lipid peroxidation. Pretreatment of the rats with vitamin E prevented the lipid peroxidation caused by PQ or CCl_4 but did not prevent the induction of MT synthesis in the liver. These results suggest that the induction of MT synthesis by radical generating agents is not directly correlated with increased lipid peroxidation. Free radicals may induce MT synthesis by direct or indirect mechanisms.

TABLE I.
Metallothionein Synthesis Induced by Oxidative Stress

Radical Generating Circumstance	Organ, Cells	Reference
CCl_4	Rat liver	Oh et al., 1978
CCl_4	Rat liver	Sato et al., 1984
High O_2 tension	Rat liver, kidney	Shiraishi et al., 1983
X-irradiation	Rat liver	Shiraishi et al., 1983
X-irradiation	Rat liver, kidney	Shiraishi et al., 1986
Paraquat	Rat liver, lung	Sato et al., 1989
Interferon-α (mRNA)	Human neuroblastoma cells	Friedman and Stark, 1985
Interleukin-I (mRNA)	Rat liver, bone marrow, thymus	Cousins and Leinart, 1988
Ultraviolet (mRNA)	Chinese hamster fibroblast	Forace et al., 1988
X-irradiation (mRNA)	Rat liver, kidney, thymus	Shiraishi et al., 1989

INTRODUCTION

Synthesis of metallothionein (MT) can be induced not only by metals but also be stress stimuli. In an early study, Bremner and Davies (1975) demonstrated that restriction of food intake led to enhanced MT synthesis in rat liver. It was subsequently shown that imposition of various types of stress such as partial hepatectomy (Ohtake et al., 1978), cold and hot stress (Oh et al., 1978), sham operation (Brady, 1981), ethanol intoxication (Waalkes et al., 1984), increased tissue MT levels. The range of treatment and agents which can stimulate MT synthesis is being continually extended. These data suggest that MT induction might be a physiological response to stress conditions.

Particular attention has been paid recently to the induction of MT synthesis by free radical generating agents or conditions such as X-irradiation, high oxygen tension (Shiraishi et al., 1983) and carbon tetrachloride (CCl_4) (Oh et al., 1978) (Table 1). In addition, the ability of MT to scavenge free radicals has been demonstrated *in vivo* and *in vitro*. Thornalley and Vašák (1985) showed the ability of Zn-MT to scavenge hydroxyl- and superoxide-radicals. Thomas et al. (1986) demonstrated that MT inhibited the enhancement of lipid peroxidation in erythrocyte ghosts. The proposed antioxidant role of MT is supported by the findings that preinduction of MT prevents the lethal toxicity and lipid peroxidation caused by adriamycin, an antitumor agent (Satoh et al., 1988). Moreover, mice injected with MT-inducing metals such as Zn exhibit marked protection against X-irradiation (Matsubara et al., 1987). In contrast, Arthur et al. (1987) demonstrated that Zn-MT had no effect on lipid peroxidation in liver microsomes. Further studies are required on the mechanism of induction of MT synthesis by radical generating agents, on the relationship to free-radical-mediated lipid peroxidation, and on the physiological role of MT *in vivo*. The aim of the present work was to clarify the role of MT as a radical scavenger by studying the induction of MT synthesis by the superoxide radical generating agent, paraquat (PQ). Attention was focused on the ability of PQ to induce MT synthesis, comparison of the effects of radical generating agents and of antioxidants like vitamin E on MT levels, and identification of factors influencing MT synthesis by radicals.

METHODS

Animals

Male Wistar rats weighing approximately 130 g were used. All rats were housed in a temperature and light controlled room with food and pure water available *ad libitum* and a 12-h light-dark cycle was maintained. Paraquat was dissolved in saline, and CCl_4 and vitamin E were mixed with corn oil, and these were subcutaneously administered to rats. Blood was collected by cardiac puncture under pentobarbital anesthesia, then rats were sacrificed. Tissues were homogenized in cold 1.15% KCl-3 mM Tris-HCl, pH 7.4 under nitrogen atmosphere. The homogenates were used for estimation of degree of lipid peroxidation and zinc (Zn) content.

Analysis

The degree of lipid peroxidation was estimated by formation of thiobarbituric acid reactive substances (TBA-RS). The TBA method for malondialdehyde (MDA) described by Uchiyama and Mihara (1978) was used. MT-I was determined by the radioimmunoassay developed by Mehra and Bremner (1983). The supernatants of the homogenates ($1500 \times g$, 15 min) were used for estimation of MT-I. Sheep anti-rat MT-I serum was kindly provided by Dr. I. Bremner, Rowett Research Institute, Scotland. Donkey anti-sheep IgG was obtained from the Scottish Antibody Production Unit (Carluke, Scotland).

RESULTS

Metallothionein Synthesis Induced by Paraquat

Paraquat (1,1'-dimethyl-4,4'-dipyridium) is widely used as a herbicide. The damage caused by PQ is manifested at first by hemorrhage and edema,

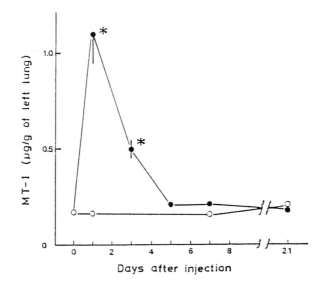

Figure 1. Concentration of pulmonary metallothionein-I (MT-I) at various times following paraquat administration. Rats were intraperitoneally injected with paraquat (22.5 mg/kg). Values are the mean ± S.E. of 4 to 5 rats. *Denotes significant difference from the control ($p < 0.05$). ○, control; ●, paraquat. (From Sato et al. [1989], *Toxicol. Lett.* 45:41. With permission.)

and then by the development of fibrosis (Faishter and Wilson, 1975). In order to determine whether PQ stimulates MT formation in the lung, rats were intraperitoneally injected with PQ (22.5 mg/kg). When compared with control rats, the pulmonary concentration of MT-I increased 7-fold by 24 h (Figure 1). Increased accumulation of MT-I was also observed at 3 d but concentrations returned to control levels by day 5. The plasma concentration of MT-I was also increased at 1 day. When rats were subcutaneously (s.c.) injected with PQ (40 mg/kg), the concentrations of MT-I began to increase 6 h after the injection (not shown). The pulmonary concentration of MT-I increased with increase in dose of PQ (20 to 40 mg/kg, s.c.).

Since PQ administration causes hepatic (Burk et al., 1980) and renal (Lock and Ishmael, 1979) damage, the effects of PQ administration on the renal and hepatic concentrations of Zn and MT were also examined. Administration of PQ resulted in an increase in Zn in the liver, but not in the kidney. The MT-I concentrations increased 7-fold in the lung, and approximately 30-fold in the liver (Figure 2). In contrast, PQ exposure did not increase renal MT concentrations, although the MT-I levels in control rats were higher in the kidney than in the liver and lung.

Mechanism of Metallothionein Synthesis Induced by Paraquat

The concentration of Zn significantly increased in the liver of the PQ-treated rats. The cytosol prepared from livers of saline- and PQ-treated rats (40 mg/kg, s.c.) was fractionated by gel filtration (Sephadex G-75®) to separate the major Zn-binding proteins. The results indicated that an induced Zn-binding protein with a retention coefficient (Ve/Vo) of an approximately 2.1 was present in the liver cytosol from PQ-treated rat. This peak, which corresponded in elution volume to authentic rat Cd-MT-I, contained no detectable copper (Cu). These data indicate that the metalloform of MT induced by PQ was Zn-MT.

When rats were injected with actinomycin D (1.0 mg/kg, s.c.) 2 h prior to injection of PQ (30 mg/kg, s.c.) or Zn (15 mg/kg, s.c.), the synthesis of hepatic MT-I was inhibited. Concentrations in the control PQ- and Zn-treated rats were 45.0 ± 2.8 and 167.5 ± 2.6 µg/g respectively, whereas they

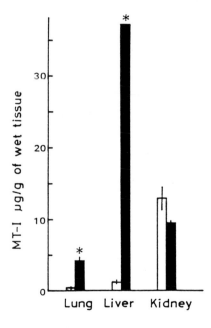

Figure 2. Tissue specific changes in metallothionein-I (MT-I) concentration following a single paraquat administration. Rats were killed 24 h after the injection of paraquat (30 mg/kg, subcutaneously). Values are mean ± S.E. of 5 rats. *Indicates significant difference from control at $p < 0.05$. ☐, saline; ■, paraquat.

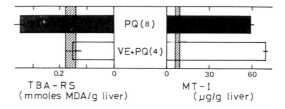

Figure 3. Effect of vitamin E pretreatment on the concentrations of metallothionein-I (MT-I) and thiobarbituric acid-reactive substances (TBA-RS), as an indicator of lipid peroxidation, in the liver of paraquat-treated rats. Rats were injected daily with ethanol (0.6 ml/kg, s.c.) or DL-α-tocopherol (VE, 400 mg/kg, s.c.) for 4 d before injection of saline (□, 5 ml/kg, s.c.) or paraquat (PQ, 30 mg/kg, s.c.). Rats were killed 16 h after the last injection. Numbers in parenthesis indicate number of rats. *Denotes significant difference from control at $p < 0.05$.

were only 23.8 ± 3.0 and 30.3 ± 4.9 μg/g respectively when the rats were pretreated with actinomycin D.

Restriction of food intake increases MT concentrations in the liver (Bremner and Davies, 1975), although the mechanism whereby this occurs remains unresolved. Since PQ exposure caused great body weight loss, starvation could be one of the factors contributing to the enhanced MT levels in tissues of PQ-treated rats. Hepatic and pulmonary concentrations of MT-I increased in both PQ-treated and starved rats, but were greater in the former. This indicates that food deprivation cannot account for the increase in MT-I concentrations in the PQ-treated rats.

Relationship Between Lipid Peroxidation and Metallothionein Synthesis

Administration of PQ caused an increase in the concentrations of Zn, MT-I and TBA-RS in the rat liver (Figures 2 and 3). In the kidney, however, PQ did not affect MT-I concentration although it did increase the concentration of TBA-RS. These results suggest that the enhancement of lipid peroxidation is not always correlated with the induction of MT synthesis.

Figure 3 shows the effect of pretreatment with vitamin E on the concentrations of MT and TBA-RS in the liver of PQ-treated rats. Three groups of rats were injected on 4 successive days with vitamin E (DL-α-tocopherol, 400 mg/kg, s.c.) or ethanol (0.6 ml/kg, s.c.). They were then subcutaneously injected with saline (5 ml/kg) or PQ (30 mg/kg). As was found previously, the concentrations of MT-I and TBA-RS increased in the livers of PQ-treated rats. Pretreatment with vitamin E did not prevent the increase in MT-I but it did prevent the enhancement of TBA-RS content in PQ-treated rats. Similar results were obtained in the lung.

The effect of pretreatment with vitamin E on the concentration of MT-I in tissues from CCl_4-treated rats was also studied. Rats were pretreated with vitamin E as in the PQ-treated animals. Hepatic concentrations of TBA-RS and MT-I significantly increased in the CCl_4-treated rats (not shown). Pretreatment with vitamin E again prevented the enhancement of TBA-RS concentration induced by CCl_4, but did not block the increase in MT-I levels.

Figure 4 shows the effect of vitamin E pretreatment on MT synthesis in starved rats. Food deprivation increased the concentrations of TBA-RS and MT-I in the liver. Pretreatment with vitamin E abolished the increase in TBA-RS in starved rats, but did not affect the ability of starvation to induce liver MT-I synthesis.

The effect of Zn pretreatment on PQ-induced MT synthesis and lipid peroxidation was also examined. Groups of rats were injected with Zn (10 mg/kg, s.c.) or saline 48 and 24 h before the injection of PQ (30 mg/kg, s.c.) or saline (5 ml/kg, s.c.). They were killed 24 h after the last injection. Pretreatment with Zn or injection of PQ each increased hepatic MT-I concentrations approximately 30-fold (Figure 5). The Zn concentration also increased in both groups. However, in the PQ-dosed rats which were pretreated with Zn, the MT-I concentrations increased by more than 300-fold. This marked synergistic interaction between Zn and PQ was also evident in the lung and kidney. The hepatic concentrations of TBA-RS were increased by PQ-administration ($p < 0.01$) but there was no effect of Zn pretreatment (not shown).

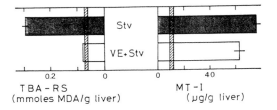

Figure 4. Effect of vitamin E pretreatment on the concentrations of metallothionein-I (MT-I) and thiobarbituric acid-reactive substances (TBA-RS) in the liver of starved rats. Rats were injected daily with ethanol (0.6 ml/kg, s.c.) or DL-α-tocopherol (VE, 400 mg/kg, s.c.) for 4 d before injection of saline (▨, 5 ml/kg, s.c.) or treatment of food deprivation for 18 h (Stv). Values are the mean ± S.E. of 4 rats. *Denotes significant difference from control at $p < 0.05$.

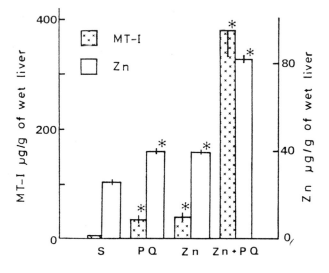

Figure 5. Effect of Zn pretreatment on MT-I concentration in the liver of paraquat-treated rats. Rats were injected daily with Zn (10 mg/kg, s.c.) for 2 d before injection of saline (S, 5 ml/kg) or paraquat (PQ, 30 mg/kg, s.c.). Rats were killed after the last injection. Values are the mean ± S.E. *Denotes significant difference from control at $p < 0.05$.

Investigation on Possible Factors Influencing Metallothionein Synthesis by Radical Generating Agents

Tissue Damage

It has been reported that partial hepatectomy causes induction of MT synthesis (Ohtake et al., 1978). Since the induction of MT and increase in hepatic Zn and Cu may function as a cellular repair mechanism after toxic exposure (Cousins, 1985), the relationship between MT synthesis and tissue damage was investigated in the CCl_4-treated rats. In CCl_4-treated rats, plasma aspartate aminotransferase (AST) activity and liver TBA-RS content were significantly increased compared to the controls. Pretreatment with vitamin E (DL-α-tocopherol, 400 mg/kg, s.c.) for 4 d prevented the increase in plasma AST activity and hepatic TBA-RS concentration but did not prevent the enhancement of MT-I synthesis induced by CCl_4 administration. It appears therefore that liver damage and its repairing process are not responsible for the induction of MT synthesis by radical generating agents.

Glucagon

Studies were carried out on the time course of MT synthesis and hormonal changes following PQ administration. Plasma glucagon levels, as measured by radioimmunoassay kit (Dinabot Corp. Ltd., Tokyo), increased at 4 and 10 h following PQ administration (not shown). However, the increase was relatively slight, indicating that the secreted glucagon does not contribute to the increase in the MT concentration in tissues. The concentration of MT-I first increased at 2.5 h in the liver and at 6 h in the lung.

Other Factors

Administration of PQ increases neutrophil counts in bronchoalveolar lavage (Martin and Howard, 1986). Since polymorphonuclear leukocytes like macrophages can produce tumor necrosis factor (TNF) (Yamazaki et al., 1989), the effect of TNF on MT synthesis was examined. When groups of rats were subcutaneously injected with recombinant TNF (10^5 U per rat), the concentrations of MT-I in the liver and lungs 16 h thereafter were 58.3 ± 7.0 and 0.82 ± 0.15 μg/g, respectively. Concentrations in the control rats were 4.7 ± 1.8 and 0.46 ± 0.01 μg/g, respectively.

DISCUSSION

It has so far been reported that MT synthesis is induced by radical generating agents and conditions such as high oxygen-tension, X-irradiation or treatment with CCl_4 (Table I). The present paper shows that MT synthesis is also induced by the superoxide radical generating agent, PQ. X-irradiation produces a large amount of hydroxyl radicals in the body. Active oxygen species of high oxygen tensions are hydrogen peroxide and superoxide radical. Carbon tetrachloride is converted to the trichlormethyl radical (CCl_3) and the trichloromethyl peroxyradical (CCl_3O_2) by a microsomal cytochrome-P-450-dependent monooxygenase system (Hodgson and Levi, 1987). Thus, most species of active oxygen seem to induce MT synthesis, although no induction was observed after X-irradiation in Chinese hamster lung fibroblast (Fornace et al., 1988).

Tissue specific synthesis of MT by various compounds has been reported at the levels of both protein and mRNA. Administration of CCl_4 to rats increased Zn-MT levels in the liver but not in the kidney (Oh et al., 1978). In X-irradiated rats, MT synthesis occurred in the liver and kidney but not in the lung (Shiraishi et al., 1986). The present study also showed tissue specificity of MT synthesis in PQ-treated rats, with an increase in the liver and lung but not in the kidney (Figure 2) and spleen (not shown). Furthermore, elevation in MT mRNA levels was observed in liver, kidney and thymus of X-irradiated rats but not in brain, spleen, lung, heart and testis (Shiraishi et al., 1989). Northern blot analysis revealed an increase in MT mRNA levels in the liver, bone marrow and thymus of rats treated with interleukin-1. However no appreciable increase in expression was detected in the kidney (Cousins and Leinart, 1988).

The cause of the tissue specificity in MT formation is still unknown, although, in the case of the PQ-treated rats, there are many possible explanations. For example there may be differences in the rates of radical formation in the tissues (Baldwin et al., 1975). The dipyridium di-cations, PQ, are thought to be reduced to the radical cations, with subsequent oxidation to di-cations by molecular oxygen; this process is essential for the toxicity of PQ. The order of radical formation among tissues is consistent with that of MT synthesis.

Although MT is thought to act as an efficient free radical scavenger, the physiological significance of stress-induced MT synthesis is uncertain. Intracellular concentrations of glutathione (GSH) are usually much higher than those of MT and this peptide is also an efficient scavenger of free radicals (Bremner, 1987). The concentration of GSH in the liver for example, is about 6.0 μmol/g of wet liver (Igarashi et al., 1983), whereas that of MT-I in starved rats was 70 μg/g (Figure 4). Assuming that MT-I accounts for half of the total liver MT, the total hepatic concentration of MT would be 0.02 μmol/g; the concentration of GSH could therefore be 300 times higher than that of MT. However, when isolated rat liver was perfused with 1 mM PQ, the GSH content was reduced to 29% of the control (Brigelius and Anwer, 1981). In addition, the *in vitro* reaction rate constants are $K_{.OH/GSH} = 8 \times 10^9$ M^{-1} S^{-1} and $K_{.OH/MT} = 3 \times 10^{12}$ M^{-1} S^{-1} (Thornalley and Vašák, 1985). Since the rate constant for interaction of MT with hydroxyl radicals is so high, the increased MT in the liver may be important as one of the radical scavengers. Further investigations are still required to establish the physiological relevance of the action of MT in the liver as a radical scavenger.

PQ is reduced by microsomal NADPH-cytochrome *c* reductase to the PQ radical, which subsequently produces the superoxide radical. Then, PQ initiates the membrane damaging process of lipid peroxidation via generation of active oxygen species (Bus and Gibson, 1984). In the present study, administration of PQ resulted in an enhancement of lipid peroxidation, as indicated by increased TBA-RS content, in body weight loss, and also in an increase in MT synthesis (Figure 3). Pretreatment with vitamin E completely prevented the enhancement of TBA-RS in the liver, but did not change either the elevated levels of MT-I or the decreased body weight. These data suggest that enhancement of lipid peroxidation is not correlated with synthesis of MT induced by PQ. Since the production of PQ radicals and superoxide radicals is essential to develop the toxicity of PQ, superoxide and/or other radicals may be responsible for MT synthesis in PQ-treated rats (Figure 6).

However, the data shown in Figure 3 are inconsistent with the report

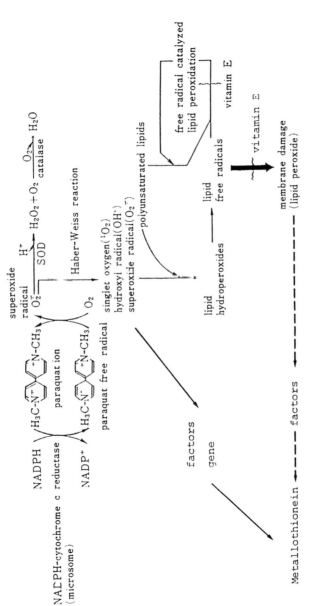

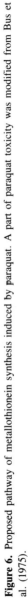

Figure 6. Proposed pathway of metallothionein synthesis induced by paraquat. A part of paraquat toxicity was modified from Bus et al. (1975).

that the enhancement by immobilization stress of MT synthesis and lipid peroxidation is decreased by vitamin E (Hidalgo et al., 1988). The reason for those differences, is, as yet, unknown. In order to investigate whether the relationship between lipid peroxidation and MT synthesis induced by PQ is a common phenomenon, the effect of vitamin E pretreatment on MT synthesis under the radical generating condition, starvation, was studied. As shown in Figure 4, food deprivation increased the concentrations of both TBA-RS and MT-I in the liver, but pretreatment with vitamin E only prevented the enhancement in TBA-RS content. Similar results were obtained with CCl_4-treated rats. Thus, the increase in MT synthesis induced under radical generating circumstances was not correlated with enhanced lipid peroxidation.

MT synthesis can be induced by hormones such as glucocorticoids, glucagon, and epinephrine and by a number of other factors including cAMP, interferon and interleukin-1 (Dunn et al., 1987). Hidalgo et al. (1986) suggested that stress-induced MT production involved more than glucocorticoid or glucagon alone. Lipopolysaccharide-induced MT synthesis is mediated by an unknown factor released from macrophages (Iijima et al., 1987). Radicals, directly or indirectly through some other factors, may induce MT synthesis (Figure 6). In the present study, possible factors such as glucagon, tumor necrosis factor or repairing process of tissue damage were investigated. Recently, Grimble and Bremner (1989) also observed an ability of TNF to induce MT synthesis in the liver.

A synergistic interaction between PQ and Zn on MT synthesis was also shown (Figure 5). Reports on similar synergistic effects between glucocorticoid and glucagon (Etzel and Cousins, 1981) and Zn and immobilization stress (Hidalgo et al., 1988) have been published, although their mechanisms remain unknown.

ACKNOWLEDGMENTS

The author is grateful to Mr. Misao Sasaki and Ms. Iwako Kanno for their skillful technical assistance. Continuous encouragement given by Dr. I. Bremner is also greatly appreciated. The author expresses appreciation to Asahi Kasei Corp. Ltd. for supplying the TNF.

REFERENCES

Arthur JR, Bremner I, Morrice PC, and Mills CF (1987): Stimulation of peroxidation in rat liver microsomes by (copper, zinc)-metallothioneins. *Free Radiat. Res. Commun.* 4: 15.

Baldwin RC, Pasi A, MacGregor JT, and Hine CH (1975): The rates of radical formation from the dipyridylium herbicides paraquat, diquat and marfamquat in homogenates of rat lung, kidney and liver: an inhibitory effect of carbon monoxide. *Toxicol. Appl. Pharmacol.* 32: 298.

Brady FO (1981): Synthesis of rat hepatic thionein in response to the stress of sham operation. *Life Sci.* 28: 1647.

Bremner I (1987): Nutritional and physiological significance metallothionein. In *Metallothionein II*, Kägi JHR and Kojima Y, Eds., Birkhäuser-Verlag, Basel, pp. 81–107.

Bremner I and Davies NT (1975): The induction of metallothionein in rat liver by zinc injection and restriction of food intake. *Biochem. J.* 149: 733.

Brigelius R and Anwer MS (1981): Increased biliary GSSG-secretion and loss of hepatic glutathione in isolated perfused rat liver after paraquat treatment. *Res. Commun. Chem. Pathol. Pharmacol.* 31: 493.

Burk RF, Lawrence RA, and Lane JM (1980): Liver necrosis and lipid peroxidation in the rat as the result of paraquat and diquat administration: effect of selenium deficiency. *J. Clin. Invest.* 65: 1024.

Bus JS, Aust SD, and Gibson JE (1975): Lipid peroxidation: a possible mechanism for paraquat toxicity. *Res. Commun. Pathol. Pharmacol.* 11: 31.

Bus JS and Gibson JE (1984): Paraquat: model for oxidant-initiated toxicity. *Environ. Health Perspect.* 55: 37.

Cousins RJ (1985): Absorption, transport, and hepatic metabolism of copper and zinc: special reference to metallothionein and ceruloplasmin. *Physiol. Rev.* 65: 238.

Cousins RJ and Leinart AS (1988): Tissue-specific regulation of zinc metabolism and metallothionein genes by interleukin 1. *FASEB J.* 2: 2884.

Dunn MA, Blalock TL, and Cousins RJ (1987): Metallothionein. *Proc. Soc. Exp. Biol. Med.* 185: 107.

Etzel KR and Cousins RJ (1981): Hormonal regulation of liver metallothionein zinc: independent and synergistic action of glucagon and glucocorticoids. *Proc. Soc. Exp. Biol. Med.* 167: 233.

Fairshter RD and Wilson AF (1975): Paraquat poisoning, manifestations and therapy. *Am. J. Med.* 59: 751.

Fornace AJ, Jr, Schalch H, and Alam I, Jr (1988): Coordinate induction of metallothioneins I and II in rodent cells by UV irradiation. *Mol. Cell. Biol.* 8: 4716.

Friedman RL and Stark GR (1985): α-Interferon-induced transcription of HLA and metallothionein genes containing homologous upstream sequences. *Nature* 314: 637.

Grimble RF and Bremner I (1989): Tumor necrosis factor enhances hepatic metallothionein-I content but reduces that of the kidney. *Proc. Nutr. Soc.* 48: 64A.

Hidalgo J, Armario A, Flos R, Dingman A, and Garvey JS (1986): The influence of restraint stress in rats on metallothionein production and corticosterone and glucagon secretion. *Life Sci.* 39: 611.

Hidalgo J, Campany L, Borras M, Garvey JS, and Armario A (1988): Metallothionein response to stress in rats: role in free radical scavenging. *Am. J. Physiol.* 255: E518.

Hodgson E and Levi PE, Eds. (1987): *A Textbook of Modern Toxicology,* Elsevier, New York, pp. 133–184.

Igarashi T, Satoh T, Ueno K, and Kitagawa H (1983): Sex-related difference in the hepatic glutathione level and related enzyme activities in rat. *J. Biochem.* 93: 33.

Iijima Y, Takahashi T, Fukushima T, Abe S, Itano Y, and Kosaka F (1987): Induction of metallothionein by a macrophage factor and the partial characterization of the factor. *Toxicol. Appl. Pharmacol.* 89: 135.

Lock ED and Ishmael J (1979): The acute toxic effects of paraquat and diquat on the rat kidney. *Toxicol. Appl. Pharmacol.* 50: 67.

Martin WJ II and Howard DM (1986): Paraquat-induced neutrophil alveolitis: reduction of the inflammatory response by pretreatment with endotoxin and hyperoxia. *Lung* 164: 107.

Matsubara J, Shida T, Ishioka K, Egawa S, Inada T, and Machida K (1986): Protective effect of zinc against lethality in irradiated mice. *Environ. Res.* 41: 558.

Mehra RK and Bremner I (1983): Development of a radioimmunoassay for rat liver metallothionein-I and its application to the analysis of rat plasma and kidney. *Biochem. J.* 213: 459.

Oh SH, Deagen JT, Whanger PD, and Weswig PH (1978): Biological function of metallothionein. V. Its induction in rats by various stresses. *Am. J. Physiol.* 234: E282.

Ohtake H, Hasegawa K, and Koga M (1978): Zinc-binding protein in the livers of neonatal, normal and partially hepatectomized rats. *Biochem. J.* 174: 999.

Sato M, Mehra RK, and Bremner I (1984): Measurement of plasma metallothionein-I in the assessment of the zinc status of zinc-deficient and stressed rats. *J. Nutr.* 114: 1683.

Sato M, Ohtake A, Takeda K, and Mizunuma H (1989): Metallothionein-I accumulation in the rat lung following a single paraquat administration. *Toxicol. Lett.* 45: 41.

Satoh M, Naganuma A, and Imura N (1988): Involvement of cardiac metallothionein in prevention of adriamycin induced lipid peroxidation in the heart. *Toxicology,* 53: 231.

Shiraishi N, Aono K, and Utsumi K (1983): Increased metallothionein content in rat liver induced by X-irradiation and exposure to high oxygen tension. *Radiat. Res.* 95: 298.

Shiraishi N, Yamamoto H, Takeda Y, Kondoh S, Hayashi H, Hashimoto K, and Aono K (1986): Increased metallothionein content in rat liver and kidney following X-irradiation. *Toxicol. Appl. Pharmacol.* 85: 128.

Shiraishi N, Hayashi H, Hiraki Y, Aono K, Itano Y, Kosaka F, Noji S, and Taniguchi S (1989): Elevation in metallothionein messenger RNA in rat tissue after exposure to X-irradiation. *Toxicol. Appl. Pharmacol.* 98: 501.

Thomas JP, Bachowski GJ, and Girotti AW (1986): Inhibition of cell membrane lipid peroxidation by cadmium- and zinc-metallothioneins. *Biochem. Biophys. Acta.* 884: 448.

Thornalley PJ and Vašák M (1985): Possible role for metallothionein in protection against radiation-induced oxidative stress. Kinetics and mechanism of its reaction with superoxide and hydroxyl radicals. *Biochem. Biophys. Acta* 827: 36.

Uchiyama M and Mihara M (1978): Determination of malonaldehyde precursor in tissue by thiobarbituric acid test. *Anal. Biochem.* 86: 271.

Waalkes MP, Hjelle JJ, and Klaassen CD (1984): Transient induction of hepatic metallothionein following oral ethanol administration. *Toxicol. Appl. Pharmacol.* 74: 230.

Yamazaki M, Ikenami M, and Sugiyama T (1989): Cytotoxin from polymorpho-nuclear leukocytes and inflammatory ascitic fluids. *Br. J. Cancer* 59: 353.

Chapter 18

Effects of Epidermal Growth Factor on Metallothionein Induction in Mammalian Cells

Shizuko Kobayashi and Junko S. Suzuki
Kyoritsu College of Pharmacy
Tokyo, Japan

Chiharu Tohyama
Environmental Health Sciences Division
National Institute for Environmental Studies
Ibaraki, Japan

SUMMARY

In order to elucidate possible physiological roles of isoforms of metallothionein (MT) in cellular growth, we have studied effects of zinc (Zn^{2+}), glucocorticoid and epidermal growth factor (EGF) on biosynthesis of isoMTs in a mouse mammary carcinoma cell line (FM3A) by anion exchange high performance liquid chromatography (HPLC).

In the presence of both Zn^{2+} (15 μM) and glucocorticoid (dexamethasone; 1 nM), MTs were either induced in very small amounts or not induced at all. Addition of EGF (10 ng/ml) to the culture medium resulted in significant induction of MTs. Most MTs were separated into three isoforms, designated as MT-1, MT-2-1, and MT-2-2. In the growing cells, the HPLC profile of isoMTs induced in the presence of EGF as well as both gluco-corticoid and Zn^{2+} showed a single Zn-associated peak, corresponding to MT-2-2 subfraction. Induction of MT-2-2 isoform may be related to cellular proliferation.

INTRODUCTION

Metallothioneins (MTs) are present in various organs of a large variety of animal species under physiological conditions. Interestingly, concentrations of MTs are low in adult tissues, whereas fetal liver harbors high levels of MT mRNA as well as significant amounts of hepatic zinc (Zn^{2+}) and/ or copper which are bound to MT polypeptides (Quaife et al., 1986). A similar finding was observed in the regenerating adult liver, in which partial hepatectomy exerted an increase in liver zinc and concomitant synthesis of MT (Ohtake et al., 1978).

Recently, it has been demonstrated that MT gene expression is regulated not only by serum cell growth factors and protein kinase C activators (Imbra and Karin, 1987), but also by cAMP (Nebes et al., 1988). Metallothionein has been localized mainly in the cytoplasm of hepatocytes of adult rats. In the fetal and neonatal kidney, however, MT has been found mainly in the nucleus and cytoplasm of the proximal tubular epithelial cells of human (Nartey et al., 1987) and rat (Banerjee et al., 1982; Nishimura et al., 1989). These results suggest a possible close association of MT synthesis with cellular proliferation although the exact functions of MT in cell metabolism are unknown.

We have studied whether MT can be induced by an additional epidermal growth factor (EGF) in the presence of physiological concentrations of Zn^{2+} and glucocorticoid.

MATERIALS AND METHODS

Cell Cultures

Mouse mammary carcinoma FM3A cells, at concentrations of 1×10^5 cells/ml in ES medium (Nissui Pharmaceutical Co., Tokyo, Japan) supplemented with 2 mM glutamine and 2.5% fetal-calf serum, were incubated at 33°C in a humidified atmosphere of CO_2/air (1:19). In the present experiment, 10 ng/ml of mouse EGF (Sigma Chem. Co., St. Louis, MO) was added to culture medium which were kept at a concentration of 1×10^6 cells/ml (exponential-phase growth) in the presence of 1 nM dexamethasone. After

24 h-incubation, Zn^{2+} was added to the medium to make its concentration 15 μM and incubation was carried out for 24 h thereafter. The treated cells were washed four times with Hanks' balanced salt solution and kept frozen at $-70°C$ until used.

Preparation of Metallothioneins

The treated cells were homogenized with a Potter-type homogenizer in 5 vol of 0.01 M Tris-HCl buffer (pH 7.5) containing 0.01 M NaHSO$_3$, 2 mM dithiothreitol, 2 μg of antipain/ml and 1 μM pepstatin at 4°C. Dithiothreitol was added to the homogenates to protect the MT from oxidation (at a final concentration of 1 mM). The homogenates were treated at 80°C for 1 min and centrifuged at $170,000 \times g$ for 60 min. The supernatants were applied to a Sephadex G-75® column (1.8 × 45 cm) equilibrated with 0.01 M Tris-HCl buffer (pH 7.5) containing 0.01 M NaHSO$_3$ and 2 mM dithiothreitol and then eluted with the same buffer at a flow rate of 10 ml/h. The concentration of Zn^{2+} in each fraction was measured by atomic absorption spectrometry. The MT fraction (Ve/Vo = 1.8 to 2.0) was pooled and concentrated with Dextran T-40® (Pharmacia Fine Chemicals AB, Uppsala, Sweden) in cellulose dialysis tubes (M$_r$ cut-off level, 1,000; Spectrum Medical Industries, Los Angeles, CA). The concentrated MT fractions were applied to a DEAE-Sephadex A-25® column (0.95 × 20 cm) equilibrated with 0.01 M Tris-HCl buffer, pH 7.5 at 4°C. After the sample was applied to the column, 0.01 M Tris-HCl buffer was used as the eluent for 30 fractions at a flow rate of 15 ml/h. Then a linear gradient of NaCl (0 to 200 mM) in 0.01 M Tris-HCl buffer, pH 7.5, was used as the eluent. The Zn-binding fractions (MT-1 and MT-2) were rechromatographed, dialysed against 10 mM NH$_4$HCO$_3$, freeze-dried and used as standard samples for analysis of isoMT by high performance liquid chromatography (HPLC) on an anion exchange column.

Analysis of MTs by HPLC

The HPLC instrument consisted of a chromatograph (Shimadzu HPLC CL-6A Gradient System; Shimadzu Co., Kyoto, Japan) and an anion exchange chromatography column (Asahipak ES-502N®, 13 ± 0.5 μm particle size; 7.6 × 100 mm column; Asahi Chemical Industries Co., Kawasaki, Japan).

An aliquot (10 μl) of the concentrated MT fraction was chromatographed with a linear gradient of 4 to 52 mM potassium phosphate buffer, pH 7.5, at a flow rate of 0.5 ml/min (Kobayashi and Suzuki, 1988a,b). The peak fractions detected by absorbance at 220 nm were collected with a Frac-100® (Pharmacia Fine Chemicals AB), and Zn^{2+} concentrations were determined by atomic absorption spectrometry.

MT Identification by Radioimmunoassay

The MT fraction obtained from an anion exchange HPLC column was identified by radioimmunoassay using rabbit antiserum against human MT-1, which completely cross-reacted with mouse MT. The immunization protocol and characteristics of the antiserum were essentially the same as described earlier (Tohyama and Shaikh, 1981).

Protein Assay

Protein concentration in the MT fraction obtained by gel filtration was measured by the dye-binding method of Bradford (1976), using a Bio-Rad® protein assay kit (Bio-Rad Laboratories, Richmond, VA).

RESULTS

As reported in our previous paper (Kobayashi and Suzuki, 1988b), mouse MTs were separated into three isoforms by anion-exchange HPLC column; mouse Zn-MT-1 and Zn-MT-2 purified by DEAE-Sephadex A-25® column chromatography showed a single peak and two peaks, respectively (Figure 1A). The designated MT-1, MT-2-1, and MT-2-2 subfractions were eluted at retention times of 13 to 14 min (4 mM potassium phosphate buffer), 26 to 27 min (7–8 mM) and 29 to 30 min (11–12 mM), respectively. A typical HPLC elution profile of MT fraction obtained from gel filtration of an adult Zn-treated mouse liver, showed three separated peaks at retention times corresponding to MT-1, MT-2-1, and MT-2-2 (Figure 1B). The Zn^{2+} amounts in each of these individual peaks accounted for 36, 8, and 30% of total amounts of Zn^{2+} applied to the column (Zn recovery), respectively. These results indicate that mouse isoMTs could be separated and analysed by applying the MT fraction, obtained from gel filtration, to an anion exchange HPLC column.

In the present experiments, mouse mammary carcinoma FM3A cells (10^6 cells per ml) were treated with dexamethasone or EGF for the first 24 h and Zn^{2+} for another 24 h. The MT fractions obtained from cells treated with 1 μM dexamethasone and 75 μM Zn^{2+} showed three peaks on the column corresponding to MT-1, MT-2-1, and MT-2-2 subfractions. The Zn recoveries for the individual peaks were: MT-1, 12%; MT-2-1, 8%; MT-2-2, 40% (Figure 2A). When cells were treated with 1 μM dexamethasone and 15 μM Zn^{2+}, a single Zn-associated peak, at a retention time of 29 to 30 min, corresponding to MT-2-2 was found whereas no detectable amounts of Zn^{2+} was eluted for other isoMTs; Zn^{2+} recovery was 60% (Figure 2B). These results suggest that the major mouse isoMT induced by glucocorticoid is an MT-2-2 isoform and a low concentration of Zn^{2+} added to the culture medium is found to bind to the induced MT.

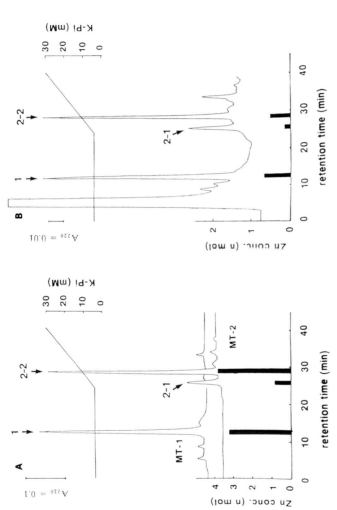

Figure 1. HPLC elution profiles of the isolated MT-1 and MT-2 (A) and the MT fraction obtained from gel filtration (B) of sample from liver of Zn-treated adult mouse. (A) Ten-week-old day female mice were given an intraperitoneal dose of 10 mg of Zn^{2-}/kg body weight and livers were removed 24 h later. Two isoMTs, MT-1 and MT-2 were isolated by gel filtration with a Sephadex G-75® column and anion-exchange chromatography with a DEAE-Sephadex A-25® column. A 10 μl sample of MT-1 or MT-2 was applied to an anion-exchange HPLC column. (B) The MT fraction was obtained by Sephadex G-75® gel filtration of supernatant from livers of Zn-treated adult mice. A 10 μl sample of the MT fraction was applied to an anion-exchange HPLC column. Chromatography was performed at 0.5 ml/min, with a gradient of 4 to 52 mM potassium phosphate buffer, pH 7.5. The peaks detected at an absorbance at 220 nm were collected and Zn^{2+} concentration in the peaks were determined by atomic absorption spectrometry.

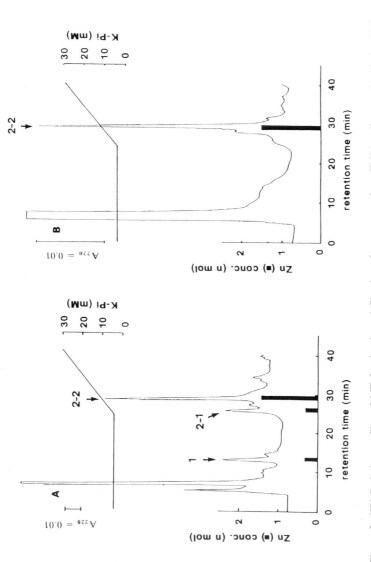
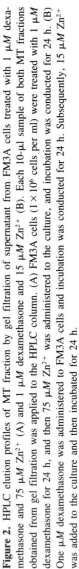

Figure 2. HPLC elution profiles of MT fraction by gel filtration of supernatant from FM3A cells treated with 1 μM dexamethasone and 75 μM Zn^{2+} (A) and 1 μM dexamethasone and 15 μM Zn^{2+} (B). Each 10-μl sample of both MT fractions obtained from gel filtration was applied to the HPLC column. (A) FM3A cells (1×10^6 cells per ml) were treated with 1 μM dexamethasone for 24 h, and then 75 μM Zn^{2+} was administered to the culture, and incubation was conducted for 24 h. (B) One μM dexamethasone was administered to FM3A cells and incubation was conducted for 24 h. Subsequently, 15 μM Zn^{2+} was added to the culture and then incubated for 24 h.

When cells treated with physiological concentration of dexamethasone (1 nM) and Zn^{2+} (15 μM) were analyzed by HPLC, no isoMT peaks were observed (data not shown), indicating that physiological concentrations of glucocorticoids and Zn^{2+} did not synthesize detectable amounts of MTs.

In the presence of physiological concentrations of glucocorticoid or Zn^{2+}, the influence of EGF on MT induction was examined. The isoMTs were not detected in the cells treated with EGF (10 ng/ml) alone for 24 to 48 h (data not shown). When the cells were treated with EGF for the first 24 hr and incubated with 15 μM Zn^{2+} for another 24 h, no peaks of MTs were found. In the cells treated with both EGF and 1 nM dexamethasone, a small peak was found at a retention time of 29 to 30 min corresponding to MT-2-2 (data not shown). When 15 μM Zn^{2+} was added to the cells after the 24 h-treatment with both EGF and 1 nM dexamethasone, the HPLC pattern showed a single Zn-associated peak at the retention time of 29 to 30 min corresponding to MT-2-2; Zn^{2+} recovery was 52% (Figure 3). These results indicated that the additional EGF to the culture medium could clearly induce MT-2-2 in the presence of 1 nM dexamethasone and 15 μM Zn^{2+}. The low level of Zn^{2+} in the culture medium is considered to be bound to the MT-2-2 polypeptide that is induced by EGF and dexamethasone.

The Zn-associated peak, corresponding to an isoform of MT-2-2, obtained from the HPLC column was analyzed by a radioimmunoassay for MT. There were no significant differences between both competition curves for an authentic rat hepatic MT-2 and MT-2-2 subfraction obtained from the HPLC column. From present results the Zn-associated MT-2-2 subfraction from HPLC column was identified as MT (data not shown).

In the presence of EGF (10 ng/ml), dexamethasone (1 nM) and Zn^{2+} (15 μM), the growth rate of FM3A cells increased by about 10% (data not shown), indicating that there might be a relationship between cellular proliferation and MT synthesis.

DISCUSSION

In the presence of either glucocorticoid (1 nM dexamethasone) or EGF (10 ng/ml), no detectable amounts of MTs were induced in FM3A cells. However, the presence of both EGF and dexamethasone resulted in a slight increase in amounts of MTs. When a physiological concentration of Zn^{2+} (15 μM) was added to the medium in addition to glucocorticoid and EGF, the induction of MTs was clearly detected. These results indicate that in the presence of physiological concentrations of glucocorticoid and Zn^{2+}, EGF induces biosynthesis of MTs. The gene expression of MTs might be induced by the combination with EGF and nanomolar concentration of dexamethasone, and physiological concentration of Zn^{2+} may be bound to the induced MT polypeptide.

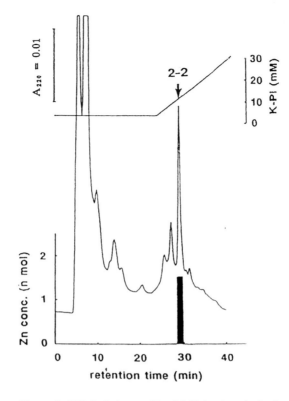

Figure 3. HPLC elution profile of MT fraction obtained by gel filtration of supernatant from FM3A cells treated with EGF, dexamethasone and Zn^{2+}. In the presence of 1 nM dexamethasone, 10 ng/ml EGF was added to the cells and subsequently incubation was carried out for 24 h. A 10-μl sample of the MT fraction obtained from gel filtration was applied to the HPLC column.

The growth rate of FM3A cells increased about 10% in response to EGF and physiological concentrations of dexamethasone and Zn^{2+}, indicating that there may be a relationship of MT induction with cellular proliferation. A high concentration of dexamethasone (1 μM) has been shown to inhibit somatic cell growth and the growth of tumors *in vivo* (Huang et al., 1984; Miya-y-Lopez, 1985) as well as suppressing proliferation of cells cultured *in vitro* (Syms et al., 1984; Smith et al., 1985). Since we used a physiological concentration of dexamethasone (1 nM) in the present experiment, the growth of FM3A cells may not be affected by the antiproliferative effect of the glucocorticoid.

It has been well known that Zn deficiency causes severe growth retardation. Addition of serum to G_1-arrested cells enhances incorporation of both Zn^{2+} and ^{3}H-thymidine, whereas depletion of serum decreases the rate of Zn^{2+} uptake (Grummt et al., 1986). These results suggest that mitogenic induction leads to an increase of Zn^{2+} uptake and that Zn^{2+} is essential for DNA synthesis. Metallothioneins are considered to be involved in Zn metabolism in both adults and embryos. Zinc-binding MT levels are increased during the late fetal or early neonatal period in a wide variety of species (Bakka and Webb, 1981). In the present experiments, the low level Zn^{2+} taken up by the growing cells (FM3A) was found to be bound to MT-2-2 induced by EGF and a low level of dexamethasone (Figure 3). Synthesis of MT may be induced to store Zn^{2+} for use in periods of high demand during cell growth and proliferation.

In the present experiments, the major isoMT induced by EGF in the presence of physiological concentrations of Zn^{2+} and dexamethasone in the growing cells was MT-2. Moreover, the major isoMT induced by the high concentration of dexamethasone was MT-2 (Figure 2B). Our previous study (Kobayashi and Suzuki, 1988b) demonstrated that in growing cells the rate of MT-2 synthesis is much greater than that of MT-1. Similar findings with regard to the presence of Zn-MT in growing cells were obtained in mouse fetal liver (Kobayashi and Suzuki, 1988b), regenerating rat liver (Cain and Griffiths, 1984) and Ehrlich tumor-bearing mouse liver (Ujjani et al., 1986). These results suggest that MT-2 synthesis may be related to cell growth or cancerous stress.

The MT-2 fraction obtained from adult mouse liver was separated into two peaks with an anion exchange HPLC column; the major (MT-2-2) and minor (MT-2-1) peaks. Similar findings were made by Suzuki et al. (1984, 1985), who analysed a rat liver MT by HPLC-atomic absorption spectrophotometry with on-line switching from gel filtration to ion-exchange columns. Immunochemical characterization of MT-2-1 is currently under investigation in our laboratories. The amounts of MT-2-1 in FM3A cells, treated with EGF in the presence of low levels of Zn^{2+} and dexamethasone, were very small or non-detectable. However, in Zn-treated ascites-sarcoma S180A cells (Figure 4), the MT-2-1 subfraction have shown a high concentration (Kobayashi and Suzuki, 1988a). The function and regulation of biosynthesis of MT-2-1 remains to be studied with a special reference to cancerous stresses.

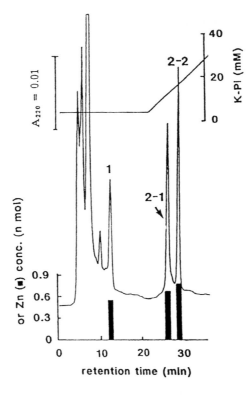

Figure 4. HPLC elution profile of the MT fraction obtained by gel filtration of supernatant from Zn-treated ascites-sarcoma S180A cells (Kobayashi and Suzuki, 1988a). Sarcoma-S180A cells at a concentration of 1×10^7 cells per ml were injected intraperitoneally into ddY mice. After 3 days, tumor-bearing mice were injected with 5 μg of Zn^{2+}/g body weight and killed 24 h after the start of metal administration. A 10 μl sample of the MT fraction of tumor cells from Zn-treated sarcoma-S180A-bearing mice was applied to the anion-exchange HPLC column.

REFERENCES

Bakka A, Samarawickrama GP, and Webb M (1981): Metabolism of zinc and copper in the neonate: effect of cadmium administration during late gestation in the rat on the zinc and copper metabolism of the newborn. *Chem.-Biol. Interactions.* 34: 161.

Banerjee D, Onosaka S, and Cherian MG (1982): Immunohistochemical localization of metallothionein in cell nucleus and cytoplasm of rat liver and kidney. *Toxicology* 24: 95.

Bradford M (1976): A rapid and sensitive method for the quantitation of microgram quantities of protein utilizing the principle of protein-dye binding. *Anal. Biochem.* 72: 248.

Cain K and Griffiths BL (1984): A comparison of isometalothionein synthesis in rat liver after partial hepatectomy and parenteral zinc injection. *Biochem. J.* 217: 85.

Grummt F, Weinmann-Dorsch C, Schneider-Schaulies J, and Lux A (1986): A zinc as a second messenger of mitogenic induction: Effects on diadenosine tetraphosphate (Ap$_4$A) and DNA synthesis. *Exp. Cell Res.* 163: 191.

Huang DP, Schwarts, CE Chiu JF, and Cook JR (1984): Dexamethasone inhibition of rat hepatoma growth and α-fetoprotein synthesis. *Cancer Res.* 44: 2976.

Imbra RJ and Karin M (1987): Metallothionein gene expression is regulated by serum factors and activators of protein kinase C. *Mol. Cell. Biol.* 7: 1358.

Kobayashi S and Suzuki JS (1988a): Zinc and copper accumulation and isometallothionein induction in mouse ascites sarcoma S180A cells. *Biochem. J.* 249: 69.

Kobayashi S and Suzuki JS (1988b): Isolation of isometallothioneins: A comparison of isometallothioneins in growing cells and post-mitotic cells. *Biochem. J.* 251: 649.

Miya-y-Lopez R, Reich E, Stolfi RL, Martin DS, and Ossowski L (1985): Coordinate inhibition of plasminogen activator and tumor growth by hydrocortisone in mouse mammary carcinoma. *Cancer Res.* 45: 2270.

Nartey NO, Barnerjee D, and Cherian MG (1987): Immunohistochemical localization of metallothionein in cell nucleus and cytoplasm of fetal human liver and kidney and its changes during development. *Pathology.* 19: 233.

Nebes VL, DeFranco D, and Morris SM, Jr. (1988): Cyclic AMP induces metallothionein gene expression in rat hepatocytes but not in rat kidney. *Biochem. J.* 255: 741.

Nishimura H, Nishimura N, and Tohyama C (1989): Immunohistochemical localization of metallothionein in developing rat tissues. *J. Histochem. Cytochem.* 37: 715.

Ohtake H, Hasegawa K, and Koga M (1978): Zinc-binding protein in the livers of neonatal, normal and partially hepatectomized rats. *Biochem. J.* 174: 999.

Quaife C, Hammer RE, Mottet NK, and Palmiter RD (1986): Glucocorticoid regulation of metallothionein during murine development. *Devel. Biol.* 118: 549.

Smith RG, Syms AJ, Nag A, Lerner S, and Norris JS (1985): Mechanism of the glucocorticoid regulation of growth of the androgen-sensitive prostate-derived R3327H-G8-A1 tumor cell line. *J. Biol. Chem.* 260: 12454.

Suzuki KT (1984): Separation of metallothionein into isoforms by column switching on gel permeation and ion exchange columns with high-performance liquid chromatography-atomic absorption spectrophotometry. *J. Chromatogr.* 303: 132.

Suzuki KT, Uehara H, Sunaga H, and Shimojo N (1985): Induction and detection of a third isometallothionein (metallothionein-II') in rat liver. *Toxicol. Lett.* 24: 15.

Syms AJ, Norris JS, and Smith RG (1984): Autocrine regulation of growth: 1. Glucocorticoid inhibition is overcome by exogenous platelet derived growth factor. *Biochem. Biophys. Res. Commun.* 122: 68.

Tohyama C and Shaikh ZA (1981): Metallothionein in plasma and urine of cadmium-exposed rats determined by a single-antibody radioimmunoassay. *Fundam. Appl. Toxicol.* 1: 1.

Ujjani B, Krakower G, Bachowski G, Krezoski S, Shaw III, CF, and Petering DH (1986): Host zinc metabolism and the Ehrlich ascites tumor; Zinc redistribution during tumor-related stress. *Biochem. J.* 233: 99.

Changes in Localization of Metallothionein in Various Tissues of Rats under Physiological Conditions

Chiharu Tohyama and Abdul Ghaffar
National Institute for Environmental Studies
Ibaraki, Japan

Hisao Nishimura and Noriko Nishimura
Aichi Medical University
Aichi, Japan

SUMMARY

In order to elucidate possible physiological roles of metallothionein (MT), we have studied immunohistological localization of MT in the developing kidney, regenerating liver and male and female reproductive organs of the rat. In the kidney of the neonate and fetus, MT was found in both the cytoplasm and the nucleus of renal tubular epithelia. Localization of MT was changed with shift of zonation in the renal cortex during development. After partial hepatectomy MT was localized first in the nucleus and then in both the nucleus and cytoplasm whereas the protein was found in the cytoplasm only after laparotomy. In the uterus and ovary, MT was found, in a cell-specific manner, in the glandular epithelium and the lutein cells and ovum. In the testis, MT was localized in the spermatogenic cells, spermatozoa and Sertoli cells but not in Leydig cells. The present result may indicate a possible association of MT in cellular proliferation and differentiation as well as storage, transport, secretion and detoxification of zinc ions.

INTRODUCTION

Metallothioneins (MTs) are a group of low-molecular-weight proteins with high affinity for heavy metals such as cadmium (Cd), copper, zinc (Zn) and mercury, and as a result, play an important role in detoxification of the heavy metals. Since MT is present in a wide variety of biological species, and can be induced not only by exposure to heavy metals but also by various endogenous factors, such as glucocorticoid, this protein is considered to be involved in physiological processes (Kägi and Nordberg, 1979; Webb, 1979; Bremner, 1987; Kägi and Kojima, 1987). However, how MTs fulfill their functions are largely unknown.

Earlier works on immunohistochemical localization of MT showed the presence of MT in specific cells of various tissues from cadmium-injected rats and from rats at various developmental stages (Banerjee et al., 1982; Danielson et al., 1982a,b). In addition to these studies, immunohistological localization of MT has been demonstrated in various organs from humans (Savino et al., 1984; Clarkson et al., 1985; Nartey et al., 1987a,b) and experimental animals (Bataineh et al., 1986; Umeyama et al., 1987; Hazelhoff et al., 1989).

Regarding a possible association of MT with development, a large amount of MT was observed in the nucleus of livers from rats in the perinatal period, while the specific staining for MT was found exclusively in the cytoplasm in the postnatal stage (Panemangalore et al., 1983). These findings suggest that distribution of MT may also change in other tissues, besides livers, during development. Since the biosynthesis of MT is known to be induced after partial hepatectomy (Ohtake et al., 1978), the regenerating rat liver could be an appropriate experimental model for clarifying regulation of biosynthesis and localization of MT. Furthermore, since the mucosa of uterus and vaginal epithelium as well as the cellular proliferation of the ovary are under a periodical control of female sex hormones based on the species-specific cycle, and the synthesis of MT was reported to be induced in response to estrogen (Nishiyama et al., 1987), a possible association of MT with these female reproductive organs need to be studied. The testis is an organ where mitosis and meiosis occurs and also a target organ of Cd toxicity. Up to present, studies on immunohistological localization of MT in the testis has been limited to Cd-injected rats (Danielson et al., 1982a; Nolan and Shaikh, 1986). In the present study, in order to elucidate possible physiological roles of MT, we have studied histological localization and changes in concentrations of MT in kidneys at various developmental stages, the regenerating liver and female and male reproductive organs of rats.

MATERIALS AND METHODS

Reagents

Biotinylated goat anti-rabbit IgG (Cat. No. BA-1000) and avidin-biotin peroxidase complex (ABC) kit were purchased from Vector Laboratories (Burlingame, CA) and, FITC-labeled sheep anti-rabbit IgG antibody and sheep control serum were purchased from Cappel Laboratories (Cat. Nos. 1212-0084 and 0112-0084, respectively; Chochranville, PA). Protein assay kit was purchased from Bio-Rad Co. (Richmond, CA). Other reagents were all analytical grade.

Animals

Male and female Wistar rats and male mice were purchased from Shizuoka Animal Center. In order to localize MT in the kidney at different developmental stages, rats at specified ages were used. For partial hepatectomy 70% of the liver was removed from male Wistar rats under ether anesthesia. Livers obtained from laparotomized rats were considered as sham-operated control. Stages of the estrous cycle of the rats were determined by both vaginal smear test and hematoxylin-eosin staining of vaginal epithelial cells. The uterus, vagina and ovaries and the testis were removed from 9-week-old female and male rats, respectively.

Immunohistochemical Staining

All the tissues were fixed in 10% buffered formalin and embedded in paraffin. Deparaffinized 5 μm thick tissue sections were stained by the ABC method (Nishimura et al., 1989b) and the indirect immunofluorescent technique (Tohyama et al., 1988). Both the ABC and indirect immunofluorescence methods resulted in indistinguishable observations on histological localization of MT. The immunohistochemical control test was carried out by replacement of the rabbit antiserum with nonimmune rabbit serum and by the use of the rabbit antiserum that had been adsorbed with rat MT-2 (Tohyama et al., 1988).

Determination of MT and Total Protein

Amounts of MT in various tissues were determined by the MT radioimmunoassay using rabbit anti-rat MT-1 antiserum (Tohyama et al., 1988). Amounts of total protein in the supernatant after centrifugation were determined by a dye-binding method (Bio-Rad® protein assay kit) using human serum albumin as standard according to the manufacturer's instructions.

RESULTS

Developing Rat Kidneys (Nishimura et al., 1989a)

Intense immunofluorescence was observed in both cytoplasm and nucleus of the tubular epithelium of the fetal rat kidney (Figure 1A). Most of the tubular epithelial cells as well as their nucleus had strong immunostaining in the inner zone of the renal cortex by Day 5, but there is no immunofluorescence in the neogenic zone of the cortex (Figure 1B). Marked immunofluorescence of MT was observed in the straight portion of proximal tubules in the zone (corresponding to the neogenic zone on Day 4) located in the outer cortex (Figure 1C, D). The tubular cells showing MT staining were mainly observed in the deepest part of the renal cortex adjacent to the medulla on Day 18 (Figure 1E), followed by disappearance of the immunostaining by Day 27 (Figure 1F). MT appeared again in the cytoplasm and brush border of limited number of proximal tubular cells in 2-month-old rats (data not shown), which was a typical distribution pattern of the adult rat kidney.

Metallothionein in the Liver after Partial Hepatectomy
(Nishimura et al., 1989a)

We have used a partially hepatectomized rat liver as a model for actively proliferating and differentiating model. Regarding a time-course of MT concentration after partial hepatectomy, the MT level in the sham-operated control varied between 50 to 90 μg/g tissue until 70 h after operation whereas the partial hepatectomy caused a considerable increase in the MT level within 6 h after operation, followed by an elevation to reach a maximum of 300 μg/g tissue at 24 h. However, the MT level decreased to a sham-operated control level 30 h after partial hepatectomy. Immunostaining of MT in the nucleus of hepatocytes was found as early as 6 h after partial hepatectomy. At 15 h after the partial hepatectomy, immunostaining in the nucleus increased in intensity. At 24 h after partial hepatectomy, strong MT immunostaining was observed in the nucleus of almost all hepatocytes as well as along the sinusoid and bile canaliculi (Figure 2A), whereas laparotomy showed MT immunofluorescence only in the cytoplasm (Figure 2B).

Metallothionein Levels in Reproductive Organs of Female Rats
(Nishimura et al., 1989b)

MT concentrations in the uterus and ovary at different stages of the estrous cycle were determined. The average MT levels in the uterus and ovary were approximately 11 and 23 μg/g tissue, respectively. From the RIA results, no marked changes in MT level depending on the estrous cycle were observed.

Rat Uterus

MT was found to localize in specific types of cells in the uterus throughout the estrous cycle (Figures 3A and B). Namely, as shown typically in Figure 3A, the epithelium of the uterine gland contained very strong immunostaining of MT and the simple columnar epithelium of the endometrium had weak immunostaining. Almost no immunostaining was observed in other parts of the uterus, such as the connective tissue and vascular endothelium of the lamina propria, the myometrium and perimetrium.

The major change in the localization of MT during the estrous cycle was observed at estrus. During diestrus (Figure 3A), proestrus and metestrus (data not shown), strong immunostaining due to MT was observed evenly in both cytoplasm and nucleus. However, at estrus, MT was found to distribute unevenly among the glandular epithelial cells; the intensity of staining in the cytoplasm of some of the cells somehow decreased whereas it completely attenuated from both cytoplasm and nucleus of other cells (Figure 3B). At this stage the epithelium became shorter in height, but higher again at metestrus (data not shown).

In the vagina at proestrus and estrus many cells harboring MT were observed in the luminal side of the epithelium as well as in the lumen. In contrast, at metestrus and diestrus the MT-positive cells were found to decrease in number and be confined to the lamina propria of mucous membrane adjacent to the epithelium (data not shown).

Rat Ovary

In the ovary strong immunostaining of MT was found in granulosa lutein cells. Some cells showed the presence of MT only in the nucleus, others only in the cytoplasm and another in both organelles (Figure 3C). Interestingly, the lutein cells which are in the process of forming the corpus luteum at diestrus were stained strongly for MT (Figure 3C). In the ovum MT was observed in the cytoplasm but not in the nucleus (Figure 3C). Furthermore, the localization of MT was also demonstrated in the germinal epithelium of the ovary and along the lumen of the oviduct (data not shown). No immunostaining of MT was detected in the granular layer of follicles that surround ova, follicular cavity and connective tissue.

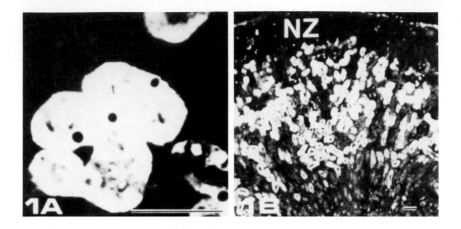

Figure 1. Immunohistochemical staining for MT in the kidney of rats at different developmental stages. Bar = 50 μm. (A) Fetus on Day 20 of gestation. Intense immunofluorescence in both cytoplasm and nucleus of the proximal convoluted epithelial cells is observed. Some nuclei did not show immunofluorescence of MT; (B) 4-day-old rat. Note absence of immunofluorescence of MT in tubules of the neogenic zone (NZ) located at outer rim of the renal cortex. The inner zone of the renal cortex appears to localize MT. No specific immunofluorescence is observed in the glomerulus (G); (C) 11-day-old rat. Straight portions (arrow) of proximal tubules in the medullary rays are strongly stained. (D) Renal cortex of 11-day-old rat. While some of the proximal convoluted tubular cells in the zone (corresponding to the neogenic zone on Day 4) are stained for MT (arrow), intensity of immunofluorescence varies among the proximal convoluted tubules beneath this zone. (E) Renal cortex of 18-day-old rat. Tubules containing MT are observed in the deepest part in the renal cortex adjacent to the medulla (M). (F) Renal cortex of 27-day-old rat. Almost all the MT immunofluorescence disappeared by Day 27. [Reproduced in part, with permission, from Nishimura et al.: Immunohistochemical localization of metallothionein in developing rat tissues. *J. Histochem. Cytochem.* 37:715 (1989).]

Metallothionein in the Testis (Nishimura et al., 1990)

Average MT and Zn concentrations in the rat testis were 30.0 μg/g tissue and 18.9 μg/g tissue, respectively. MT immunoreactivity was present in spermatogenic cells, spermatozoa and Sertoli cells, but not in Leydig cells. Seminiferous tubules which have mature spermatozoa exhibited weak MT staining whereas the tubules which consist of differentiating spermatogenic cells but do not contain spermatozoa showed strong MT staining (data not shown).

DISCUSSION

The present study not only has demonstrated a considerable change in the localization of MT during development of rat kidney, but also suggests

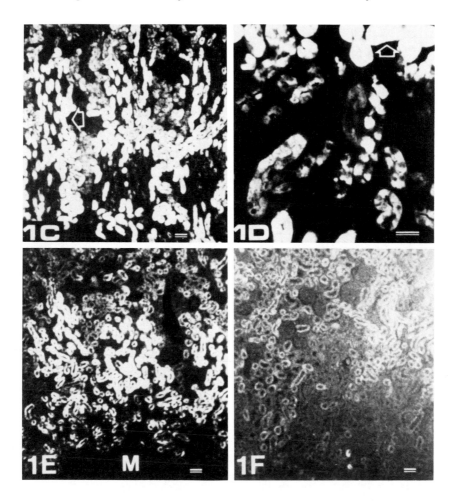

Figure 1. (continued.)

a possible involvement in cellular proliferation and differentiation in the regenerating rat liver. Since a remarkable increase in MT was demonstrated at the time when active development and differentiation occurred in the perinatal period, partial hepatectomy was chosen as an experimental model to investigate physiological roles of MT during development. One of the most interesting findings was the presence of MT in the nucleus and cytoplasm in regenerating liver after 70% partial hepatectomy (Figure 2B), but only in the cytoplasm after laparotomy (Figure 2A). The regenerating rat liver actively grows, recovers and returns to a normal size within 10 d. In contrast to this length of recovering period, MT level of the partially-hepatectomized liver reached a maximum 24 h after operation and started to decrease to a laparotomized control level at 30 h, and nuclear MT was found as early as 6 h in the partially-hepatectomized liver only (unpublished

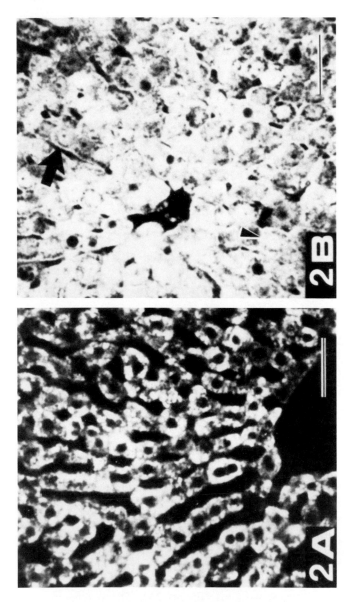

Figure 2. Immunohistochemical staining for MT in the liver after partial hepatectomy. Bar = 50 μm. (A) MT localization in the liver at 24 h after laparotomy. Immunofluorescence is observed throughout the cytoplasm but not in the nuclei of hepatocytes. (B) MT localization in regenerating liver at 24 h after 70% partial hepatectomy. MT appears not only in the nucleus and cytoplasm but also in sinusoids (arrow) and bile canaliculi (arrowhead). [Reproduced, with permission, from Nishimura et al.: Immunohistochemical localization of metallothionein in developing rat tissues. *J. Histochem. Cytochem.* 37:715 (1989).]

result). Partial hepatectomy is known to induce a dramatic increase in hepatic mitosis followed by a peak of its mitotic index around 28 h (Bucher, 1963), leading to the notion that the presence of MT in the nucleus is not the consequence of proliferation, but may function as an essential element at the very early step of proliferation. A similar trend of the fate of MT was observed in mouse skin to which a tumor promoter, 12-*O*-tetradecanoyl-phorbol-13-acetate, was topically applied. The induced synthesis of MT in the basal cell layer, to which ^{3}H-thymidine was found to be incorporated, paralleled with the hyperplasia caused by these agents (Karasawa et al., 1988; Nishimura et al., 1988). It needs to be further studied whether MT found in the nucleus is newly synthesized in the cytoplasm and transported to the nucleus or MT already present in the cytoplasm is transferred to the nucleus. It is conceivable that MT, if it is involved, is associated with a relatively early period of cellular proliferation and differentiation.

Another interesting observation is a developmental change in the zonal distribution of MT in the renal cortex. MT was mainly detectable in the inner cortex, but not in the neogenic zone on Day 4 (Figure 1B) but appeared on Day 11 (Figure 1C and D) in the zone where renal tubules got more mature and started functioning (Baxter and Yoffey, 1948). With further gradual postnatal development tubular cells containing MT, as a phenomenon, appeared to move down to the deepest zone of the renal cortex on Day 18 (Figure 1E). The neogenic zone located at the outer rim of the cortex is known to comprise immature tubules and to be easily distinguishable by histological staining from other parts that have amply differentiated tubules (Baxter and Yoffey, 1948). Therefore, the stage-specific changes in the zonal distribution of MT presented here may reflect the constructive process of the nephron, indicating the physiological demand for MT. This idea is also supported by the fact that MT disappeared on Day 27 (Figure 1F) when nephrogenesis is known to complete in the rat kidney (Baxter and Yoffey, 1948).

The present study is the first to show the immunohistological localization of MT in the female reproductive organs, i.e., the uterus, ovary, and vagina (Figure 3). In the glandular epithelium of the uterus, a marked difference in MT localization between estrus and other stages is a considerable decrease in cytoplasmic MT at estrus. A drastic change in distribution and intensity of MT staining during the estrous cycle was also found in the vaginal epithelium (Nishimura et al., 1989b). The presence of MT was also found in lutein cells in the corpus luteum, after cell proliferation (Figure 3C), that is transformed from the ovulated folliculi. Nishiyama et al. (1987) reported that the administration of estradiol to rats evoked the elevation of Zn-MT concentrations in the liver and kidney 10- and 2-fold over control organs, respectively. This and the present results suggest that estrogen which regulates the estrous cycle through other growth factors may be involved in the induction of MT biosynthesis.

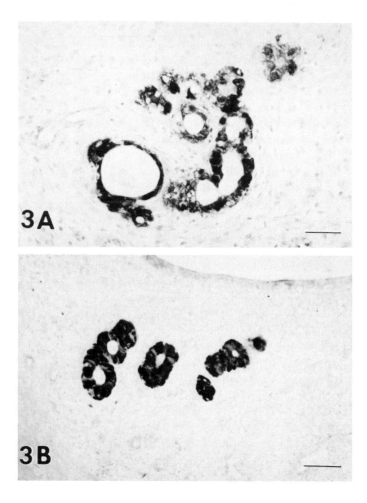

Figure 3. Immunohistochemical localization of MT in the uterus (A and B) and ovary (C) from rats. The glandular epithelium exhibits strong immunostaining and the simple columnar epithelium shows weak immunostaining. The cytoplasm of the glandular epithelial cells at the estrus (B) does not appear to contain as much immunostaining for MT as diestrus (A) and those of other stages (data not shown). In the ovary, all the different stages of ovarian change, in the process from the formation of ovum to ovulation, were observed in a tissue section since the histological observation could not be differentiated by each stage of the estrous cycle. Bar = 50 μm. (A) Uterus at the diestrus; (B) Uterus at the estrus; (C) The corpus luteum shows the presence of immunostaining for MT. It is clear that MT antigenicity is present both in the nucleus and cytoplasm of some cells and either the nucleus or cytoplasm of other cells. The cytoplasm of the ovum shows strong immunostaining for MT. [Reproduced in part, with permission from Nishimura et al. Localization of metallothionein in female reproductive organs of rats and guinea pigs. *J. Histochem. Cytochem.* 37:1601 (1989b).]

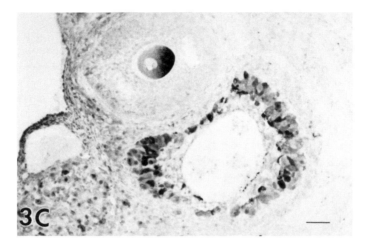

Figure 3. (continued.)

MT determination by a radioimmunoassay revealed that the ovary and uterus from non-pregnant rats contain MT at 23 µg/g wet tissue and 11 µg/g wet tissue, respectively, the values of which are similar to the reported MT values of the liver (Onosaka and Cherian, 1981; Tohyama et al., 1988). In the rat liver MT was found in the entire region of lobes (Tohyama et al., 1988) and, on the other hand, the localization of MT was cell-specific in the ovary and uterus (Figure 3), supporting the notion that actual amounts of MT in the specific cells are greater than the levels of MT on an organ basis. In addition, it should be stressed here that immunohistological techniques have an advantage over biochemical and immunochemical methods in terms of visualizing and detecting the presence of MT in specific cell types and tissues.

MT may be involved in detoxification of excess Zn ions by binding them and also play roles of storage and transport of bound Zn to other macromolecules depending on necessity (Cousins, 1985; Bremner 1987). The glandular epithelial cells of the uterus from rats during non-proliferative period (Figure 3A), the mammary gland from non-pregnant guinea pigs (Nishimura et al., 1989b) and cells comprising of seminiferous tubules (Nishimura et al., 1990) were found to contain appreciable amounts of MT. In these tissues MT may play a role of storage of Zn ions that are needed for the growth of these tissues during pregnancy or spermatogenesis.

In each seminiferous tubule of the testis, MT was found to localize in the supporting cells or, Sertoli cells, and all the spermatogenic cells including spermatogonia. In seminiferous tubules of the rat the spermatogenic cells accomplish the entire period of 48 days for spermatogenesis through a mitosis and meioses (Bloom and Fawcett, 1986). Portions of each seminiferous tubule harbor different stages of spermatogenesis along its long axis, and thus a cross-section of seminiferous tubules of tissue preparation showed various differentiation stages of spermatogenesis (Hemminki et al., 1985). In the seminiferous tubules where spermatogenesis is accomplished, only weak MT staining was observed in all the spermatogenic cells whereas strong MT staining was observed in these cells of the seminiferous tubules that were in the process of spermatogenesis (Nishimura et al., 1990). A difference in staining pattern between seminiferous tubules may be relevant to the present observation that localization of MT migrates, in a zonal fashion, in the renal cortex according to development of nephron from fetal to adult period of the rat (Figure 1). Brady and Webb (1981) reported that the testis of the rat linearly increases in weight until Day 35 after birth and that a testicular MT binds Zn and a concentration of MT is highest among various organs, and suggested the possibility that MT may be involved in the cell division by supplying Zn ions to actively growing tissues such as the testis. Different immunohistological localization of MT among various seminiferous tubules observed in the present study may be related to this notion.

It is still a controversial matter whether MT exists in the testis or not. Two groups of workers reported that a Zn-binding protein isolated from the testis of the rat is a novel protein different from MT and that the testis lacks MT (Waalkes et al., 1984; Deagen and Whanger, 1985; Waalkes and Perantoni, 1986). However, even the studies of the above two groups showed that physicochemical properties of the testicular Zn-binding proteins are very similar to authentic MTs in terms of molecular weight, electric charge, heat stability and metal-binding ability and only drawback against the presence of MT is the amino acid composition. Our present study revealed testicular MT concentrations to be approximately 30 μg/g tissue, which is similar to reported values (Nolan and Shaikh, 1986) as well as the immunohistochemical localization of MT in spermatogenic cells, spermatozoa and Sertoli cells (Nishimura et al., 1990). Furthermore, MT mRNA was highly expressed in a constitutive manner in the mouse and rat (Durnam and Palmiter, 1981; Shiraishi et al., 1989), and specimens of supernatant from testicular homogenate completely cross-reacted with sheep anti-rat MT antiserum (Mehra and Bremner, 1987). In addition, when we partially isolated Zn-binding proteins by anion-exchange high performance column chromatography, two separate peaks similar in retention time to authentic liver MT-1 and 2 were observed in terms of MT antigenicity, Zn and protein (Tohyama et al., 1990). MT was also immunohistochemically localized in the testis of Cd-treated rats (Danielson et al., 1982a; Nolan and Shaikh, 1986) and of control rats (Nishimura et al., 1990). To solve the apparent controversy, a more intensive study is currently being carried out in our laboratories.

In summary, the present study has demonstrated a possible involvement of MT in the proliferation and differentiation of cells and in the secretion, storage and transport of metals. We believe that the immunohistochemical technique offered valuable information on intracellular localization of MT which is difficult to exhibit only by the biochemical analysis. How MT participates during developmental processes will require further studies.

REFERENCES

Bakka A and Webb M (1981): Metabolism of zinc and copper in the neonate: changes in the concentrations and contents of thionein-bound Zn and Cu with age in the livers of the newborn of various mammalian species. *Biochem. Pharmacol.* 30: 721.

Banerjee D, Onosaka S, and Cherian MG (1982): Immunohistochemical localization of metallothionein in cell nucleus and cytoplasm of rat liver and kidney. *Toxicology* 24: 95.

Bataineh ZM, Hediger PM, Thompson SN, and Timms BG (1986): Immunocytochemical localization of metallothionein in the rat prostate gland. *Prostate* 9: 397.

Baxter JS and Yoffey JM (1948): The postnatal development of renal tubules in the rat. *J. Anatomy* 82: 189.

Bloom WW and Fawcett DW, Eds., (1976): *A Textbook of Histology,* 10th ed. W.B. Saunders, Philadelphia, p. 829.

Brady FO and Webb M (1981): Metabolism of zinc and copper in the neonate. (Zinc, copper)-thionein in the developing rat kidney and testis. *J. Biol. Chem.* 256: 3931.

Bremner I (1987): Nutritional and physiological significance of metallothionein. In, *Metallothionein II. Experientia Supplementum* Vol. 52, Kägi JHR and Kojima Y, Eds., Birkhäuser-Verlag, Basel.

Bucher NLR (1963): Regeneration of mammalian liver. *Int. Rev. Cytol.* 15: 245.

Clarkson JP, Elmes EM, Jasani B, and Webb M (1985): Histological demonstration of immunoreactive zinc metallothionein in liver and ileum of rat and man. *Histochem. J.* 17: 343.

Cousins RJ (1985): Absorption, transport, and hepatic metabolism of copper and zinc: special reference to metallothionein and ceruloplasmin. *Physiol. Rev.* 65: 238.

Danielson KH, Ohi S, and Huang PC (1982a): Immunochemical detection of metallothionein in specific epithelial cells of rat organs. *Proc. Natl. Acad. Sci. U.S.A.* 79: 2301.

Danielson KH, Ohi S, and Huang PC (1982b): Immunochemical localization of metallothionein in rat liver and kidney. *J. Histochem. Cytochem.* 30: 1033.

Deagan JT and Whanger PD (1985): Properties of cadmium-binding proteins in rat testes: characteristics unlike metallothionein. *Biochem. J.* 231: 279.

Durnam DM and Palmiter RD (1981): Transcriptional regulation of the mouse metallothionein-I gene by heavy metals. *J. Biol. Chem.* 256: 5712.

Hazelhoff RW, Tohyama C, Nishimura H, Nishimura N, and Morselt AFW (1989): Quantitative immunohistochemistry of metallothionein in rat placenta. *Histochemistry* 90: 365.

Hemminki K, Sorsa M, and Vainio H (1985): *Occupational Hazards and Reproduction.* Hemisphere Publishing, Washington, D.C., p. 3.

Kägi JHR and Nordberg M, Eds. (1979): *Metallothionein: Experientia Supplementum* Vol. 34, Birkhäuser-Verlag, Basel.

Kägi JHR and Kojima Y, Eds., (1987): *Metallothionein II: Experientia Supplementum* Vol. 52, Birkhäuser Verlag, Basel.

Karasawa M, Tohyama C, Nishimura N, Hashiba H, and Kuroki T (1988): Possible role of metallothionein in epidermal hyperplasia. *Proc. 47th Ann. Meet. Jpn. Cancer Assoc.* p. 133.

Mehra RK and Bremner I (1987): Induction of synthesis and degradation of metallothionein-I in the tissues of rats injected with zinc. In, *Metallothionein II: Experientia Supplementum* Vol. 52, Kägi JHR and Kojima Y, Eds., Birkhäuser-Verlag, Basel, pp. 565–572.

Narty NO, Cherian MG, and Banerjee D (1987a): Immunohistochemical localization of metallothionein in human thyroid tumors. *Am. J. Pathol.* 129: 177.

Narty NO, Banerjee D, and Cherian MG (1987b): Immunohistochemical localization of metallothionein in cell nucleus and cytoplasm of fetal human liver and kidney and its changes during development. *Pathology* 19: 233.

Nishiyama S, Taguchi T, and Onosaka S (1987): Induction of zinc-thionein by estradiol and protective effects on inorganic mercury-induced renal toxicity. *Biochem. Pharmac.* 36: 3387.

Nishimura N, Nishimura H, Tohyama C, Karasawa M, and Kuroki T (1988): Localization of metallothionein in epidermal hyperplasia caused by topical application of tumor promoter, 12-O-tetradecanoylphorbol-13-acetate, on the mouse skin. *J. Histochem. Cytochem.* 36: 945.

Nishimura H, Nishimura N, and Tohyama C (1989a): Immunohistochemical localization of metallothionein in developing rat tissues. *J. Histochem. Cytochem.* 37: 715.

Nishimura N, Nishimura H, and Tohyama C (1989b): Localization of metallothionein in female reproductive organs of rats and guinea pigs. *J. Histochem. Cytochem.* 37: 1601.

Nishimura H, Nishimura N, and Tohyama C (1990): Localization of metallothionein in the genital organs of the male rat. *J. Histochem. Cytochem.* 38: 927.

Nolan CV and Shaikh ZA (1986): An evaluation of tissue metallothionein and genetic resistance to cadmium toxicity in mice. *Toxicol. Appl. Pharmacol.* 85: 135.

Ohtake H, Hasegawa K, and Koga M (1978): Zinc-binding protein in the livers of neonatal, normal, and partially hepatectomized rats. *Biochem. J.* 174: 999.

Onosaka S and Cherian MG (1981): The induced synthesis of metallothionein in various tissues of rat in response to metals. I. Effect of repeated injection of cadmium salts. *Toxicology* 22: 91.

Panemangalore M, Banerjee D, Onosaka S, and Cherian MG (1983): Changes in the intracellular accumulation and distribution of metallothionein in rat liver and kidney during postnatal development. *Dev. Biol.* 97: 95.

Savino W, Huang PC, Corrigan A, Berrih S, and Dardenne M (1984): Thymic hormone-containing cells. V. Immunohistological detection of metallothionein within the cells bearing thymulin (a zinc-containing hormone) in human and mouse thymuses. *J. Histochem. Cytochem.* 32: 942.

Shiraishi N, Hayashi H, Hiraki Y, Aono KM, Itano Y, Kosaka F, Noji S, and Taniguchi S (1989): Elevation in metallothionein messenger RNA in rat tissues after exposure to X-irradiation. *Toxicol. Appl. Pharmacol.* 98: 501.

Tohyama C, Nishimura H, and Nishimura N (1988): Immunohistochemical localization of metallothionein in the liver and kidney of cadmium- or zinc-treated rats. *Acta Histochem. Cytochem.* 21: 91.

Tohyama C, Ghaffar A, Nishimura N, and Nishimura H (1990): Presence and localization of a zinc-binding protein reactive with metallothionein antibody in the rat restis. *Toxicologist* 10: 213.

Umeyama T, Saruki K, Imai K, Yamanaka H, Suzuki K, Ikei N, Kodaira T, Nakajima K, Saitoh H, and Kimura M (1987): Immunohistochemical demonstration of metallothionein in the rat prostate. *Prostate.* 10: 257.

Waalkes M, Chernoff SB, and Klaassen CD (1984): Cadmium-binding proteins of rat testes: characterization of a low-molecular-mass protein that lacks identity with metallothionein. *Biochem. J.* 220: 811.

Waalkes MP and Perantoni A (1986): Isolation of a novel metal-binding protein from rat testes: characterization and distinction from metallothionein. *J. Biol. Chem.* 261: 13097.

Webb M, Ed. (1979): The metallothioneins: the chemistry, biochemistry and biology of cadmium. Elsevier/North Holland, Amsterdam, pp. 195–266.

Chapter

20

Studies on Induction of Zinc Metallothionein by Sensory and Psychological Stresses in Rat Liver

Tadashi Niioka and Yutaka Kojima
Department of Environmental Medicine
Graduate School of Environmental Science
Hokkaido University
Kita-ku, Sapporo, Japan

ABSTRACT

The induction of zinc-metallothionein biosynthesis was investigated in rat liver under the following stresses; electric stimuli on tail and through grid floor, restraint, cold environment, immersion under restraint, noise and vibration. The quantity of metallothionein was evaluated by measurement of the zinc content in the metallothionein fraction separated by Sephadex G-75® gel filtration. Among the stresses tested, strong induction of metallothionein synthesis was observed after both electric stimuli. After immersion or after the uninterrupted bell noise stimulus, metallothionein content was twice as much as that of the control. These results indicate that sensory and psychological stresses can also induce the biosynthesis of metallothionein in rat liver.

INTRODUCTION

The biological significance of metallothionein (MT) has mainly been deduced from analysis of factors by which this protein is induced. Soon after the discovery (Margoshes and Vallee, 1957) and characterization (Kägi and Vallee, 1960, 1961) of metallothionein, a cysteine-rich, low molecular weight metal-binding protein occurring ubiquitously in nature, Piscator found that this protein was inducible by cadmium (Piscator, 1964). The induction of metallothionein biosynthesis was first observed to be induced by a variety of metal ions and subsequently by stress conditions which change zinc metabolism. Whanger's group reported metallothionein induction by physical and metabolic stresses (Oh et al., 1978) and Hidalgo et al. (1986) by restraint, a psychological stress. Recently, the issue has been complicated since biosynthesis can be elicited by a large number of different agents and pathophysiological conditions (Bremner, 1987; Kägi and Kojima, 1987). The most important inducers are metal salts, especially cadmium, but also hormones, tumor promoters, and a great many cytotoxic substances have similar effects, as summarized by Bremner (1987).

Their inducibility by a number of factors has, of course, generated a strong interest in many fields and suggests that metallothioneins play not only an important role in heavy metal metabolism as postulated soon after their discovery, but also a pivotal role in self-defense mechanism. In this article, we report the study on induction of metallothionein biosynthesis by various sensory and psychological stresses (Niioka and Kojima, 1988).

EXPERIMENTAL PROCEDURES

Animals

Male Sprague-Dawley rats (Shizuoka Laboratory Animal Center, Hamamatsu, Japan, 5 weeks old) were housed in groups of three per cage in a controlled room (light on 5 to 19 h, temperature $20.5 \pm 0.5°C$, white noise constant) for at least one week before starting experiments. Food and water were available *ad libitum*.

Treatments of Animals

Animals were randomly assigned and exposed to stress before sacrifice. The stress conditions are listed in Table I. After the stresses all animals were sacrificed with ether. The livers were rapidly removed and stored at $-20°C$ until use.

TABLE I. Condition of Stresses

		Exposure Time (h)	On/Off Time Ratio	Duration Time (min)
Electric stimuli	Tail, 6 mA DC pulse	8	—	—
Electric stimuli	Grid floor, 2 mA DC pulse	8	—	—
Immersion	34°C water, polyethylene net	8	—	—
Noise	Bell, 100 dB, uninterrupted	8	—	—
Noise	Bell, 100 dB, interrupted	3	1:9	6
Noise	Bell, 100 dB, interrupted	48	1:9	6
Noise	White noise, 100 dB, interrupted	3	1:9	1
Noise	White noise, 100 dB, interrupted	72	1:9	1
Vibration	Horizontal 1 cm, 100 rpm	8	—	—
Cold	4°C	24	—	—
Restraint	Tube (6 × 12 cm)	2	—	—

Purification of Metallothionein

All steps were performed at 4°C. Livers were thawed and divided into 10-g sections. A portion was cut into small pieces and homogenized in 2 volumes of 50 mM Tris-25 mM HCl buffer solution (pH 8.1) using a Polytron®, Type PT 10-35 for 30 s, three times. The homogenate was centrifuged at 10,000 × g for 30 min with a Kubota® centrifuge. Approximately 20 ml of the fat-free supernatant was recentrifuged at 30,000 rpm (105,000 × g) for 60 min with a Hitachi® ultracentrifuge. The liver cytosol was applied to a Sephadex G-75® column, 3.0 cm × 100 cm, equilibrated with 10 mM Tris-5 mM HCl buffer solution (pH 8.1) and eluted with the same buffer solution at a flow rate of approximately 30 ml/h maintained with an Atto peristalic pump, Model SJ-1211. The eluate was collected in 10 ml fractions and analyzed for metals. The fractions containing metallothionein were pooled.

Chemical Analyses

Zinc and copper concentrations were determined with a Hitachi® atomic absorption spectrophotometer, Model 180-30®. The quantity of metallothionein was evaluated by zinc content in metallothionein fraction of Sephadex G-75® gel filtration.

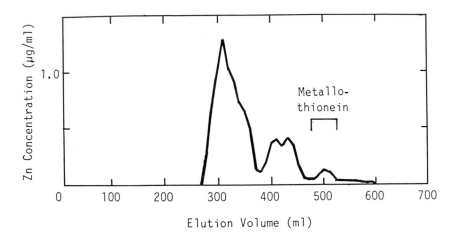

Figure 1. Gel filtration of metallothionein.

TABLE II.
Effect of Various Stresses on Induction
of Metallothionein

	Metallothionein	
	μg/g Liver	-Fold Increase
Control	3.73	1
Electric stimuli, tail	31.8	8.5
Electric stimuli, grid floor	30.1	8.1
Restraint	10.0	2.7
Cold	9.46	2.5
Immersion	7.31	2.0
Bell noise, uninterrupted, 8 h	6.73	1.8
Vibration	4.87	1.3
White noise, interrupted, 3 h	3.87	1.0
Bell noise, interrupted, 3 h	3.73	1.0
White noise, interrupted, 72 h	2.87	0.8
Bell noise, interrupted, 48 h	2.01	0.5

RESULTS AND DISCUSSION

A representative gel filtration profile is shown in Figure 1 and the results are listed in Table II.

Among the stresses tested, strong induction of metallothionein synthesis was observed after both electric stimuli (more than 8-fold increase). After immersion, metallothionein content was twice as much as that of the control. Cold stress was reported to be stimulated metallothionein synthesis approximately 3-fold. The induction of metallothionein was stimulated 1.8 times under 8-h bell noise, although it was not observed by interrupted noises which were reported to cause the increase of serum glucocorticoid concentration. The increase of metallothionein content after vibration condition was 30%. These values can be compared with 4 or 14-fold increase caused by the peritoneal administration of Zn^{2+}, 2 mg/kg body weight, two times or 10 mg/kg four times, respectively.

These results indicate that in addition to physical stresses reported previously, sensory and psychological stresses can also induce the biosynthesis of metallothionein in rat liver.

ACKNOWLEDGMENT

This study was supported by Grant-in-Aid from the Ministry of Education, Science and Culture of Japan.

REFERENCES

Bremner I (1987): Nutritional and physiological significance of metallothionein. *Metallothionein II. Experientia, Suppl.* 52: Kägi JHR and Kojima Y, Eds., Birkhäuser-Verlag, Basel, pp. 81–107.

Hidalgo J, Armario A, Flos R, and Garvey JS (1986): Restraint stress induced changes in rat liver and serum metallothionein and in Zn metabolism. *Experientia* 42: 1006–1010.

Kägi JHR and Vallee BL (1960): Metallothionein: a cadmium- and zinc-containing protein from equine renal cortex. *J. Biol. Chem.* 235: 3460–3465.

Kägi JHR and Vallee BL (1961): Metallothionein: a cadmium- and zinc-containing protein from equine renal cortex. II. Physicochemical properties. *J. Biol. Chem.* 236: 2435–2442.

Kägi JHR and Kojima Y (1987): Chemistry and biochemistry of metallothionein. *Metallothionein II. Experientia, Suppl.* 52: Kägi JHR and Kojima Y, Eds., Birkhäuser-Verlag, Basel, pp.25–61.

Margoshes M and Vallee BL (1957): A cadmium protein from equine kidney cortex. *J. Am. Chem. Soc.* 79: 4813–4814.

Niioka T and Kojima Y (1988): Studies on induction of metallothionein by sensory and psychological stresses in rat liver. *Abstracts, 14th International Congress of Biochemistry,* IV: 104.

Oh SH, Deagen JT, Whanger PD, and Weswig PH (1978): Biological function of metallothionein. V. Its induction in rats by various stresses. *Am. J. Physiol.* 234: E282–E285.

Piscator M (1964): Om kadmium i normala människonjurar samt redogörelse för isolering av metallothionein ur lever från kadmiumexponerade kaniner (On cadmium in normal human kidneys together with a report on the isolation of metallothionein from livers of cadmium-exposed rabbits). *Nord. Hyg. Tidskr.* 45: 76–82.

Induction of Metallothionein by Emotional Stress

Koji Arizono, Akiko Tanahe,
and Toshihiko Ariyoshi
School of Pharmaceutical Sciences
Nagasaki University
Nagasaki, Japan

Minehiro Moriyama
Daiichi College of
Pharmaceutical Sciences
Fukuoka, Japan

INTRODUCTION

Metallothionein (MT) is a small molecular weight, cystein-rich metal-binding protein. Involvement of the protein in binding toxic metals such as cadmium (Cd) and mercury (Hg) has been widely studied, whereas involvement with metabolism of physiologically required metals such as zinc (Zn) and copper (Cu) has only more recently come under scrutiny (Kägi and Nordberg, 1979; Kägi and Kojima, 1987). The diverse aspects of MT research have been well reviewed (Brady, 1982; Hamer, 1986; Kägi and Schäffer, 1988).

Liver is the richest source of MT after exposure of exogenous metal to animals. In recent years the modulation of hepatic zinc thionein (Zn-MT) levels by a variety of physical, chemical, and environmental stresses has been reported (Oh et al., 1978; Sugawara et al., 1983; Hidalgo et al., 1986, 1988).

The method of physiological stress used by Ogawa and Kuwabara (1966) employed the communication box method which utilized purely emotional (psychological) stress and excludes physical stimulation.

Although the involvement of glucocorticoid on hepatic Zn-MT induction in this stress response is clear (Etzel and Cousins, 1981; Hidalgo et al., 1986; Bremner, 1987), it is possible that hepatic Zn-MT induction through this stress response could also be mediated by catecholamine (Brady and Helvig, 1984).

In the present study, we have investigated the induction ability of MT (Zn-MT) in mouse or rat liver by emotional stress, based on the communication box method. In addition, using several adrenoceptor-related blockers we examined whether catecholamine relates to the induction of MT by emotional stress.

MATERIALS AND METHODS

Animals: male Wistar rats (180 to 220 g) and ddy male mice (30 to 35 g) were used in this study. Animals in the light and temperature controlled room were maintained with food and water available *ad libitum* for 1 week, before being used for experiments.

Room temperature was maintained at 25 ± 2°C during each stress exposure.

Communication Box Stress

Apparatus
As the apparatus for the transmission of emotional stimulus, the communication box described by Ogawa and Kuwabara (1966) was used. This apparatus was characterized by complete removal of physical stimulus such as electric stimulus to set up the form of communication between animals.

Mice. The apparatus consisted of a wooden box measuring 32 cm longitudinally, 32 cm transversally and 32 cm in height, with the floor or grid made of stainless steel 5 mm in diameter spaced at 1 cm intervals as shown in Figure 1. The inside of the box was divided into 9 compartments each measuring 10 cm longitudinally, 10 cm transversally and 32 cm in height. One animal was placed in each compartment. In the white portion (4 rooms), it was possible to pass direct current through the grid on the floor (0 to 10 mA) by means of an apparatus for electric stimulation from the outside, to induce foot shock in the animals. The animals in those rooms were called senders. In the shaded portion (4 rooms), the grid was covered with plastic to prevent the transmission of the electric stimulation to the animals. The animals in these rooms were called responders. In this apparatus, sender

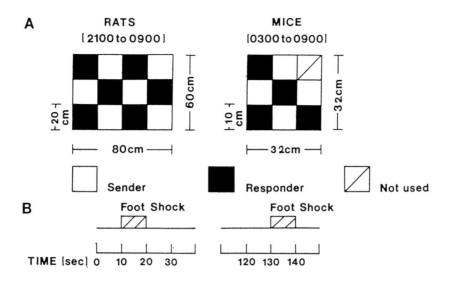

Figure 1. (A) Arrangement of senders and responders in a communication box. (B) Schedule of emotional stimuli. Animals suffering from foot shock through the grids are called senders, and those not suffering from foot shock are called responders. Compartments for the sender (open square) or responder (closed square) are alternately arranged.

animals exposed to electrical stimulation exhibited emotional reactions such as abnormal crying, increased jumping, piloerection, and odor. Such reactions were transmitted to responder animals via visual, aural, and olfactory sensations.

Rats. The apparatus consisted of a wooden box measuring 60 cm longitudinally, 80 cm transversally and 50 cm in height. The inside of the box was divided into 12 compartments measured 20 cm longitudinally, 20 cm transversally and 50 cm in height.

Procedures

Mice. Animals were divided into four experimental groups such as control, starvation, sender and responder. Each group was i.p. injected with psychotropic drugs such as diazepam, chlorpromazine at −1 h with stresses beginning at 0 h. All injection solutions (0.1 mg/ml) were prepared in distilled water before injection. Foot shock (2 mA) was given for 10 s. This cycle was repeated with an interval of 120 s for 6 h, as shown in Figure 1.

Rats. Animals were divided into four experimental groups such as control, starvation, sender and responder. Each group (except for sender) was i.p. injected with several chemicals such as phentolamine, propranolol, atropine, reserpine and cimetidine at −1 h and +6 h with stresses beginning at

0 h. All injection solutions (1 mg/2 ml) were prepared in distilled water before injection. Foot shock (8 to 10 mA) was given for 10 s. This cycle was repeated with an interval of 120 s for 12 h, as shown in Figure 1.

Restraint Stress

Procedures

Animals were divided into three experimental groups such as control, starvation and restraint. Restraint group rats were tied at their limbs with a string attached to a wire net frame (2100-0900). Starvation group rats were deprived of food and water for 12 h (2100-0900). Each group was i.p. injected with atropine and phentolamine at -1 h and $+6$ h with stresses beginning at 0 h. Doses of the chemicals used were as follows: atropine (1 or 5 mg/kg) and phentolamine (1 or 10 mg/kg). All injection solutions (2 ml/kg) were prepared in distilled water before injection.

The animals were sacrificed by decapitation, and blood was collected in glass tubes for determination of serum Zn concentration. Livers were perfused *in situ* with cold 0.9% NaCl solution and then removed, washed and weighed. The tissues were homogenized with 4 volumes of 0.25 M sucrose in a Potter-Elvehjem homogenizer with a teflon pestle. Hepatic cytosols were prepared by the method described previously (Arizono et al., 1985). To obtain serum, blood was centrifuged at $1,000 \times g$ for 10 min. The MT concentration was determined according to Onosaka et al. (1978). The concentrations of cytosol and serum Zn were also measured. Stomach lesions of animals were observed in the gastric mucosa as index of stress.

At least three animals in each group were processed individually. Data is presented as the mean $\pm$ SE. Statistical comparisons between groups were performed using the student's t-test.

RESULTS

Communication Box Stress

Mice

Induction of MT by Communication Box Stress. Mice were given a stress period of 6 h and were killed immediately. Three types of stresses, such as starvation, sender, and responder, significantly increased the hepatic Zn-MT levels as compared with control (Table I). The induced hepatic Zn-MT levels in the responder was more than that in the sender. However, no

TABLE I.
Effects of Physiological Stress on Cytosol Zinc and Metallothionein Concentrations

Groups	Mice		Rats	
	Cytosol Zn[a]	MT[b]	Cytosol Zn[a]	MT[b]
Control	3.86 ± 0.37	0.16 ± 0.02	5.43 ± 0.19	0.13 ± 0.03
Starvation	3.80 ± 0.04	0.75 ± 0.27*	9.36 ± 0.53*	0.98 ± 0.11*
Sender	3.97 ± 0.06	1.07 ± 0.11*	8.54 ± 0.92*	1.69 ± 0.10*
Responder	3.91 ± 0.05	1.26 ± 0.11*	6.94 ± 0.39*	1.16 ± 0.11*

Animals were exposed to each stress for 6 h (mice) and 12 h (rats).
Each value represents the mean $\pm$ S.E. of 3 to 5 animals.
Significantly different from corresponding mean of control group, *$p < 0.01$.
[a]μg/ml.
[b]μg/mg protein.

significant changes were observed in the cytosol Zn levels by these stresses.

Gastric mucosal lesions (petechica bleeding) were observed in both sender and responder mice.

Effects of Psychotropic Drugs. We have also tested the effect of tranquilizers on the induction of mouse hepatic Zn-MT in sender and responder (Figure 2).

In the responder group, Zn-MT levels were decreased by the pretreatment with chlorpromazine (major tranquilizer) but not by diazepam (minor tranquilizer) at 1 h before the exposure to these stresses. In the sender group, in contrast, MT levels were significantly increased by the pretreatment with both tranquilizer, as compared with those of starved control. These effects are expressed as percent inhibition in Table II.

The incidences of gastric lesions in both sender and responder were reduced by each drug pretreatment, respectively.

Rats

Induction of MT by Communication Box Stress. The ability to induce hepatic Zn-MT by emotional stress (responder), as compared with physical stresses (sender), was examined with the communication box method.

Rats were given three types stresses (starvation, sender, and responder) for a period of 12 h, and were killed immediately after 12-h stresses. The load of these stresses resulted in an increase of hepatic Zn-MT and cytosol Zn levels in rats (Table I). A modest increase in Zn-MT level was seen with responder as compared to sender. The Zn-MT level in responder did not indicate the significant enhancement to starvation.

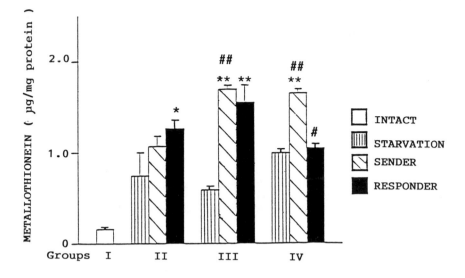

Figure 2. Induction of metallothionein by communication box method in mice. Group I, Saline; Group II, 6-h Stress; Group III, Diazepam pretreatment; Group IV, Chlorpromazine pretreatment. Chemicals were given (i.p.) at -1 h with stress beginning at 0 h and animals were killed immediately after 6-h stress. Each value represents the mean $\pm$ S.E. of 6 to 8 mice. *: $p < 0.02$, **: $p < 0.01$ as compared with starved mice of each group. #: $p < 0.02$, ##: $p < 0.01$ as compared with corresponding mice of Group II.

TABLE II.
Percent Inhibition of Physiological Stress Induced Metallothionein Levels by Tranquilizers

Treatments	% Inhibition
Sender + Diazepam	-250.1[a]
+ Chlorpromazine	-93.8[a]
Responder + Diazepam	-88.2[b]
+ Chlorpromazine	94.1

[a] $100-[(\text{sender}+@)-(\text{starvation}+@)]/(\text{sender})-(\text{starvation})$.
[b] $100-[(\text{responder}+@)-(\text{starvation}+@)]/(\text{responder})-(\text{starvation})$.
$@ = $ Chemical treatment.

Gastric mucosal lesions (petechica bleeding) were observed in both sender and responder rats.

Effects of Receptor Blockers. Figure 3 presents the results of an experiment in which several receptor blockers (each at 1 mg/kg i.p.) were administered to responders at −1 h and +6 h with stresses beginning at 0 h. Hepatic Zn-MT levels were apparently depresed by adrenoceptor blockers, such as phentolamine (α-blocker) and propranolol (β-blocker), while little decrease was seen with atropine (anticholinergic drug) or cimetidine) histamine H_2 receptor antagonist). A modest decrease in MT synthesis was seen with reserpine (antihypertensive agent:norepinephrine re-uptake blocker). These results are represented as percent inhibition (Table III). Phentolamine and propranolol, showed good MT synthesis inhibition compared to the responders (68.0%, 65.0%), and starvation (25.9%, −5.9%) respectively. Reserpine also showed an inhibition effect compared to the responders (57.3%).

The incidences of gastric lesions in both sender and responder were reduced by all drug pretreatments.

Restraint Stress

Induction of MT by Restraint Stress

Rats were given a restraint stress for a period of 12 h, and killed immediately. The concentration of Zn-MT was increased about 15.8 fold 12 h after restraint stress treatment as compared with the control (Table IV). In addition, an increase in cytosol Zn concentration (1.6-fold) and the decrease in serum Zn concentration (0.7-fold) was observed.

Gastric mucosal lesions (hemorrhagic erosion) were observed in the restraint stress group.

Effects of Phentolamine or Atropine on Restraint Stress

No significant alteration was observed in the concentration of hepatic Zn-MT by the treatment of either atropine (1 mg/kg) or phentolamine (1 mg/kg) compared to the control rat groups, respectively. Induction of hepatic Zn-MT by restraint stress was greatly depressed by atropine pretreatment, while the pretreatment of phentolamine at a dose of 1 mg/kg did not affect Zn-MT concentration (Figure 4). Ten mg/kg pretreatment of phentolamine resulted in a depression of hepatic Zn-MT induction by restraint stress in rats.

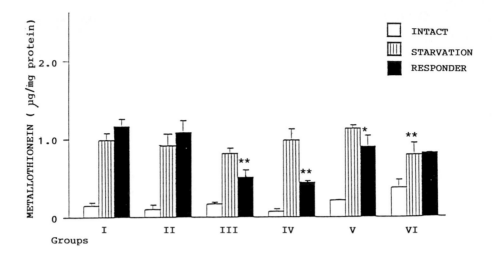

Figure 3. Induction of metallothionein by starvation or emotional stress in rats. Group I, Saline; (Control) 12 h Starvation; 12 h Responder; Group II, Atropine treatment; Group III, Phentolamine treatment; Group IV, Propranolol treatment; Group V, Cimetidine treatment; Group VI, Reserpine treatment. Chemicals were given (i.p.) at −1 h and +6 h with stress beginning at 0 h and animals were killed immediately after 12-h stress. Each value represents the mean ± S.E. of 3 to 5 rats. *: $p < 0.02$, ** $p < 0.01$ as compared with corresponding rats of Group I.

TABLE III.
Percent Inhibition of Physiological Stress Induced Metallothionein Levels by Several Chemicals

	% Inhibition	
Treatments	A	B
Atropine	−76.5	4.9
Phentolamine	25.9	68.0
Propranolol	−5.9	65.0
Reserpine	49.4	57.3
Cimetidine	−22.4	−23.3

[a]100-[(sender + @) − (starvation + @)]/(sender) − (starvation).
[b]100-[(responder + @) − (starvation + @)]/(responder) − (starvation).
@ = Chemical treatment.

TABLE IV.
Concentrations of Zinc in Serum, Hepatic Cytosols, and Metallothionein After Stress Treatment in Rats

	Control	Restraint Stress
Metallothionein (μg/mg protein)	100[0.15 ± 0.03]	1580 ± 67**
Zn		
Serum (μg/ml)	100[2.06 ± 0.09]	72 ± 8*
Cytosol (μg/ml)	100[5.43 ± 0.19]	164 ± 5**

Animals were exposed to restraint stress for 12 h. Each value represents % of control group and the mean ± S.E. to 3 to 5 rats. Significantly different from corresponding mean of control group, *p <0.02, **p <0.01, [ ]: control value.

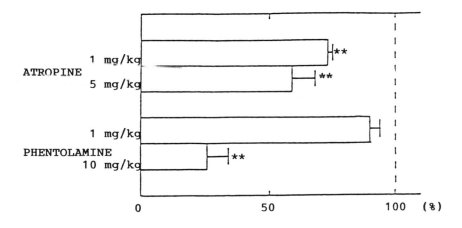

Figure 4. Effects of atropine or phentolamine on the content of hepatic metallothionein by restraint stress. Atropine (1 or 5 mg/kg) or Phentolamine (1 or 10 mg/kg) was i.p. injected at − 1 h and +6 h with restraint stress beginning at 0 h. Animals were killed immediately after 12 h restraint stress. Each value represents percent of restraint stress-treated group and the mean ± S.E. of 3 to 5 rats. Significantly different from corresponding mean of restraint stress treated group. ** p <0.01.

DISCUSSION

It has been reported that MT levels are increased in response to a variety of physiological stresses. In this study, we examined the MT inducibility in mice and rats by emotional stresses based on the communication box method and by the restraint stress method.

As a method of emotional transmission between animals, the communication box method has recently been used, for observing the change of general behavior and the appearance of stress ulcers, as the typical indexes. This communication box method is very useful to study purely emotional (psychological) stress, while excluding physical stimulation.

When the communication box method was applied to mice, hepatic Zn-MT levels were significantly enhanced in the emotional stress group (responder) as well as in the physical stress group (sender) after each 6 h stress exposure. The concentrations of hepatic Zn-MT in both stresses (responder, sender) showed higher levels than starved stress group.

We examined whether the administration of the psychotropic drugs (chlorpromazine: major tranquilizer and diazepam: minor tranquilizer) could affect the inducibility of Zn-MT by emotional stress in the mouse liver.

Chlorpromazine, which is an antipsychotic drug, prevented induction of Zn-MT by emotional stress, but diazepam, which is an anti-anxiety drug did not prevent induction of Zn-MT by emotional stress. The emotional stresses caused by communication box method enhances norepinephrine turnover in specific brain regions such as hypothalamus and amygdala which are closely related to emotions in rats (Iimori et al., 1982). Chlorpromazine depresses both hypothalamus and amygdala regions directly. In addition, Longo (1972) reported that chlorpromazine blocks both dopamine receptor and adrenoceptors in brain.

Iimori et al. (1982) also reported that repeated physical stress such as restraint stress and foot shock stress produces a decrease of the sensitivity to catecholamines in rat brain. On the other hand, this phenomenon (adaptation) has not been observed in rat brain exposed to emotional stress based on the communication box method. There is a significant difference between the physical stress and the emotional stress in brain. Chronic foot shock stress has also been found to reduce the sensitivity of the norepinephrine-cyclic AMP generating system in the cerebral cortex and hypothalamus (Stone and Platt, 1982). The next study was conducted to investigate an experiment procedure that can be applied to rats.

After 12 h of the psychological stress in rats, hepatic Zn-MT levels were enhanced but Zn-MT levels did not show a significant increase when compared to the starvation groups. It has been demonstrated that rats indicate more weak level of stress ulcer as the index of emotional stress condition than mice (Ogawa et al., 1984). Our experiment also showed similar results.

Brady and Helvig (1984) reported that catecholamines can induce rat hepatic Zn-MT to high levels via adrenoceptors. Furthermore, prior administration of adrenoceptor blockers prevented induction of Zn-MT by catecholamines.

When emotional stress takes place, an increase of turnover rate of catecholamines is also seen (Iimori et al., 1982).

To confirm the action of catecholamine, we attempted to use adrenoceptor blockers to peripheral tissues. Adrenoceptor blockers, phentolamine and propranolol, significantly prevented the effect of psychological stress on the induction of Zn-MT. Several emotional stresses (acute anxiety, terror, and anger) lead to an increase in catabolic hormone secretion and a decrease in anabolic hormone secretion (Mason, 1971).

The ability of adrenoceptor antagonists to block the increase of Zn-MT levels by emotional stress may support the hypothesis that catecholamine acts via adenylate cyclase or protein kinase to induce hepatic Zn-MT.

Reserpine which is monoamine (norepinephrine, serotonin, and dopamine) re-uptake blocker also reduced Zn-MT level in responder. These results suggest that the sympathetic nervous system can induce Zn-MT via emotional stress based on communication box. Atropine and cimetidine did not indicate a significant effect to Zn-MT level in responder.

Restraint stress confirmed large Zn-MT induction effect as previously reported (Hidalgo et al., 1986, 1988). It is known that emotional stress facilitates both sympathetic nervous and parasympathetic nervous system, function simultaneously. Induction of hepatic Zn-MT by restraint stress was very significantly depressed by atropine (1 mg/kg) pretreatment, while phentolamine treatment (1 mg/kg) showed only a weak inhibition effect on hepatic Zn-MT level induction as compared to atropine treatment in restraint stress rats. However, high dose treatment (10 mg/kg) of phentolamine demonstrated a significant depressive effect on hepatic Zn-MT levels in restraint stress rats. These data suggested that the predominant effect of adaptation to norepinephrine release in restraint stress reveals in brain and peripheral nervous system. Torda et al. (1981) reported that chronic restraint stress has been shown to reduce the density of adrenergic receptors in the cortex, cerebellum, hypothalamus, and brainstem.

As atropine treatment showed an inhibition effect on hepatic Zn-MT levels in restraint stress in rats, the parasympathetic nervous system may be involved in induction of hepatic Zn-MT by physical stress.

REFERENCES

Arizono K, Ito T, Yamaguchi M, and Ariyoshi T (1982): Induction of zinc metallothionein in the liver of rats by lead. *Eisei Kagaku.* 28: 94–98.

Bremner I (1987): Nutritional and physiological significance of metallothionein. In, *Metallothionein II.* Kägi JHR and Kojima Y, Eds., Birkhäuser-Verlag, Basel. pp. 81–107.

Brady FO (1982): The physiological function of metallothionein. *Trends Biochem. Sci.* 7: 143–145.

Brady FO and Helvig B (1984): Effect of epinephrine and norepinephrine on zinc thionein levels and induction in rat liver. *Am. J. Physiol.* 247: E318–E322.

Etzel KR and Cousins RJ (1981): Hormonal regulation of liver metallothionein zinc: independent and synergistic action of glucagon and glucocorticoids. *Proc. Soc. Exp. Biol. Med.* 167: 233–236.

Hamer DH (1986): Metallothionein. *Ann. Rev. Biochem.* 55: 913–951.

Hidalgo J, Armario A, Flos R, Dingman A, and Garvey JS (1986): The influence of restraint stress in rats on metallothionein production and corticosterone and glucagon secretion. *Life Sci.* 39: 611–616.

Hidalgo J, Giralt M, Garvey JS, and Armario A (1988): Physiological role of glucocorticoids on rat serum and liver metallothionein on basal and stress conditions. *Am. J. Physiol.* 254: E71–E78.

Iimori K, Tanaka M, Kohno Y, Ida Y, Nakagawa R, Hoaki Y, Tsuda A, and Nagasaki N (1982): Psychological stress enhances noradrenaline turnover in specific brain regions in rats. *Pharmacol. Biochem. Behav.* 16: 637–640.

Kägi JHR and Nordberg M, Eds. (1979): *Metallothionein*, Birkhäuser-Verlag, Basel.

Kägi JHR and Kojima Y, Eds. (1987): *Metallothionein II*, Birkhäuser-Verlag, Basel.

Kägi JHR and Schäffer A (1988): Biochemistry of metallothionein. *Biochemistry* 27: 8509–8515.

Longo VG (1972): Antipsychotic drugs. *Neuropharmacology and Behavior*, WH Freeman, San Francisco, pp. 7–46.

Mason JW (1971): A re-evaluation of the concept of non-specificity in stress theory. *J. Psychiatr. Res.* 8: 323–333.

Ogawa N and Kuwabara H (1966): Psychophysiology of emotion-communication of emotion, *J. Jap. Psychosom. Soc.* 6: 352–357.

Ogawa N, Yoshimura H, Pack SJ, and Tsunekawa K (1984): A new experimental model of stress ulcers. *Ann. Rep. Pharmacopsychia. Res. Found.* 15: 22–29.

Oh SH, Deagen JT, Whanger PD, and Weswig PH (1978): Biological function of metallothionein V, its induction on rats by various stress. *Am. J. Physiol.* 234: E282–E285.

Onosaka T, Tanaka K, Doi M, and Okahara K (1978): A simplified procedure for determination of metallothionein in animal tissues. *Eisei Kagaku.* 24: 128–131.

Stone EA and Platt JE (1982): Brain adrenergic receptors and resistance to stress. *Brain Res.* 237: 405–414.

Sugawara N, Sugawara C, Maehara N, Sadamoto T, Harabuchi, and Yamamura K (1983): Effect of acute stresses on Zn-thionein production rat liver. *Eur. J. Appl. Physiol.* 51: 365–370.

Torda T, Yamaguchi I, Hirata F, Kopkin IJ, and Axelroad I (1981): Mepacrine treatment prevents immobilization-induced desensitization of beta-adrenergic receptors in rat hypothalamus and brain stem. *Brain Res.* 205: 441–444.

Hormonal Induction of Metallothionein Synthesis: Its Effect on Zinc Kinetics in the Rat

Michael A. Dunn
*Department of Food Science
and Human Nutrition
University of Hawaii
Honolulu, Hawaii*

INTRODUCTION

In intact animals, metallothionein (MT) gene expression is increased by a number of physiological and endocrine factors unrelated to metal exposure. These factors include stress, trauma, endotoxins, glucocorticoids, cAMP and the cytokines interleukin 1 (IL-1) and interleukin 6 (IL-6). These same factors also greatly affect zinc (Zn) metabolism. For example, the polypeptide cytokine IL-1, produced by monocytes and activated macrophages in response to a variety of stresses, has been shown to increase liver zinc concentrations and to transiently decrease plasma zinc by half (Cousins and Leinart, 1988). Additionally, two of the above mentioned physiological factors, cAMP and IL-1 have been shown to cause a redistribution of ^{65}Zn between body tissues (Cousins and Leinart, 1988; Dunn and Cousins, 1989). The physiological significance of the redistribution of tissue zinc is presently uncertain, but may be a part of the body's defense mechanism against infection, inflammation, injury or other types of stress. This paper summarizes data from MT gene expression and ^{65}Zn kinetic studies which indicate that the mechanism for altering zinc metabolism is related to tissue-specific enhancement of metallothionein synthesis at the level of MT gene transcription.

REGULATION OF TISSUE SPECIFIC METALLOTHIONEIN GENE EXPRESSION

Experiments by Cousins et al. (1986) and Cousins and Leinart (1988) have shown that intraperitoneal injections of cAMP or human recombinant IL-1 induce MT gene expression in a tissue-specific fashion. In these studies, tissue MT gene expression was monitored by measuring the MTmRNA levels using oligonucleotide hybridization probes specific for MTmRNAs. Both cAMP and IL-1 markedly increase liver MTmRNA levels, but levels in kidney and small intestine remain unchanged. IL-1 has also been shown to increase MTmRNA levels in thymus and bone marrow as well as the liver.

Recently, Schroeder and Cousins (1989) working at the cellular level, i.e., with isolated hepatocytes, showed that IL-1 had little effect on MT gene expression, but IL-6 in the presence of dexamethasone and zinc markedly stimulated MT gene expression. This suggests that at the level of the cell, at least in hepatocytes, IL-6 and not IL-1 is the primary inducer and that synergistic effects of various inducers (e.g. IL-6 and dexamethasone) are possible. Whether cAMP acts at the cellular level as an inducer is not yet clear.

METALLOTHIONEIN GENE EXPRESSION AND TISSUE ^{65}Zn DISTRIBUTION

The concentration of MT in the liver (and presumably MT levels in other tissues) generally parallels MTmRNA levels when concentrations are determined by either the cadmium binding method (Eaton and Toal, 1982) or gel filtration chromatography of tissue cytosol fractions followed by Zn or ^{65}Zn analysis of column fractions eluting at a Ve/Vo of 1.8. These changes in tissue MT concentrations resulting from tissue-specific gene induction are associated with a concomitant redistribution of body zinc.

Cousins and Leinart (1988) compared the kinetics of ^{65}Zn distribution in rats injected with IL-1 and control rats injected with saline. Six hours after IL-1 was administered MTmRNA levels were increased in liver, thymus and bone marrow. The percentage of a pulse dose of i.v. administered ^{65}Zn recovered in tissues was also measured. More ^{65}Zn was recovered in those tissues in which MT had been induced, i.e. liver, bone marrow and thymus when compared to control tissues. The ^{65}Zn content of plasma, bone,

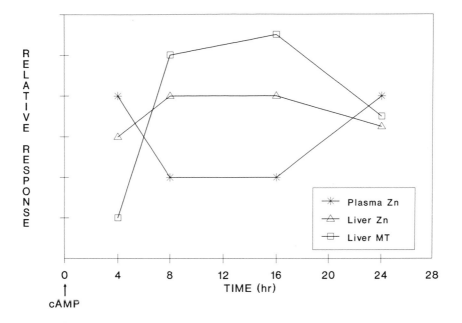

Figure 1. Effect of intraperitoneal injections of dibutyryl cAMP on plasma zinc, liver zinc, and liver metallothionein (MT) levels over time.

skin and intestine, however, was reduced by IL-1. Thus, IL-1 produced a dramatic shift in ^{65}Zn distribution among various tissues possibly related to tissue-specific induction of MT synthesis and subsequent zinc binding.

METALLOTHIONEIN GENE EXPRESSION AND ^{65}Zn KINETICS

Dunn and Cousins (1989) used compartmental kinetic analysis to investigate the effects of MT induction on rates of zinc exchange between tissues and within subcellular compartments of the liver, including hepatic metallothionein. In these studies intraperitoneal injections of dibutyryl cAMP (cAMP) were used to induce hepatic MT gene expression; control rats were injected with saline.

The temporal relationships between hepatic MT, serum zinc and liver zinc levels after cAMP injection are shown in Figure 1. Eight hours after cAMP treatment, hepatic MT levels had increased four-fold and plasma zinc was reduced by half. These levels then remained fairly constant until hour 16, after which they began to revert back to pretreatment (control) levels. In control rats, no change was seen in MT, plasma, or liver zinc levels over time.

At hour 8, when MT levels were clearly increased in cAMP-treated rats, a pulse dose of tracer amounts of ^{65}Zn was injected intrajugularly. The time course of ^{65}Zn distribution (percent of dose) in tissues and fecal excretions was measured and comparisons were made between cAMP and saline-treated rats. The observed data (percent of dose) for plasma, liver, liver MT and fecal excretions are shown as symbols (open or closed circles) in Figure 2. The lines through the data points are compartmental-model based computer simulations of the kinetic distributions (described below).

The disappearance of ^{65}Zn from the plasma of MT induced rats was faster than that in control rats (Figure 2A). However, by 24 h the ^{65}Zn content was the same in both groups. The accelerated disappearance of plasma ^{65}Zn was related in part to a greater uptake of ^{65}Zn by the liver of MT-induced rats (Figure 2B). Bone marrow and spleen were also found to contain increased amounts of ^{65}Zn in cAMP treated rats (data not shown). Most other tissues sampled contained less ^{65}Zn due to cAMP treatment. Most notable reductions were in skin, marrow-free bone, small intestine, pancreas (data not shown) and fecal excretion of ^{65}Zn (Figure 2D).

Within the liver, the subcellular distribution of ^{65}Zn was also altered by treatment with cAMP (Figure 3). Three crude subcellular fractions were assayed for ^{65}Zn content: a cytosolic MT fraction isolated by gel filtration of liver cytosol, a high-molecular-weight cytosolic fraction consisting of the pooled proteins from all gel filtration fractions of molecular weight greater than MT, and a crude, insoluble, pelleted fraction remaining after the high-speed centrifugation of liver homogenate in the preparation of cytosol.

In control rats, the cytosolic MT fraction accumulated little ^{65}Zn (never more than 5% of the dose). Most liver ^{65}Zn rapidly accumulated in the insoluble pellet (up to 14% of the dose) and intermediate amounts were found in the pooled, high-molecular-weight, cytosolic proteins (Figure 3).

In cAMP treated rats, the induction of MT resulted in a four-fold increase in the amount of ^{65}Zn bound to hepatic cytosolic metallothionein, so that now MT accumulated a large proportion of liver ^{65}Zn. More ^{65}Zn also accumulated in the insoluble pelleted fraction due to cAMP treatment (Figure 3). However, there did not appear to be any significant difference in the amount of ^{65}Zn bound to the high-molecular-weight protein fraction due to cAMP treatment early in the experimental period. This suggests that the increase in ^{65}Zn found in the insoluble pellet was not due to a general increase in nonspecific binding of ^{65}Zn to intracellular binding sites. Rather, it suggests that cAMP treatment altered the intracellular kinetics of ^{65}Zn.

The alterations in whole body and hepatic ^{65}Zn kinetics discussed above were analyzed further by compartmental analysis (Foster and Boston, 1983) in an effort to understand the kinetic mechanisms underlying zinc redistribution and the role of metallothionein in zinc kinetics. This kinetic analysis was used to describe pathways of zinc exchange between tissues and between

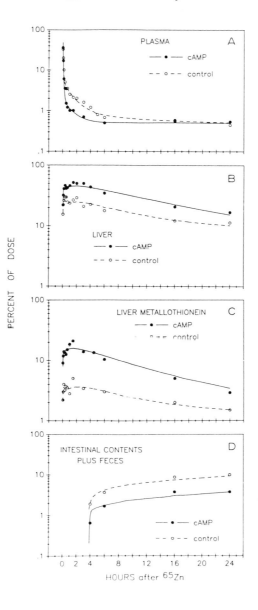

Figure 2. Comparison of observed (symbols) with model-calculated values (lines) for ⁶⁵Zn activity in plasma (A), liver (B), liver metallothionein (C), and intestinal contents plus feces (D) of rats administered either saline (control) or dibutyryl cAMP prior to ⁶⁵Zn injection. Model calculated ⁶⁵Zn activity in liver includes sum of activity in compartments 7, 8, and 9 in the control model and compartments 7, 8, 9 and 17 in the cAMP model.

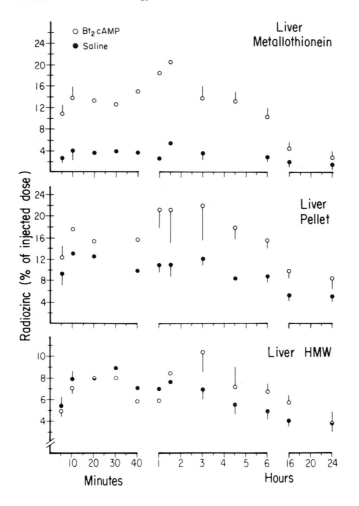

Figure 3. Amount of ^{65}Zn in subcellular fractions of liver at selected times after ^{65}Zn injection into rats administered either dibutyryl cAMP (Bt$_2$cAMP) or saline. Metallothionein and high-molecular weight (HMW) fractions of liver cytosol were obtained by gel filtration, the liver pellet by high speed centrifugation of liver homogenates. Points are means of 2 to 4 rats, vertical bars represent S.D. Points without error bars represent n = 1.

subcellular compartments of the liver and to identify which pathways were altered by cAMP induction of MT. The results support the hypotheses that MT induction results in the net uptake of zinc from the plasma and that cytosolic MT exchanges zinc with other zinc ligands within hepatocytes.

The method of compartmental analysis resulted in two compartmental kinetic models that simulate the temporal and spatial distribution of ^{65}Zn as observed experimentally in the distribution data shown in Figure 2. First, a model was constructed (Figure 4) that could simulate the control rat data. The changes in the control rat model that were needed to simulate the altered kinetics of the cAMP treated rats were then investigated and a second model for cAMP treated rats was developed. All model development was done using the SAAM 27 and CONSAM modeling programs (Foster and Boston, 1983) run on a VAX® 11/780 computer. The details of model development have been described elsewhere (Dunn and Cousins, 1989).

The model of zinc kinetics in control rats shown in Figure 4 represents the simplest arrangement of transfer pathways and zinc compartments (pools)

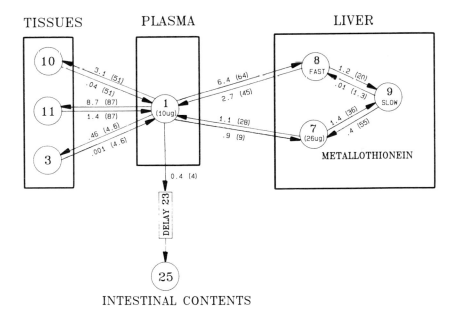

Figure 4. Model of zinc metabolism in control rats. Circles represent compartments, arrows represent transfer pathways. Large numbers within circles indicate compartment number. Number in parentheses within circles are model-predicted steady-state masses of zinc in micrograms. Mass of plasma zinc (compartment 1) was fixed at 10 μg. Numbers by arrows are fractional rate constants which represents fraction of compartment J transferred to compartment I per h. Numbers in parentheses by arrow are steady-state transfer rates which represent mass (μg) of zinc transferred from compartment J to compartment I per h. Small rectangle represents a delay element.

that could simulate or "fit" all the observed ^{65}Zn time course data shown in Figure 2A-D simultaneously. The model consists of a single, homogeneous, plasma zinc pool that exchanges zinc with compartments in the liver and extrahepatic tissues and is the source of zinc appearing in the intestinal contents and feces.

Within the liver plasma zinc exchanges with two distinct hepatic pools (pools 7 and 8), one of which (pool 7) simulates the kinetics of ^{65}Zn in cytosolic metallothionein. The physiological identity of the nonmetallothionein pool (pool 8) is unknown. Other models which had plasma zinc exchanging with liver zinc solely via the MT pool of the liver were tested. None of these models could be fit to the plasma, whole liver, and MT observed data simultaneously indicating that plasma zinc rapidly exchanges with at least one other pool besides MT in the liver (i.e. pool 8). Furthermore, the model in Figure 4 suggests that most plasma zinc enters the liver of control rats via this nonmetallothionein exchangeable pool (pool 8).

Both hepatic pools that exchange zinc with plasma also had to exchange zinc with a slow turnover pool within the liver in order to fit the observed data (pool 9). This necessary kinetic feature of the model implies that MT zinc is exchanged with zinc on other ligands in the cell.

The kinetic mechanisms that caused the redistribution of ^{65}Zn due to MT induction by cAMP were investigated using the above described compartmental model for control rats. Basically, this involved altering the model structure and rates of zinc transfer between compartments until a new model was developed that could simulate the observed data for cAMP treated rats shown in Figure 2A-D. The model in Figure 5 shows the major changes in the control model necessary to simulate the altered kinetics of ^{65}Zn due to cAMP. Broad arrows indicate an increase in the fractional rate of zinc transfer between compartments compared to control transfer rates, and a dashed arrow indicates a decrease.

The increase in ^{65}Zn uptake by the total liver and liver MT fraction could be simulated by a four-fold increase in the fractional rate of plasma ^{65}Zn uptake into metallothionein in combination with an 85% reduction in the fractional rate of release of MT bound ^{65}Zn back to plasma. No change was needed in the exchange of plasma zinc with the nonmetallothionein hepatic pool 8 to fit the data. The ^{65}Zn not released to plasma from MT was redirected to an additional compartment in the cAMP treated liver, compartment 17, which received ^{65}Zn from MT. This pathway may represent the movement of MT with its bound ^{65}Zn into a new cellular compartment possibly due to partial degradation or polymerization of MT or, alternatively, the transfer of MT zinc to a new ligand in cAMP treated rats.

The induction of hepatic MT also appeared to increase the rate of exchange of ^{65}Zn with the slow turnover liver compartment. The physiological significance of this is unknown but suggests that the induction of MT may affect the transfer of zinc to other ligands in the cell.

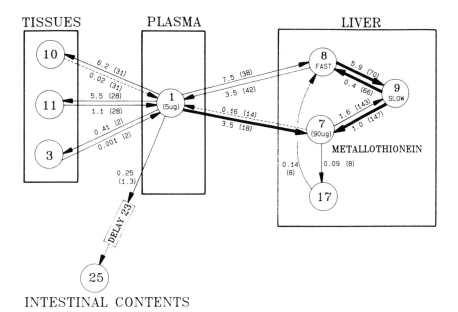

TISSUES   PLASMA   LIVER

INTESTINAL CONTENTS

Figure 5. Model of Zn metabolism in cAMP-treated rats. See Figure 4 for definitions of circles, numbers within circles, arrows, and numbers by arrows. Compartment masses and fractional rate constants shown represent values during the steady-state period (hour 0 to 6 after ^{65}Zn injection) before the system began to return to the control state. Broad arrows and dashed arrows represent sites of regulation of Zn metabolism due to cAMP administration. Broad arrows represent an increase in fractional rate constant over control values and dashed arrows represent a decrease. Additional compartment 17, not required in the control model (Figure 4), represents an added turnover mechanism for metallothionein Zn.

The greater rate of ^{65}Zn disappearance from plasma in cAMP treated rats could not be totally explained (simulated) just by altering the exchange rates between plasma and hepatic MT as described above. The rate constant for release of ^{65}Zn from extrahepatic tissue compartment 10 back to plasma also needed to be reduced by half. This reduction in release of tissue zinc back to plasma is consistent with the induction of MT in extrahepatic tissues as judged by the similar kinetic effect of MT induction in the liver.

Tissue compartments 10, 11, and 3 could not be assigned to individual tissues. Rather, tissues are thought to consist of different proportions of each compartment. Compartment 10 may represent extrahepatic MT. Bone marrow and spleen, then, may have accumulated more ^{65}Zn in their compartment 10 due to increased MT levels in these two tissues after cAMP injection.

Before summing up the conclusions from this kinetic analysis some comments on computer modeling and the kinetic models presented here should be made. Computer models are indeed only models that simulate kinetics observable in real systems and predict kinetics that are not directly observable, such as the *in vivo* kinetics between MT and other intracellular ligands. Obviously, the pathways of zinc transfer in intact animals are much more complex than that represented in the models described here. Nevertheless, these relatively simple models do accurately simulate short term ^{65}Zn kinetics in plasma, liver and liver MT. When a homogeneous pool of zinc like MT zinc or plasma zinc can be observed (sampled), their kinetic relationship to each other and to other pools in the model can be simulated even though the physiological identity of other compartments in the model are unknown. The models do not prove that the kinetic relationships exists, only that the observed data can be explained by such relationships.

In the development of these models, many simpler models were tried but discarded because they could not simulate the data. It is possible to simulate the data with a more complex model but until other zinc pools are sampled (for example ^{65}Zn in hepatic nuclei) there is little justification for adding additional hepatic pools.

The models presented here are steady state models that simulate zinc kinetics in control rats and the steady state kinetics in cAMP treated rats evident over the period of hours 8 to 16 in Figure 1 (i.e. when the amount of zinc in plasma, liver and liver MT remains relatively constant over time). The altered rate constants in the steady-state cAMP model, then, represent transport rates that have been altered by increased MT synthesis, MT concentrations and the appearance of zinc transfer to compartment 17. It is assumed that these altered rates are responsible for the redistribution of zinc evident during hours 4 to 8 after cAMP injection (Figure 1). However, to substantiate such assumptions the values of these rate constants should be varied over time from their values in the control model to their values in the cAMP model and this should produce an effect on the amount of zinc in the plasma and MT zinc pools in the model that is consistent with that observed *in vivo*. This simply means that modeling the transition between two steady states (non-steady state modeling) gives more information about the mechanisms causing the transition than steady-state modeling.

Dunn and Cousins (1989) used non-steady state modeling to try and simulate the increase of plasma zinc back to control values evident between hours 16 and 24 after cAMP injection (Figure 1). To do this they made the rate constants in the cAMP model revert back to their control values over the period of hours 16 to 24. This did result in an appropriate decrease in the zinc content of the MT compartment and an increase in plasma zinc in the model. However, the increase in the zinc content of the plasma pool in the model was only half that needed to be consistent with the increase observed *in vivo*. This indicates that the body has other mechanisms to return plasma zinc to normal besides the release of MT bound zinc back to plasma. This unknown mechanism for controlling plasma zinc may explain why plasma zinc is only transiently reduced by IL-1 injection even though MT levels and presumably zinc levels continue to rise in the liver (Cousins and Leinart, 1988).

Dunn and Cousins (1989) investigated whether the rise of plasma zinc back to control levels could result from the secretion of zinc bound to alpha-2 macroglobulin, a protein thought to contain non-exchangeable zinc and known to be secreted by rats in response to inflammation (Parisi and Vallee, 1970; Schreiber et al., 1982). Sodium dodecyl sulfate polyacrylamide gel electrophoresis of serum from cAMP injected rats did demonstrate that alpha-2 macroglobulin levels are elevated 24 h after cAMP treatment. But, gel filtration of the same serum through Sephadex G-200® showed that no ^{65}Zn or zinc could be detected with the alpha-2 macroglobulin fractions (unpublished observations). Thus, the mechanisms for the return of plasma zinc to normal 24 h after cAMP or 12 h after IL-1 injection remain unknown.

SUMMARY AND CONCLUSIONS

The hormonal or cytokine induction of MT gene expression is tissue specific. The specific tissues affected and the degree of induction may depend on the profile of hormones and cytokines presented to the cells. IL-6 in the presence of glucocorticoids and zinc appears to be the most potent inducer in isolated hepatocytes. The liver is always a primary target organ but IL-1 has been shown to increase MTmRNA in bone marrow and thymus as well. Kinetic evidence (^{65}Zn uptake) suggests that cAMP induces MT gene expression in liver, bone marrow and spleen.

Those tissues in which MT is induced have been shown to take up more zinc or ^{65}Zn from the plasma. This results in a reduction in plasma zinc and zinc redistribution in the body. The increase in zinc in the liver is greater than what can be accounted for by the reduction in plasma zinc indicating that some extrahepatic tissues lose zinc to the liver. ^{65}Zn uptake studies indicate that skin, marrow-free bone and intestine are probably sites of zinc loss. The physiological significance of the redistribution of zinc between tissues is unknown but may relate to host defense mechanisms. Increased zinc in the thymus and bone marrow may promote thymic function and hematopoiesis while decreased plasma zinc may help control infection. Schroeder and Cousins (1989, 1990) showed that MT induction in isolated hepatocytes resulted in the zinc uptake into the cells and afforded cytoprotection against carbon tetrachloride toxicity.

The transport mechanisms that cause the redistribution of body zinc are not completely understood. They may relate to MT synthesis in that the filling of zinc binding sites on hormonally induced apometallothionein may draw zinc into cells from the plasma and, it may reduce the transfer of zinc from MT binding sites back to plasma. Additionally, some zinc brought into the cytosolic MT pool of the liver may be directed to other intracellular compartments. Both the steady-state and non-steady state kinetic models mentioned above support these mechanisms.

It appears that one of the biological roles of hormonal MT induction is to cause shifts in zinc transport between tissues. This role, coupled with the kinetic evidence for the exchange of MT zinc with other intracellular ligands, raises the question of the significance of MT in intracellular zinc transport. For example, if apometallothionein is synthesized or present in the nucleus, or any organelle, would this draw zinc into the organelle? Can the intact zinc-MT molecule or degradation products move into different cellular compartments? Do changes in nuclear MT levels alter the exchange rates of zinc among intranuclear ligands? These questions keep the potential biological roles for metallothionein intriguing.

REFERENCES

Cousins RJ, Dunn MA, Leinart AS, Yedinak KC, and DiSilvestro RA (1986): Coordinate regulation of zinc metabolism and metallothionein gene expression in rats. *Am. J. Physiol.* 251: E688.

Cousins RJ and Leinart AA (1988): Tissue-specific regulation of zinc metabolism and metallothionein genes by interleukin 1. *FASEB J.* 2: 2884.

Dunn MA and Cousins RJ (1989): Kinetics of zinc metabolism in the rat: effects of dibutyryl cAMP. *Am. J. Physiol.* 256: E420.

Eaton DL and Toal BF (1982): Evaluation of the Cd/hemoglobin affinity assay for the rapid determination of metallothionein in biological tissues. *Toxicol. Appl. Pharmacol.* 66: 134.

Foster DM and Boston RC Eds., (1983): *Compartmental Distribution of Radiotracers,* CRC Press, Boca Raton, FL, pp. 73–142.

Parisi AF and Vallee BL (1970): Isolation of a zinc α-$_2$-macroglobulin from human serum. *Biochemistry* 9:2421.

Schreiber G, Howlett G, Nagashima M, Millership A, Martin H, Urban J, and Kotler L (1982): The acute phase response of plasma protein synthesis during experimental inflammation. *J. Biol. Chem.* 237: 10271.

Schroeder JJ and Cousins RJ (1989): Interleukin 6 (interferon B$_2$) regulates metallothionein gene expression and zinc metabolism in hepatocyte monolayer culture. *FASEB J.* 3: A458 (abstract no. 1344).

Schroeder JJ and Cousins RJ (1990): Metallothionein induction and zinc accumulation in hepatocytes stimulated by interleukin 6, glucocorticoids and zinc correlate with cytoprotection against carbon tetrachloride toxicity. *FASEB J.* 4: A388 (abstract no. 706).

Chapter 23

Metallothionein Gene Family in *Candida glabrata*

R.K. Mehra and D.R. Winge
University of Utah Medical Center
Salt Lake City, Utah

INTRODUCTION

Cells exposed to elevated concentrations of essential as well as non-essential metal ions are susceptible to metal-induced cytotoxicity. In response to these stress conditions, cells have evolved a variety of mechanisms to resist metal-induced cytotoxicity. Sequestration and reduced uptake and/or facilitated efflux of potentially toxic metal ions are among the most commonly used mechanisms. Prokaryotes generally limit the intracellular concentrations of the metal ions by regulating uptake or facilitating efflux (Silver et al., 1982, 1989; Silver and Misra, 1988). Eukaryotes typically detoxify heavy metal ions by sequestering the ions within stable complexes (Hamer, 1986; Kägi and Kojima, 1987; Grill et al., 1985; and Hayashi et al., 1986).

MOLECULES INVOLVED IN METAL ION RESISTANCE

Two families of molecules, one represented by cysteine-rich polypeptides functionally designated metallothioneins (Hamer, 1986; Kägi and Kojima, 1987) and the other by enzymatically synthesized glutathione-related peptides of general structure $(\gamma\text{-EC})_n G$ (Grill et al., 1985; Hayashi et al.,

1986; Winge et al., 1989) are involved in the cellular sequestration of toxic metal ions in eukaryotes. Animals use metallothioneins (MT) as the main metal ion sequestering molecules while plants utilize $(\gamma EC)_n G$ peptides for the same purpose. Metallothioneins are known to function in metal ion resistance, but additional physiological functions have been proposed (Bremner, 1987). Certain plant species have been reported to contain MT molecules, but it is unclear whether these molecules function primarily in metal ion detoxification or in other processes such as zinc ion storage within the plant embryo (Lane et al., 1987).

Fungi are known to synthesize either MT-like polypeptides or $(\gamma EC)_n G$ peptides (Hayashi et al., 1986; Beltramini and Lerch, 1983; Winge et al., 1985). For example, *Saccharomyces cerevisiae* and *Neurospora crassa* respond to the intracellular Cu(I) ion concentration by synthesizing MT-like polypeptides, whereas $(\gamma EC)_n G$ peptides are the major metal-binding species in *Schizosaccharomyces pombe*. We recently demonstrated that the yeast *Candida glabrata* uses both MTs and $(\gamma EC)_n G$ peptides to detoxify metal ions and the synthesis of each is regulated in a metal-specific manner (Mehra et al., 1988). Cadmium ions induce the synthesis of $(\gamma EC)_n G$ peptides whereas MTs are synthesized in response to copper ions.

Metal ions are sequestered within metallothioneins as metal:thiolate polynuclear clusters (Kägi and Kojima, 1987). Mammalian MT typically contains 20 cysteinyl thiolates within a 61 residue polypeptide and binds a variety of metal ions within two polynuclear clusters enfolded by distinct domains. The type and stoichiometry of the polynuclear cluster is dictated by the metal ion bound (Nielson et al., 1985). The structure of the Cd,ZnMT molecule consists of a monolayer of polypeptide wrapped around a core consisting of the metal:thiolate clusters (Braun et al., 1986; Furey et al., 1986).

A variety of nondescriptive names have been used in reference to the $(\gamma EC)_n G$ peptides including cadystin and phytochelatin (Hayashi et al., 1986; Grill et al., 1985). Typically a heterogeneous mixture of peptides varying in the number of dipeptide repeats (from n_2 to n_4) are synthesized. An enzyme has recently been described that catalyzes the elongation of the $(\gamma EC)_n G$ peptides and the catalytic activity of this enzyme appears to be metalloregulated (Grill et al., 1989). The peptides bind metal ions in a metal:cysteine thiolate cluster involving an oligomer of $(\gamma EC)_n G$ peptides (Reese et al., 1988).

Cd(II)-$(\gamma EC)_n G$ peptide complexes from *S. pombe* and *C. glabrata* contain sulfide ions as an additional component of the cluster (Murasugi et al., 1984; Mehra et al., 1988; Reese et al., 1988). The sulfide-containing clusters consists of cadmium:sulfide mineral lattice coated with $(\gamma EC)_n G$ peptides (Dameron et al., 1989). The cluster from *C. glabrata* contains a lattice of 85 cadmium:sulfide pairs with nearly 30 $(\gamma EC)_n G$ peptides as the coating sheath. The metabolic production of sulfide ions is part of the cellular repertoire of eukaryotic cells to resist the adverse effects of metal ions. Some species precipitate metal ions as metal:sulfide particles on the cell surface or in the growth medium (Naiki and Yamagata, 1976; Minney and Quirk, 1985).

Glutathione also functions as an initial defense against metal-induced cytotoxicity in most if not all species. Depletion of mammalian and plant cells of glutathione by the use of an inhibitor of the enzyme γ-glutamylcysteine synthetase sensitizes cells to toxic effects of metal ions (Singhal et al., 1987; Ochi et al., 1988). Metal complexes with glutathione have been observed in some systems (Freedman et al., 1989; Dameron et al., 1989). Cd(II)-glutathione appears to be the initial sequestration complex in *C. glabrata* prior to formation of the Cd(II)-(γEC)$_n$G peptide clusters (Barbas and Winge, 1991). Under certain growth conditions, sulfide ions are incorporated within the Cd-glutathione complex to yield CdS lattices coated with a mixture of glutathione and the γ-glutamylcysteine dipeptide (Dameron et al., 1989).

COPPER-METALLOTHIONEINS IN *C. GLABRATA*

C. glabrata responds to copper toxicity by synthesizing a family of metallothioneins (Mehra et al., 1988). Two members of this family, designated MT I and MT II, have been cloned and sequenced (Mehra et al., 1989). Southern analyses indicate multiple MT II genes but a single MT I gene. This result is consistent with the observed microheterogeneity in the purified MT II protein sequence (Mehra et al., 1988). It is noteworthy that the overall organization of the *C. glabrata* MT gene family is very similar to MT gene families seen in higher vertebrates as each family consists of two principle genes and only one of these is typically present in multiple isoforms.

The MT family in vertebrates consists of highly conserved polypeptides. The positions of cysteinyl residues involved in metal-binding are invariant (Hamer, 1986; Kägi and Kojima, 1986). In contrast, the two MT genes in the invertebrate *Drosophila* encode proteins that show little sequence homology to each other (Lastowski-Perry et al., 1985; Mokdad et al., 1987). *C. glabrata* MTs, likewise, exhibit limited sequence homology with each other as indicated by alignment of the two sequences shown below. Neither of the *C. glabrata* MTs shares any appreciable sequence similarity with known vertebrate, invertebrate, or fungal MTs.

```
         1                                                  50
MT II PEQVNCQYDCHCSNCACENTCNC--CAKPACACTN-SASNECSCQTCKCQTCKC
         1  : : : : :  ::  .: :           :: :   ::: 50
MT I       ANDCKCPNGCSCPNCANGGCQCGDKCECKKQSCHGCG-EQCKCGSHGSSCH
MT I cont. GSCGCGDKCECK
```

Despite a lack of sequence similarity, the two *C. glabrata* MTs exhibit the typical metallothionein sequence motif Cys-X-Cys (where X is any other amino acid). The role played by these sequence motifs in the formation of metal clusters in MTs is well recognized. Both *C. glabrata* MT I and MT II contain seven Cys-X-Cys sequences. MT I has 18 cysteines in a polypeptide of 62 residues whereas MT II has 16 cysteines in a molecule of 51 residues. The presence of His and Tyr in *C. glabrata* MTs is rare in this protein family. Cyanobacterium MT (Olafson, 1986) and *C. glabrata* MT II are the only MTs known to contain tyrosine. Histidine has been observed only in MTs from chicken, *S. cerevisiae,* and cyanobacterium (Winge et al., 1985; Olafson, 1986; Fernando et al.,1989). Both *C. glabrata* MT I and MT II contain histidine, MT I has three whereas MT II has a single residue of this amino acid. It is not clear whether the histidinyl residues participate in metal ligation in MT I.

A significant feature of the primary structures of *C. glabrata* MTs, not usually seen in MT, is the presence of internal sequence repeats. The pentapeptide Gln-Thr-Cys-Lys-Cys is repeated in MT II. MT I has two sequence repeats: the pentapeptide Cys-X-Cys-Pro-Asn and the octapeptide sequence Cys-Gly-Asp-Lys-Cys-Glu-Cys-Lys. These repeats may be indicative of gene duplications leading to elongation of the protein chain.

C. glabrata produces a processed MT II designated MT II' with Gln_7 of the full length protein as the amino terminus. The truncated molecule does not derive from an unique MT gene as shown by Southern analyses with a oligonucletide probe direct at the N-terminal sequence of MT II. It appears likely that MT II' is produced by proteolytic cleavage of MT II at the junction of Cys_6 and Gln_7. Similar post translational processing has been observed in *S. cerevisiae* MT (Winge et al., 1985). The fact that the peptide cleaved from *C. glabrata* MT II contains a cysteine (Cys_6) may indicate lack of involvement of this particular residue in the formation of metal clusters, although this was not observed in alkylation studies using iodoacetate.

The metal composition of vertebrate MTs depends on factors such as age, sex, nutritional conditions, and metal exposure (Webb, 1987). A variety of metals ions including cadmium, zinc, copper and mercury have been found associated with animal MTs (Hamer, 1986; Kägi and Kojima, 1987). In contrast, fungal MTs have been found to contain only copper (Beltramini and Lerch, 1983; Winge et al., 1985) and this is true also with *C. glabrata* MTs (Mehra et al., 1988). Both native and reconstituted samples of *C. glabrata* MT II show luminescence characteristic of Cu(I)-thiolate clusters (Byrd et al., 1988) indicating that the metal is bound to the protein in its monovalent state. This finding is consistent with previous studies on all copper-containing MTs (Abrahams et al., 1986; Smith et al., 1986; George et al., 1988). MT II binds 10 mol. eq. of copper. This stoichiometry is observed in native samples and in Cu(I)-reconstituted samples. Analysis of the native MT I suggested that approximately 11–12 mol. eq. of copper were bound, although the limited availability of MT I precluded a detailed investigation of metal-binding stoichiometry of this protein (see below).

The Cu(I)-thiolate coordination complex in CuMT is extremely stable. Proton displacement studies have shown that the pH at which 50% of bound Cu(I) ions dissociate from rat and probably other mammalian MTs is 2.7. The pH of half dissociation of Cu(I) binding to $(\gamma EC)_n G$ peptides and *S. cerevisiae* MT is 1.3 and 0.3, respectively. The corresponding value for *C. glabrata* MT II is pH 0.8.

EXPRESSION OF METALLOTHIONEIN GENES IN *CANDIDA GLABRATA*

The expression of MT genes in *C. glabrata* is regulated at the transcriptional level (Mehra et al., 1989). The mRNA content of both MT I and MT II is increased in cells exposed to copper and silver salts, but not cadmium salts. MT II mRNA is induced far more extensively than MT I mRNA. This result is consistent with the finding that copper-treated cells produced very small amounts of MT I protein. In the absence of added copper salts a small basal signal was observed. The basal amounts of both MT I and MT II mRNA were reduced when the cells were treated with cadmium sulfate. It is unclear whether the basal level of MTs implies basal regulatory elements or low levels of copper ions in the growth medium components.

The transcriptional activation of the *S. cerevisiae* MT gene is mediated by a transcriptional activation protein which binds promoter DNA sequences only as the Cu(I):protein complex (Furst et al., 1988; Welch et al., 1989). It is postulated that Cu(I) interacts with the transcription factor, called ACE1 or *CUP2*, causing a conformational change in the molecule enabling it to bind to upstream activating DNA sequences. A similar mechanism of MT gene regulation in *C. glabrata* cells is likely. The treatment of *C. glabrata* cells with cadmium salts decreased the levels of both MT I and MT II mRNA, an observation which may imply that cadmium binding to the cysteinyl thiols in the putative transcription factor(s) confers a tertiary fold unsuitable for interaction with upstream activating sequences. Current investigations in our laboratory are focused on the delineation of upstream activating sequences that may be present in the *C. glabrata* MTII gene and the factor(s) that activate these sequences.

DIFFERENTIAL AMPLIFICATION IN THE METALLOTHIONEIN GENE FAMILY

There are multiple restriction fragments of genomic DNA that contain MT II sequences form different *C. glabrata* strains. One of the MT II genes (MT II$_a$) consists of tandemly amplified copies. The copy number of this gene varied from 3 to 8 in four wild-type isolates of *C. glabrata*. In the same strains the MT I gene is always present as a single copy as is the case with two other MT II genes. Differential amplification of MT genes has been observed only in *Drosophila melanogaster* (G. Maroni, personal communication), mammalian MT genes have been shown to undergo co-ordinate amplification (Crawford et al., 1985; Durnam and Palmiter, 1987; Hamer, 1986).

The MT gene copy number was determined in highly copper-resistant (Cu^R) strains isolated by EMS mutagenesis and by repeated culturing of the wild-type cells in medium containing high concentrations of copper sulfate. The concentration of copper sulfate required to inhibit growth of the cells by 50% was 0.8 mM for the parental strains 2001 and 67, and this EC$_{50}$ increased to 7 mM and 3 mM, respectively in the resistant cells. Analysis of these Cu^R strains for the MT gene copy number revealed no noticeable change in the dosage of MT I gene but a fourteen-fold increase in the copy number of the MT II$_a$ gene in strain 2001. The amplified copies were arranged tandemly. The increase in the number of tandem repeats in Cu^R strains was apparent in the size of the MT II-containing chromosome. Nine to ten chromosomal bands were resolved by pulsed field electrophoresis in different wild-type strains of *C. glabrata*. The MT I and MT II genes are associated with different chromosomes. The lack of amplification of single copy MT genes in *C. glabrata* is analogous to the situation in *S. cerevisiae*. The strains of the later harboring a single MT gene never show amplification at the *CUP1* locus (Fogel et al., 1984).

The intensity of the MT II band in Cu^R cells of strain 67 was only twice that of parental strain. It was determined that the entire locus was duplicated in this strain without affecting the size of the chromosome. One mechanism by which the MT II locus may be duplicated is through chromosomal disomy. Likewise, *S. cerevisiae* has been shown to become disomic for the MT-containing chromosome in some Cu^R strains (Fogel et al., 1984).

Drugs that inhibit DNA synthesis have been shown to enhance the frequency of amplification of certain genes (Schimke, 1988). Carcinogens induce amplification of the *CUP1* MT gene in *S. cerevisiae* and yield a Cu^R phenotype (Aladjem et al., 1988). Ethylmethanesulfonate treatment of *C. glabrata* strain 2001 increased the frequency of copper-resistant clones 11-fold and one EMS Cu^R clone exhibited a increase in the number of tandem repeats of MT II.

Acquisition of metal resistance in *S. cerevisiae* and a variety of cultured mammalian cells has been correlated to amplification of MT genes (Palmiter, 1987; Grady et al., 1987; Butt and Ecker, 1987). Amplification of MT genes in response to metal stress has also been observed in whole animals (Koropatnick et al., 1985). The present observations on increased copper resistance in strains of *C. glabrata* exhibiting amplification of MT II_a locus further support the thesis that MT is directly involved in metal detoxification. However, mechanisms other than MT gene expression are involved in metal detoxification reactions. The chelation of metals by glutathione presents an early event in metal detoxification (Singhal et al., 1987; Ochi et al., 1988). The generation of inorganic sulfide appears to be a significant metal detoxification mechanism in yeast (Naiki and Yamagata, 1976; Murasugi et al., 1984; Minney and Quirk, 1985). It is known that some strains of *S. cerevisiae* become copper resistant without amplification of *CUP1* locus (Aladjam et al., 1988). There is suggestive evidence that sulfide generation in these strains may be a major mechanism of copper detoxification (Naiki and Yamagata, 1976). Glutathione and sulfide are both involved in copper detoxification reactions in *C. glabrata*. The level of metal resistance in strains 2001 and 67 is nearly the same, although they differ significantly in the size of MT II locus. It appears likely that glutathione, sulfide and other mechanisms probably involving membrane transport may compensate for the low copy number of MTII gene in strain 2001. It can be concluded that *C. glabrata* elaborates multiple pathways for detoxification of copper ions, although the product of the MT II_a locus is the main sequestering molecule.

REFERENCES

Abrahams IL, Bremner I, Diakun GP, Garner CD, Hasnain SS, Ross I, and Vašák M (1986): Structural study of the copper and zinc sites in metallothioneins by using extended X-ray absorption fine structure. *Biochem. J.* 236: 585.

Aladjem MI, Koltin Y, and Lavi S (1988): Enhancement of copper resistance and *CUP1* amplification in carcinogen-treated yeast cells. *Mol. Gen. Genet.* 211: 88.

Barbas J and Winge DR (1991): In preparation.

Beltramini M. and Lerch K (1983): Spectroscopic studies on *Neurospora* metallothionein. *Biochemistry* 22: 2043.

Braun W, Wagner G, Wörgötter E, Vašák M, Kägi JHR, and Wüthrich K (1986): Polypeptide fold in the two metal clusters of metallothionein-2 by nuclear magnetic resonance in solution. *J. Mol. Biol.* 187: 125.

Bremner I (1987): Nutritional and physiological significance of metallothionein. *Experientia Supplementum* 52: 81.

Butt TR and Ecker DJ (1987): Yeast metallothionein and applications in biotechnology. *Microbiol. Rev.* 51: 351.

Byrd J, Berger RM, McMillin DR, Wright CR, Hamer D, and Winge DR (1988): Characterization of the copper-thiolate cluster in yeast metallothionein and two truncated mutants. *J. Biol. Chem.* 263: 6688.

Crawford BD, Enger MD, Griffith BB, Griffith JK, Hanners JL, Longmire JL, Munk AC, Stallings RL, Tesmer JG, Walters RA, and Hildebrand CE (1985): Coordinate amplification of metallothionein I and II genes in cadmium-resistant Chinese hamster cells. *Mol. Cell Biol.* 5: 320.

Dameron CT, Reese RN, Mehra RK, Kortan AR, Carroll PJ, Steigerwald ML, Brus LE, and Winge DR (1989): Biosynthesis of cadmium sulphide quantum semiconductor crystallites. *Nature* 338: 596.

Dameron CT, Smith BR, and Winge DR (1989): Glutathione-coated cadmium-sulfide crystallites in *Candida glabrata*. *J. Biol. Chem.* 264: 17355.

Durnam DM and Palmiter RD (1987): Analysis of the detoxification of heavy metal ions by mouse metallothionein. *Experientia Supplementum* 52: 457.

Fernando LP, Wei D, and Andrews GK (1989): Structure and expression of chicken metallothionein. *J. Nutr.* 119: 309.

Fogel S and Welch JW (1982): Tandem gene amplification mediates copper resistance in yeast. *Proc. Natl. Acad. Sci. U.S.A.* 79: 5342.

Fogel S, Welch JW, and Louis EJ (1984): Meiotic gene conversion mediates gene amplification in yeast. *Cold Spring Harbor Symp. Quant. Biol.* 49: 55.

Freedman JH, Ciriolo RM, and Peisach J (1989): The role of glutathione in copper-metabolism and toxicity. *J. Biol. Chem.* 264: 5598.

Furey WF, Robbins AH, Clancy LL, Winge DR, Wang BC and Stout CD (1986): Crystal structure of Cd,Zn-metallothionein. *Science* 231: 704.

Furst P, Hu S, Hackett R, and Hamer D (1988): Copper activates metallothionein gene transcription by altering the conformation of a specific DNA binding protein. *Cell* 55: 705.

George GN, Byrd J, and Winge DR (1988): X-ray absorption studies of yeast copper metallothionein. *J. Biol. Chem.* 263: 8199.

Grady DL, Moyzis RK, and Hildebrand CE (1987): Molecular and cellular mechanisms of cadmium resistance in cultured cells. *Experientia Supplementum* 52: 447.

Grill E, Winnacker EL, and Zenk MH (1985): Phytochelatins, the principle heavy-metal complexing peptides of higher plants. *Science* 230: 674.

Grill E, Loffler S, Winnacker EL, and Zenk MH (1989): Phytochelatins, the heavy-metal binding peptides of plants, are synthesized from gluthatione by a specific γ-glutamylcysteine dipeptidyl transpeptidase (phytochelatin synthase). *Proc. Natl. Acad. Sci. U.S.A.* 86: 6838.

Hamer DH (1986): Metallothionein. *Ann. Rev. Biochem.* 55: 913.

Hayashi Y, Nakagawa CW, and Murasugi A (1986): Unique properties of Cd-binding peptides induced in fission yeast, *Schizosaccharomyces pombe* 65: 13.

Kägi JHR and Kojima Y (1987): Chemistry and biochemistry of metallothionein. *Experientia Supplementum* 52: 25.

Koropatnick J, Winning R, Weise E, Heschl M, Gedamu L, and Duerksen J (1985): Mouse hepatic metallothionein-I gene cleavage by micrococcal nuclease is enhanced after induction by cadmium. *Nucl. Acids Res.* 13: 5423–5439.

Lane B, Kajioka R, and Kennedy T (1987): The wheat-germ E_c protein is a zinc-containing metallothionein. *Biochem. Cell Biol.* 65: 1001.

Lastowski-Perry D, Otto E, and Maroni G (1985): Nucleotide sequence and expression of a *Drosophila* metallothionein. *J. Biol. Chem.* 260: 1527.

Mehra RK, Tarbet BE, Gray WR, and Winge DR (1988): Metal-specific synthesis of two metallothioneins and γ-glutamyl peptides in *Candida glabrata. Proc. Natl. Acad. Sci. U.S.A.* 85: 8815.

Mehra RK, Garey JR, Butt TR, Gray WR, and Winge DR (1989): *Candida glabrata* metallothioneins: cloning and sequence of the genes and characterization of proteins. *J. Biol. Chem.* in press.

Minney SF and Quirk AV (1985): Growth and adaptation of *Saccharomyces cerevisiae* at different cadmium concentrations. *Microbios* 42: 37.

Mokdad R, Debec A, and Wegnez M (1987): Metallothionein genes in *Drosophilia melanogaster* constitute a dual system. *Proc. Natl. Acad. Sci. U.S.A.* 84: 2658.

Murasugi A, Wada-Nakagawa C, and Hayashi Y (1984): Formation of cadmium-binding allomorphs in fission yeast. *J. Biochem.* 96: 1375.

Naiki N and Yamagata S (1976): Isolation and some properties of copper-binding proteins found in a copper-resistant strain of yeast. *Plant and Cell Physiol.* 17: 1281.

Nielson KB, Atkin CL, and Winge DR (1985): Distinct metal-binding configurations in metallothionein. *J. Biol. Chem.* 260: 5342.

Ochi T, Otsuka F, Takahashi K, and Ohsawa M (1988): Glutathione as a cellular defense against cadmium toxicity in cultured Chinese hamster cells. *Chem.-Biol. Interactions* 65: 1.

Olafson RW (1986): Primary and secondary structural analysis of a unique prokaryotic metallothionein from a *Synechococcus* sp. cyanobacterium. *Biochem. J.* 251: 691.

Palmiter RD (1987): Molecular biology of metallothionein gene expression. *Experientia Supplementum* 52: 63.

Reese RN, Mehra RK, Tarbet EB, and Winge DR (1988): Studies on the γ-glutamyl Cu-binding peptide from *Schizosaccharomyces pombe. J. Biol. Chem.* 263: 4186.

Schimke RT (1988): Gene amplification in cultured cells. *J. Biol. Chem.* 263: 5989.

Silver S, Budd K, Leahy KM, Shaw WV, Hammond D, Novick RP, Willsky GR, Malamy MH, and Rosenberg H (1982): Inducible plasmid-determined resistance to arsenate, arsenite and antimony(III) in *Escherichia coli* and *Staphyloccus aureus. J. Bacteriol.* 146: 983.

Silver S and Misra TK (1988): Plasmid-mediated heavy metal resistances. *Ann. Rev. Microbiol.* 42: 717.

Silver S, Nucifora G, Chu L, and Misra TK (1989): Bacterial resistance ATPases: primary pumps for exporting toxic cations and anions. *Trends Biochem. Sci.* 14: 76.

Singhal RK, Anderson ME, and Meister A (1987): Glutathione, a first line of defense against cadmium toxicity. *FASEB J.* 1: 220.

Smith TA, Lerch K, and Hodgson KO (1986): Structural study of the Cu sites in metallothionein from *Neurospora crassa. Inorg. Chem.* 25: 4677.

Webb M (1987): Toxicological significance of metallothionein. *Experientia Supplementum* 52: 109.

Welch J, Fogel S, Buchman C, and Karin M (1989): The *CUP2* gene product regulates the expression of the *CUP1* gene coding for yeast metallothionein. *EMBO J.* 8: 255.

Winge DR, Nielson KB, Gray WB, and Hamer DH (1985): Yeast metallothionein: sequence and metal-binding properties. *J. Biol. Chem.* 260: 14464.

Winge DR, Reese RN, Mehra RK, Tarbet BE, Hughes AK, and Dameron CT (1989): In *Metal Ion Homeostasis: Molecular Biology and Chemistry. UCLA Symposium on Molecular and Cellular Biology* 98: 301.

Effect of Preinduction of Metallothionein Synthesis on Toxicity of Free Radical Generating Compounds in the Mouse

Akira Naganuma, Masahiko Satoh,
and Nobumasa Imura
School of Pharmaceutical Sciences
Kitasato University
Tokyo, Japan

INTRODUCTION

The physiological roles of metallothionein (MT) is not well understood, although there are some evidences that MT may function in the detoxification of heavy metals and in tissue storage of Zn (Webb, 1979). Recently, radical scavenging activity of MT has been observed in *in vitro* experiment (Shiraishi et al., 1982; Thornalley and Vasak, 1985). Moreover, protective effects of induction of MT against lethal and bone marrow toxicity of γ-ray irradiation in mice have been reported (Matsubara et al., 1988; Satoh et al., 1989). This prompted us to examine the possibility that preadministration of MT inducers prevents toxic effects of free radical inducing chemicals in mice. In the present study, we examined the effects of preinduction

TABLE I.
Effect of Pretreatment with Metal Compounds on Lethal Toxicity
of Adriamycin (ADR) in Mice

| Pretreatment | | | No. of Survivals | | | | | | Survival rate[a] (%) |
| | | | Days after ADR Injection | | | | | | |
Metal	Dose (μmol/kg/d)	Injection of ADR	0	4	6	8	10	20	
Control		−	7	7	7	7	7	7	100
—	0	+	7	4	1	0	0	0	0
$ZnCl_2$	400 × 2	+	7	5	4	4	4	4	57
$CuSO_4$	40 × 2	+	7	5	2	0	0	0	0
$Bi(NO_3)_3$	50 × 2	+	7	7	6	6	5	5	71
$CoCl_2$	300 × 2	+	7	4	2	1	1	1	14
$CdCl_2$	5 × 2	+	7	6	4	4	4	4	57
$HgCl_2$	4 × 2	+	7	5	3	2	2	2	28

Mice were preinjected with a metal compound once a day for 2 d. ADR (35 μmol/kg, s.c.) was injected 24 h after the last injection of each metal compound.
[a]Determined 20 d after ADR injection.

of MT synthesis against toxicity of adriamycin and other radical generating agents, bleomycin, paraquat, cephaloridine, menadione, and carbon tetrachloride, in mice.

EFFECT OF MT-INDUCING METALS ON ADRIAMYCIN TOXICITY

First of all, we examined the effect of pretreatment of mice with several metal compounds on lethal toxicity of adriamycin which is a free radical generating antitumor drug (Satoh et al., 1988). We used 6 metal compounds, zinc chloride, copper sulfate, bismuth nitrate, cobalt chloride, cadmium chloride and mercuric chloride as MT inducers. Treatments with these metal compounds except copper were effective to a greater or lesser degree in depressing the adriamycin toxicity (Table I). The protective effects of pretreatment with zinc, bismuth, and cadmium were especially remarkable. Since adriamycin is considered to cause cardiotoxicity by generating free-radicals, lipid peroxidation in the heart of mice administered adriamycin with or without preadministration of the MT inducers was examined. Values of both malondialdehyde and conjugated dienes were determined as indicators of lipid peroxidation in the heart. These values were increased markedly by adriamycin administration. Table II shows the level of MT in the heart, liver and kidney at 24 h after the last injection of each metal compound, that is at the time of adriamycin administration. MT concentration was determined by the ^{203}Hg-binding assay (Naganuma et al., 1987). The highest MT concentration was observed in the liver of mice receiving zinc, copper, cobalt or cadmium, and in the kidney of those treated with bismuth or Hg. The MT concentration in the heart was also increased significantly by treatment with zinc, bismuth or cadmium, although the increased level of MT was lower than those in the liver and kidneys. Figures 1 and 2 show the relation between the protective effect of metal-pretreatment and MT contents in the heart, liver, and kidneys of mice treated with metals. The survival rate of mice was significantly correlated only with cardiac MT levels (Figure 1). The levels of malondialdehyde and conjugated dienes in the heart showed a clear inverse correlation with the cardiac MT concentration (Figure 2). These results suggest that the preinduced MT might prevent the lipid peroxidation probably by scavenging free radicals generated from adriamycin.

EFFECT OF MT INDUCTION ON TOXICITIES OF SEVERAL RADICAL-INDUCING COMPOUNDS

Table III shows effect of pretreatment of mice with zinc on lethal toxicity of several radical inducing compounds, such as paraquat, bleomycin, cephaloridine, menadione, carbon tetrachloride and adriamycin. Under the experimental condition used, the lethal toxicity induced by all of those compounds were significantly depressed by the pretreatment with zinc probably through the induction of MT scavenging free radicals formed in the tissues of mice. Since tissue specific MT inductions by various metals have been

TABLE II.
Metallothionein (MT) Content in Heart,
Liver, and Kidneys of Mice Treated
with Metal Compounds

Metal	Dose (μmol/kg/d)	MT (Hg bound nmol/g tissue)		
		Heart	Liver	Kidney
Control	—	18 ± 4	23 ± 4	21 ± 2
ZnCl$_2$	400×2	39 ± 6^a	278 ± 66^a	108 ± 47^a
CuSO$_4$	40×2	19 ± 4	269 ± 61^a	22 ± 7
Bi(NO$_3$)$_3$	50×2	42 ± 3^a	32 ± 6	157 ± 21^a
CoCl$_2$	300×2	19 ± 1	229 ± 64^a	30 ± 7
CdCl$_2$	5×2	32 ± 4^a	186 ± 32^a	46 ± 3^a
HgCl$_2$	4×2	21 ± 2	31 ± 5	254 ± 16

Mice were injected with a metal compound once a day for 2 d. MT was determined 24 h after the last injection of each metal compounds. The values are mean $\pm$ S.D. for 4 mice.
[a]Significantly different from the control ($p < 0.01$).

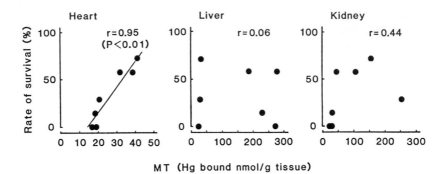

Figure 1. Correlation between the protective effect of metal pretreatment against lethal toxicity of ADR and MT contents in the heart, liver, and kidney of mice treated with metals.

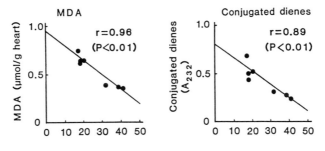

Figure 2. Correlation between ADR-induced lipid peroxidation and MT contents in the hearts of mice pretreated with metals.

TABLE III.
Effect of Pretreatment with ZnCl$_2$ on Lethal Toxicity of Radical Inducing Compounds in Mice

Compound	Dose	Survival Rate on Day 20 (%)	
		None	ZnCl$_2$
Control	—	100	100
Adriamycin	35 μmol/kg	0	57
Bleomycin	300 mg/kg	0	71
Paraquat	200 μmol/kg	0	86
Cephaloridine	4 mmol/kg	0	71
Menadione	400 μmol/kg	0	86
Carbon tetrachloride	30 mmol/kg	0	43

Mice were pretreated with ZnCl$_2$ (200 μmol/kg; s.c.) once a day for 2 d. Radical inducers were injected i.p. 24 h after the last administration of ZnCl$_2$.

TABLE IV.
Induction of Metallothionein (MT) in Mouse Tissues by
Administration of Free-Radical Inducers

Compound	MT (Hg bound nmol/g tissue)			
	Liver	Kidney	Heart	Lung
Control (saline)	12 ± 3	11 ± 2	11 ± 2	6 ± 1
Adriamycin[a]	$78 \pm 27*$	14 ± 2	$37 \pm 3*$	8 ± 1
Bleomycin[a]	$158 \pm 14*$	$18 \pm 1*$	$22 \pm 5*$	$11 \pm 2*$
Paraquat[a]	$114 \pm 35*$	16 ± 2	$22 \pm 7*$	$21 \pm 3*$
Cephaloridine[a]	$38 \pm 11*$	$33 \pm 6*$	15 ± 3	8 ± 3
Control (olive oil)	40 ± 12	13 ± 1	11 ± 1	7 ± 1
Menadione[b]	$86 \pm 10*$	14 ± 1	13 ± 3	$10 \pm 2*$
Carbon tetrachloride[b]	$159 \pm 12*$	$40 \pm 10*$	$22 \pm 6*$	$12 \pm 2*$

MT was determined 24 h after the injection (i.p.) of each compounds. The
values are mean $\pm$ S.D. for 4 mice.
[a]Dissolved in saline.
[b]Dissolved in olive oil.
*Significantly different from the control ($p < 0.005$).

observed so far, appropriate MT inducer rather than Zn may protect much
more effectively against lesions caused by a certain inducer.

INDUCTION OF MT SYNTHESIS BY RADICAL GENERATING AGENTS

Finally we examined MT levels in tissues of mice after administration
of the radical inducers. Table IV shows MT concentration in the liver,
kidney, lung and heart of mice determined 24 h after administration of
adriamycin, bleomycin, paraquat, cephaloridine, menadione or carbon tetrachloride. All radical inducers used in this experiment significantly increased MT level in the liver. And some of them also increased MT
concentration in the kidney, lung, or heart.

Some investigators could not observe the radical scavenging effects of
MT in *in vitro* experiments (Arthur et al., 1987). In the present study,
however, it is clearly shown that MT prevents the toxicity of radical inducing
compounds in mice. Although precise mechanism of the protective action
of MT against the toxicity of those compounds is still obscure, the findings
seem to support the hypothesis that MT plays a role in scavenging free
radicals formed in animal bodies. Moreover, MT induction by radical inducer itself confirmed in the present study may suggest a self defense mechanism functioning on the exposure to oxidative stresses.

REFERENCES

Arthur JR, Bremner I, Morrice PC, and Mills CF (1987): Stimulation of peroxidation in rat liver microsomes by (copper, zinc)-metallothioneins. *Free Rad. Res. Comms.* 4: 15–20.

Matsubara J, Tajima Y, Ikeda A, Kinoshita T, and Shimoyama T (1988): A new perspective of radiation protection by metallothionein induction. *Pharmac. Ther.* 39: 331–333.

Naganuma A, Satoh M, and Imura N (1987): Prevention of lethal and renal toxicity of *cis*-diamminedichloroplatinum(II) by induction of metallothionein synthesis without compromising its antitumor activity in mice. *Cancer Res.* 47: 983–987.

Satoh M, Naganuma A, and Imura N (1988): Involvement of cardiac metallothionein in prevention of adriamycin induced lipid peroxidation in the heart. *Toxicology* 53: 231–237.

Satoh M, Miura N, Naganuma A, Matsuzaki N, Kawamura E, and Imura N (1989): Prevention of adverse effects of γ-ray irradiation after metallothionein induction by bismuth subnitrate in mice. *Eur. J. Cancer Clin. Oncol.* 25: 1727–1731.

Shiraishi N, Utsumi K, Morimoto S, Joja I, Iida S, Takeda Y, and Aono K (1982): Inhibition of nitroblue tetrazolium reduction by metallothionein. *Physiol. Chem. Phys.* 14: 533–537.

Thornalley PJ and Vašák M (1985): Possible role for metallothionein in protection against radiation-induced oxidative stress. Kinetics and mechanism of its reaction with superoxide and hydroxyl radicals. *Biochim. Biophys. Acta* 827: 36–44.

Webb M (1979): Metallothionein. In, *The Chemistry, Biochemistry and Biology of Cadmium.* Webb M, Ed., Elsevier, Amsterdam, pp. 195–266.

Chapter 25

Proximal Tubule Cell Injury

B.A. Fowler
Program in Toxicology and
Department of Pathology
University of Maryland
Medical School
Baltimore, Maryland

R.E. Gandley and M. Akkerman
University of Maryland
Program in Toxicology
Baltimore, Maryland

M.M. Lipsky and M. Smith
Department of Pathology
University of Maryland
Medical School
Baltimore, Maryland

ABSTRACT

Previous studies have demonstrated that parenteral administration of cadmium metallothionein (CdMT) produces a marked renal calcuria which is prevented by prior Zn-induction of the renal MT pool and rapid binding of Cd^{2+} ions released from the absorbed CdMT. These data indicate that Cd^{2+} intereferes with proximal tubule cell (PTC) handling of calcium, but the mechanism is presently unknown. This information is of potentially great significance since both Cd^{2+} and Ca^{2+} activate calmodulin (CaM) *in vitro* and Cd^{2+} activation of CaM has been hypothesized as the mechanism underlying Cd^{2+}-induced proximal tubule cell injury. Previous investigations from this laboratory found no change in the permeability of renal cell membranes to external $^{45}Ca^{2+}$ until the onset of PCT necrosis. Preliminary data from the present studies showed no measurable change in internal Ca^{2+} concentrations using the fluorescent dye Fura-2. These data support the hypothesis that Cd^{2+} ions could act directly within cells by CaM activation and that MT prevents initiation of this process by binding Cd^{2+} content from internal or external sources.

INTRODUCTION

Cadmium-induced nephrotoxicity is commmonly encountered in a variety of occupational circumstances but the *mechanisms* by which these agents produce injury to renal proximal tubule cells or the biological factors which influence target cell toxicity are not completely understood. Metallothionein (MT) is a low molecular weight (6800), cysteine-rich, metal-binding protein (Kägi and Nordberg, 1979; Kägi and Kojima, 1987) which binds a number of both toxic and essential metals including both mercury (Hg) and cadmium (Cd). Radioimmunoassay studies (Garvey and Chang, 1981; Garvey et al., 1982; Mehra and Bremner, 1982; Lee et al., 1983) have shown that both HgMT and CdMT are excreted in the urine and that MT carries a number of metals (Cd, Cu, Zn) in the blood following chronic exposure and, as such, represents a major biochemical mechanism for delivery of these metals to proximal tubule cells of the kidney. As a low molecular weight protein, MT is readily filtered by the glomerulus and reabsorbed from the urinary filtrate by endocytosis with rapid degradation and release of metal ions from the protein (Cherian and Shaikh, 1975; Webb and Etienne, 1977; Squibb et al. 1984; Cain and Holt, 1983). For Cd, this process results in the selective destruction of renal proximal tubule cells from the first and second (S_1-S_2) segments due to reabsorption of MT in these segments, but no damage to cells in the third segment (S_3). The initiation of cellular necrosis is preceded by a characteristic vesiculation and disruption of lysosomal biogenesis which produces an attendant tubular proteinuria. (Squibb et al., 1984.) Such data are consistent with early studies using Cd^{2+} ions which showed interference with heterolysosome formation in mice (Mego and Cain, 1975). The observed proximal tubule cell injury is due to the release of Cd^{2+} ions which are eventually re-bound to renal MT following induction of this protein. Prior induction of MT by zinc (Zn) markedly attentuates this nephrotoxic process by apparently providing vacant and/or displaceable binding sites for released Cd^{2+} ions and thus preventing their interaction with sensitive target molecules such as *calmodulin* (CaM) which has been shown to be activated by Cd^{2+} *in vitro* (Chao et al., 1984; Suzuki et al., 1985; Mills and Johnson, 1985). Activation of CaM would lead to damage to the cytoskeleton which is thought to play a major role in lysosome biogenesis. While the actual nature of the intracellular target site (S) for Cd^{2+} ions *in vitro* is currently unknown, calmodulin (CaM) is a likely candidate based on these data. It is clear, in any event, that MT plays a central role in mediating the toxicity of this metal by regulating its intracellular availability to these molecules within renal target cell populations. It should be noted that injection of Cd^{2+} ions does not produce the renal toxicity described above since most of the administered dose is taken up by the liver, resulting in binding to MT and followed by a slow release into the circulation of CdMT with subsequent handling by the kidney as described above.

The hypothesized mechanism by which Cd^{2+} ions could produce the widely observed effects of Cd on renal proximal tubule cells via calmodulin activation is shown in Figure 1. The specific hypothesis is as follows:

Hypothesis—Cd^{2+} ions released from reabsorbed/degraded TM interact with CaM to produce attendant changes in the cytoskeleton which in turn produce disruption of primary lysosomal fusion with endocytic vesicles leading to the observed attendant tubular proteinuria. The renal MT pool regulates the availability of Cd^{2+} ions to CaM and prevents this process from occurring until its capacity to bind Cd^{2+} ions is exceeded.

In addition, evaluation of relationships between cadmium and renal calcium metabolism is important since previous studies (Goering et al., 1986; Fowler et al., 1987; Jin et al., 1987) have demonstrated that parenteral administration of CdMT produces a calcuria which is similar to that observed in workers with prolonged Cd exposure (Adams et al., 1969) suggesting that Cd^{2+} produces a disturbance in the renal handling of Ca^{2+} at the level of the proximal tubule. Data from Fowler et al., 1987 suggest that there were no overt alterations in the membrane transport of Ca^{2+} until the onset of cellular necrosis but changes in the intracellular compartmentation of Ca^{2+} were not examined. Such data are of clear importance to understanding both the mechanism of the calcuria and the possible role of Ca^{2+} in the mediating Cd-induced proximal tubule cell injury tubule cell injury with regard to the hypothesized mechanism of Cd^{2+} activation of calmodulin previously described.

The present studies were undertaken to measure possible changes in *internal* renal proximal tubule cell Ca^{2+} content during Cd-induced cell injury. These data are clearly essential to testing the above hypothesis since changes in intracellular Ca^{2+} (Trump et al., 1984, 1989) could obfuscate interpretation of data regarding Cd^{2+} activation of cellular CaM. The data are also essential to determining whether possible alterations in intracellular calcium stores within proximal tubule cells play a role in the development of the observed calcuria. In order to evaluate these parameters, this report reviews data from both the *in vivo* CdMT administration model (Squibb et al., 1984; Goering et al., 1986; Fowler et al., 1987) and presents more recent preliminary data from *in vitro* CdMT exposure studies of renal proximal tubule cells in culture using a modification of model systems described by Cherian (1984, 1985).

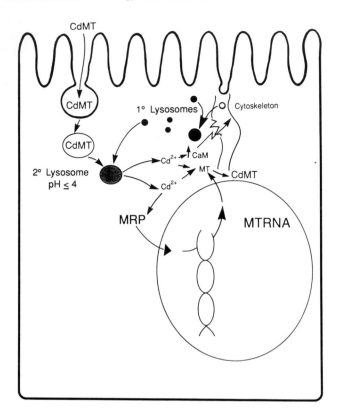

Figure 1. Hypothesized mechanism for Cd^{2+} ion induced renal proximal tubule cell injury following uptake and degradation of reabsorbed CdMT. According to this hypothesis, released cd^{2+} ions are available to react with effector molecules, such as calmodulin (CaM), until they are re-bound by metallothionein (MT) which is induced by action of the as yet unidentified metal-regulatory protein (MRP) which binds to regulatory/promoting regions of the metallothionein genes. The activation of CaM by Cd^{2+} under this hypothesis occurs prior to sufficient induction of MT and results in alterations in the cytoskeleton which in turn mediate the observed disruption of lysosomal biogenesis leading to tubular proteinuria.

MATERIALS AND METHODS

In Vivo Studies

Data from these studies have been previously published (Goering et al., 1986; Fowler et al., 1987) but briefly, purified rat liver CdMT was prepared and administered to rats via intraperitoneal injection (0.6 mg Cd/kg) as previously reported (Squibb et al., 1984) and urine samples collected at 1, 4 and 8 h. ^{45}Ca uptake into renal slices was performed as previously described (Fowler et al., 1987).

In Vitro Studies

CdMT Exposures

For these studies, rat kidney proximal tubule cells were prepared according to the method of Trifillis et al., 1985 and allowed to come to confluence at 5 d. The cells were incubated for time periods of 1, 4 and 8 h with rabbit kidney CdMT (Sigma) following passage of the CdMT over a Sephadex G-25® column (1×10 cm) to remove any unbound Cd^{2+} ions. The concentration of Cd in the cultures as well as CdMT in these cultures, was 10^{-4} M since this concentration has been previously reported (Cherian et al., 1984, 1985) to produce toxicity in similar primary rat kidney tubule cell cultures. Cell cultures used in the studies reported below appeared clear of bacterial contamination but other cell cultures used in this series were observed to contain bacteria by electron microscopy so that all data presented here should be regarded as preliminary and in need of replication.

MEASUREMENT OF CYTOSOLIC IONIZED CALCIUM

In order to delineate the precise time course of changes in intracellular ionized calcium for this model *in vitro*, primary cultures of rat kidney proximal tubule cells will be loaded with the fluorescent dye Fura-2. Quantitative measurement of ionized cytosolic calcium will be conducted on proximal tubule cell primary cultures incubated with CdMT (10^{-4} M) for 1, 4, or 8 h and loaded with Fura-2 as described by Smith et al. (1989). Changes in Fura-2 fluorescence will be monitored as described by Smith et al. (1989) using a Perkin-Elmer® MPF-66 spectrofluorimeter. The technique is briefly as follows:

Cytosolic Calcium Determinations

The Fura-2 fluorescence of $(0.2$ to $0.4) \cdot 10^6$ cells/ml was measured at 25°C on a Perkin Elmer MPF-66 spectrofluorometer by monitoring the 510 nm emission with continuous 340 nm excitation. Cells were held on ice and allowed to settle; prior to each assay the supernatant was replaced with fresh medium. Estimation of $[Ca^{2+}]$ was based on the formula:

$$[CA^{2+}]_i = \frac{(F - F_{min})}{(f_{max} - F)} K_d$$

Computerized Digitizing Fluorescent Imaging of Cells *In Vitro*

For these studies, computerized digitized images of kidney proximal tubule cells in culture was performed at 1, 4, and 8 hours using the fluorescent microscope system described by Trump et al. (1989).

RESULTS

In Vivo Studies

Previously reported investigations, (Goering et al., 1986; Fowler et al., 1987; Jin et al., 1987) showed no changes in membrane ATPase activities, ATP content, $^{45}Ca^{2+}$ uptake into renal slices, brush border or basolateral membrane transport until 24 h after parenteral administration of CdMT during the initial stages of cell death. No changes were observed in these parameters within the 8-h interval during which time cellular vesiculation occurred.

In Vitro Studies

Results of preliminary *in vitro* studies showed no change in Fura-2 fluorescence as measured by either spectrofluorimetry (Figures 2A and 2B) or computerized digitizing image analyses of individual cells (data not shown). The apparent absence of changes in internal Ca^{2+} following CdMT treatment is significant since the characteristic vesiculation phenomenon was observed in parallel cultures of cells examined by electron microscopy (Figures 3 and 4) suggesting that this morphological phenomenon is *not* linked to changes in intracellular ionized calcium.

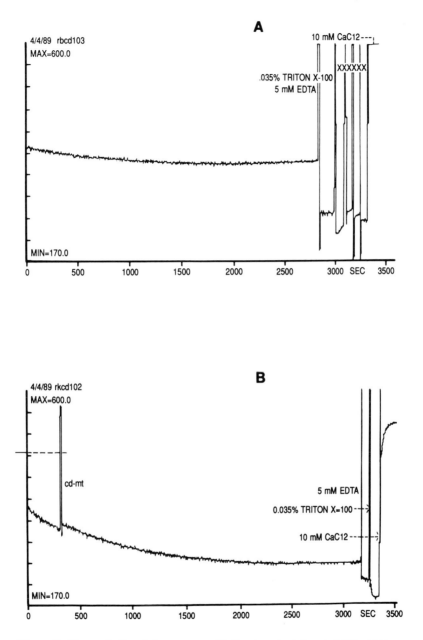

Figure 2. Changes in Fura-2 fluorescence with time in untreated control (A) rat kidney proximal tubule cells and (B) cells exposed to 10^{-4} M CdMT for 8 h. The data show no appreciable difference in fluorescence, indicating an absence of change in internal Ca^{2+} ionic content as a result of this treatment during the time period studied.

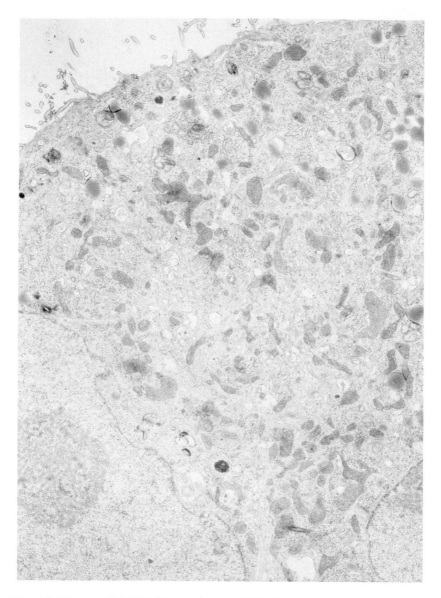

Figure 3. Electron micrograph of a renal proximal tubule cell from an untreated control culture. Original magnification. × 13,913.

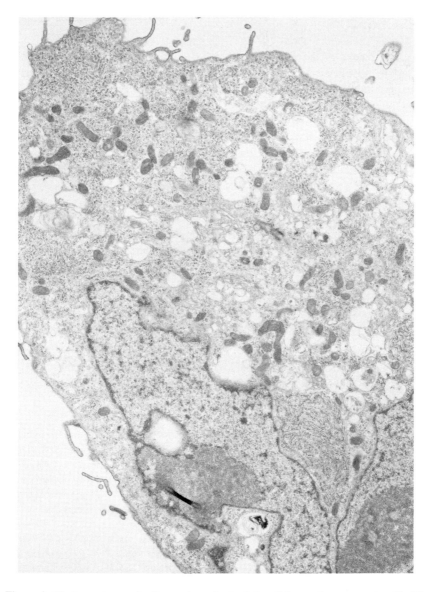

Figure 4. Electron micrograph of a renal proximal tubule cell from culture exposed to 10^{-4}M CdMT for 8 h showing characteristic vesiculation. Original magnification. $\times 13,913$.

DISCUSSION

The results of the preliminary studies conducted to date are consistent with the hypothesis (Figure 1) that cadmium-induced alterations in renal proximal tubule cell lysosome biogenesis *are* directly mediated by Cd^{2+} ions rather than secondary to changes in cellular calcium (Ca^{2+}) homeostasis from external *or* internal cellular pools. It is likely that the Cd^{2+} ions within these cells interact with a number of non-MT binding sites which are capable of producing alterations in cellular metabolism. The hypothesized interaction of Cd^{2+} ions with CaM and subsequent activation of this important intracellular effector molecule in the absence of changes in cellular Ca^{2+} pools is attractive since it would explain the observed changes in lysosomal biogenesis via alterations in the cytoskeleton which is thought to play an important role in the primary lysosome-pinocytotic vesicle fusion process.

These data also suggest that he observed calcuria is *not* due to release of calcium from internal cellular stores prior to cell death. They are hence consistent with our previous hypothesis that the calcuria is secondary to proteinuria (Fowler, 1987).

Further studies are currently in progress within this laboratory to evaluate these hypotheses in greater depth and to evaluate the relationship(s) between the observed morphological-biochemical changes and alterations in renal proximal tubule cell gene expression during these processes.

REFERENCES

Adams RG, Harrison JF, and Scott P (1969): The development of cadmium-induced proteinuria impaired renal function and osteomalacia in alkaline battery workers. *Quart. J. Med.* 38: 425.

Cain K and Holt DE (1983): Studies of cadmium-induced mephropathy: Time-course of cadmium-thionein uptake and degradation. *Chem.-Biol. Interact.* 43: 223.

Chang CC, Vander Mallie RJ, and Garvey JS (1980): A radioimmunoassay for human metallothionein. *Toxicol. Appl. Pharmacol.* 55: 94.

Chao S-H, Suzuki Y, Ztsk JR, and Cheung WY (1984): Activation of calmodulin by various metal cations and as a function of ionic radius. *Mol. Pharmacol.* 26: 75.

Cherian MG and Shaikh ZA (1975): Metabolism of intravenously injected cadmium-binding protein. *Biochem. Biophys. Res. Commun.* 65: 863.

Cherian MG (1982): Studies on toxicity of metallothionein in rat kidney epithelial cell culture. In, *Biological Roles of Metallothionein.* Faulkner EC, Ed., Elsevier/North Holland, New York, p. 193.

Fowler BA, Goering PL, and Squibb KS (1987): Mechanism of cadmium-metallothionein-induced nephrotoxicity: relationship to altered renal calcium metabolism. In, *Metallothionein, Second International Meeting on Metallothionein and Other Low Molecular Weight Metal-Binding Proteins.* Kägi, JHR and Kojima Y, Eds., Birkhäuser-Verlag, Basel, pp. 661–668.

Garvey JS and Chang CC (1981): Detection of circulating metallothionein in rats injected with zinc or cadmium. *Science* 211: 805.

Goering PL, Squibb KS, and Fowler BA (1986): Increased renal calcium excretion during cadmium-induced proximal tubule cell injury. In, *Trace Substances in Environmental Health-XIX*, Hemphill DD, Ed., University of Missouri Press, Columbia, pp. 22–36.

Jin T, Leffler P, and Nordberg GF (1987): Cadmium-metallothionein nephrotoxicity in the rat: transient calcuria and proteinuria. *Toxicology* 45: 307.

Kägi JHR and Nordberg M, Eds., (1979): *Metallothionein and Other Low Molecular Weight Metal-Binding Proteins.* Proc. First Internat. Symp on Metallothionein. Birkhäuser-Verlag, Basel, pp. 378.

Kägi JHR and Jojima Y, Ed. (1987): *Metallothionein and Other Low Molecular Weight Metal-Binding proteins.* Second Internat. Conf. on Metallothionein. Birkhäuser-Verlag, Basel.

Lee Y-H, Shaikh ZA, and Tohyama C (1983): Urinary metallothionein and tissue metal levels of rats injected with cadmium, mercury, lead, copper, or zinc. *Toxicology* 27: 337.

Mego JL and Cain JA (1975): An effect of cadmium on heterolysosome formation and function in mice. *Biochem. Pharmacol.* 24: 1227.

Mehra FK and Bremner I (1983): Development of a radio-immunoassay for metallothionein I and its application to the analysis of rat plasma and kidneys. *Biochem J.* 213: 459.

Mills JS and Johnson JD (1985): Metal ions as allosteric regulators of calmodulin. *J. Biol. Chem.* 260: 15100.

Smith MW, Ambudkar IS, Phelps PC, Regec AL, and Trump BF (1987): $HgCl_2$-induced changes in cytosolic Ca^{2+} of cultured rabbit renal tubular cells. *Biochem. Biophys. Acta* 931: 130.

Squibb KS, Pritchard JB, and Fowler BA (1984): Cadmium metallothionein nephropathy: ultrastructural/biochemical alterations and intracellular cadmium binding. *J. Pharmacol. Exper. Therap.* 229: 311.

Suzuki Y, Charo S-H, Zysk JR, and Cheung WY (1985): Stimulation of calmodulin by cadmium ion. *Arch. Toxicol.* 57: 205.

Trifillis AL, Reges AL, and Trump BF (1985): Isolation, culture, and characterization of human renal tubular cells. *J. Urology.* 133: 324.

Trump BF, Berezesky IK, Sato T, Laiho KU, Phelps PC, and DeClaris N (1984): Cell calcium, cell injury, and cell death. *Environ. Health Perspec.* 57: 281.

Trump BF, Berezesky IK, Smith MW, Phelps PC, and Elliget KA (1989): The relationship between cellular ion deregulation and acute and chronic toxicity. *Toxicol. Appl. Pharmacol.* 97: 6.

Webb M and Etienne AT (1977): Studies on the toxicity and metabolism of cadmium-thionein. *Biochem. Pharmacol.* 26: 25.

Assessment of Nutritional Status by Immunoassay of Metallothionein

Ian Bremner and Anne M. Wood
Rowett Research Institute
Aberdeen, Scotland

Nancy A. Noble
Department of Medicine
University of Utah
School of Medicine
Salt Lake City, Utah

Aileen Robertson
Department of Nutrition and Dietetics
Raigmore Hospital
Inverness, Scotland

INTRODUCTION

Although health problems associated with malnutrition are endemic in many developing countries, it is not always appreciated that they can also occur, with serious consequences, in the Western world. Growth may be impaired, susceptibility to infection and disease increased, and intellectual development compromised. Unfortunately considerable difficulties are still encountered in the assessment of the nutritional status of individuals. The standard anthropometric tests lack sensitivity and specificity and are unsuitable for monitoring short-term responses to therapy. Biochemical tests, such as analysis of specific plasma proteins, may also lack sensitivity and can be difficult to interpret because of the influence of trauma or other disease states.

Particular problems occur in the diagnosis of imbalances in trace element status, especially when they do not result in characteristic clinical lesions. There is still reliance on the measurement of metal concentrations in urine or blood components, despite the fact that there are severe limitation to this technique. These include the lack of sensitivity and the occurrence of disturbances of metal metabolism in many other conditions. Another approach has been to assess the functional activity of the metals by assay of metal-dependent enzymes. However, this is not always satisfactory and, in the case of diagnosis of zinc deficiency, does not offer significant advantages over measurement of plasma zinc. Since plasma metal concentrations tend to decrease only after depletion of tissue reserves of the element, they do not provide any warning of developing problems. Liver biopsies or bone marrow aspirations can be used in animal or human studies to assess body stores of copper and iron respectively, but such invasive procedures are unsatisfactory for routine screening purposes. More satisfactory is the measurement of ferritin, the principal iron storage protein, in serum or erythrocytes, since there is a close correlation between the concentration of this protein in blood and liver.

Unfortunately no specific copper- or zinc-binding storage proteins have yet been identified. However, the tissue concentrations of metallothionein are often related to zinc and, to a lesser extent, copper status, suggesting that assay of this protein in some accessible body fluid might be of value in the assessment of trace-element status (Bremner, 1987). In this paper, the effects of changes in dietary zinc and copper intake on metallothionein levels in urine, blood cells and plasma are described. Attention is also directed to the effects of changes in general nutritional status on the presence of the protein in circulating blood cells, particularly in reticulocytes.

ASSAY OF METALLOTHIONEIN

The determination of metallothionein concentrations in blood and urine samples is only possible by immunoassay procedures (Garvey et al., 1982; Mehra and Bremner, 1983). The most sensitive and precise methods appear to be the radioimmunoassays, which have detection limits of 1 to 2 ng/ml and are suitable for analysis of blood plasma and erythrocytes, urine, and bile. In most of the radioimmunoassays, the major isoproteins of metallothionein from several mammalian species cross-react to equal extents (Garvey et al., 1982) but the assay described by Mehra and Bremner (1983) is specific for rat (and mouse) metallothionein-I and moreover cannot be used to measure any form of human metallothionein. Enzyme-linked immuno-sorbent assays (ELISA) offer advantages in terms of speed and the fluorometric ELISA described by Thomas et al. (1986) has a sensitivity similar to that of the radioimmunoassays. However the assay of Grider et al. (1989) is only sufficiently sensitive to measure tissue metallothionein concentrations. An indirect ELISA developed by us for human metallothionein, based on reaction of the bound metallothionein-primary antibody complex with an anti-sheep IgG-peroxidase conjugate, has a detection limit of about 7 ng/ml, takes only a few hours to complete and is suitable for analysis of tissues, urine and erythrocytes from most mammalian species (Ghaffar et al., 1989). However, concentrations recorded for rat plasma are far in excess of those recorded by radioimmunoassay, implying some nonspecific reaction. Conversely negative values are recorded for polymorphonuclear cells, possibly because of reaction of endogenous peroxidase with the substrate used in the ELISA (Branca, 1989). Care is therefore needed in interpreting the results obtained when mixed blood cells are analyzed, as they may be spuriously low; selective removal of leukocytes can result in an apparent increase in the metallothionein concentrations in the erythrocytes.

EFFECT OF METAL STATUS ON METALLOTHIONEIN CONCENTRATIONS

Plasma metallothionein concentrations, as measured by radioimmunoassay, decrease rapidly in growing rats maintained on a zinc-deficient diet (Sato et al., 1984). They also decrease in plasma from rat pups whose mothers are given zinc-deficient diets during pregnancy and lactation (Morrison and Bremner, 1987). Similar decreases occur in metallothionein concentrations in lysed blood cells from zinc-deficient neonatal and growing rats, with the concentrations being directly related to dietary zinc intake (Bremner et al., 1987; Morrison and Bremner, 1987). No such decreases occur in blood cells from copper-deficient rats, implying that a decrease in blood cell metallothionein concentration might be specific for zinc deficiency.

Increases in plasma, blood cell and urinary metallothionein concentrations occur after parenteral administration of zinc, cadmium or copper, although the effect of copper on blood-cell concentrations is slow to appear (Bremner et al., 1987; Williams et al., 1989). Dietary supplementation with copper also results in substantial increases in metallothionein-I concentrations in plasma and urine (Bremner et al., 1986). The concentrations in plasma and liver are frequently related, indicating that the liver is the main source of plasma metallothionein. This view is supported by the changes recorded with time in the immunolocalization of metallothionein in copper-injected rats (Williams et al., 1989). It is likely that measurement of plasma metallothionein levels could be of value in the detection of copper-overload conditions, such as Wilson's disease, Indian Childhood Cirrhosis or Primary Biliary Cirrhosis, where hepatic concentrations of the protein are elevated.

Assay of urinary metallothionein levels has also been proposed as a means of identifying renal disorders in individuals occupationally exposed to cadmium (Nordberg et al., 1982; Falck et al., 1983). It is possibly less sensitive than measurement of β_2-microglobulin excretion but has the advantage that it is a more specific test.

EFFECT OF STRESS FACTORS ON METALLOTHIONEIN CONCENTRATIONS

Synthesis of metallothionein is induced not only by metals but also by a variety of hormones, growth factors and "stress factors" (Cousins, 1985; Bremner, 1987). Most types of physical and inflammatory stress result in increased metallothionein production, particularly in the liver, indicating that metallothionein is an acute phase protein. In most instances, stress-induced synthesis of hepatic metallothionein is accompanied by increased hepatic uptake of zinc and a reduction in plasma zinc concentrations (Sobocinski et al., 1978; Cousins and Leinart, 1988; Hidalgo et al., 1988). Since the occurrence of stress-induced hypozincemia is one of the principal reasons why measurement of plasma zinc cannot be used for the unequivocal diagnosis of zinc deficiency, the effect of a variety of stress factors and of cytokines on blood and urine metallothionein concentrations has been established. Treatment of rats with agents such as endotoxin, turpentine, carbon tetrachloride, dextran sulphate, interleukin-I and recombinant tumor necrosis factor invariably increases both hepatic and plasma metallothionein-I concentrations (Sato et al., 1984; Morrison et al., 1988a; Bremner, Shenkin and Grimble, unpublished observations). However, restriction of food intake and physical stress do not always result in increased plasma metallothionein levels, although synthesis of the protein in the liver is induced (Sato et al., 1984; Hidalgo et al., 1988). Endotoxin also increases urinary excretion of the protein but none of the "stress" treatments has any major effect on blood cell metallothionein concentrations. In some cases the concentrations decrease slightly whereas in others there is a minor and non-significant increase.

These findings suggested therefore that assay of blood cell metallothionein levels would be of particular value in the diagnosis of zinc deficiency, since concentrations would be decreased regardless of the possible concurrence of stress or infection (Bremner et al., 1987). This is of particular importance as zinc deficiency adversely affects immunocompetence and the children in underdeveloped countries who are the most likely to develop zinc deficiency frequently suffer from various types of infection (Golden and Golden, 1981).

DISTRIBUTION OF METALLOTHIONEIN IN BLOOD CELLS

The first demonstration that metallothionein can occur in blood cells was made by Nordberg et al. (1971), working with cadmium-dosed mice. Tanaka et al. (1985, 1986) subsequently reported that the protein is present in the erythrocytes of cadmium-dosed mice, that it is synthesized in the precursor cells and that it remains within the erythrocytes until they come to the end of their life-span. However, metallothionein can also be synthesized in leukocytes, with both monocytes and lymphocytes producing more metallothionein when grown in cadmium-containing medium (Peavy and Fairchild, 1987; Harley et al., 1989). Lymphocytes which are stimulated by PHA also produce more metallothionein when grown in zinc-supplemented medium (Alexander et al., 1982).

Nevertheless, fractionation of blood cells from normal rats on Percoll gradients showed that only trace amounts of metallothionein are associated with the leukocytes (Morrison et al., 1988b). Most of the protein is present in the red cells, and particularly in the fraction containing the lightest and therefore by implication the youngest cells. This fraction is greatly enriched in reticulocytes.

Injection of rats with zinc causes a rapid but transient increase in blood cell metallothionein concentrations, with concentrations reaching a maximum after only 24 h and returning to normal after 4 days (Morrison et al., 1988b). Fractionation of the cells on Percoll gradients again showed that the protein is concentrated in the fraction rich in reticulocytes, suggesting that the protein is synthesized in the precursor cells but is relatively unstable and is degraded or lost from these cells before they mature into erythrocytes. This contrasts with the findings in cadmium-dosed mice, where the protein is considerably more stable and resists degradation (Tanaka et al., 1986).

DEGRADATION OF METALLOTHIONEIN IN RETICULOCYTES

The relative instability of metallothionein in reticulocytes from normal or zinc-injected rats has been confirmed in studies with cells maintained in culture. By a combination of phlebotomy and temporary implantation of thiamphenicol in rats, it is possible to induce reticulocytosis and the generation of cells of relatively uniform age. These cells can be harvested,

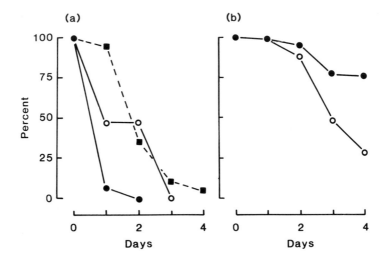

Figure 1. Maturational change in rat reticulocytes *in vitro*. (a) ●, metallothionein-I; ○, transferrin receptors; ■, cells staining as reticulocytes. (b) ○, pyruvate kinase; ●, glucose-6-phosphate dehydrogenase. All values are presented
as the percentage of those at the start of the incubation. Details of the isolation
and culture of the cells are given in Noble et al. (1989).

separated from erythrocytes and leukocytes, and maintained in culture for
several days, with no significant loss of viability (Noble et al., 1989). It is
therefore possible to study the changes in these cells during their maturation
under closely controlled conditions. Noble et al. (1989) showed that there
is a gradual decrease in the activity of glycolytic and other enzymes, including pyruvate kinase and glucose-6-phosphate dehydrogenase; activities
of these enzymes after 4 d were only 50 and 76% of the initial values
(Figure 1). The decrease in reticulocyte counts was more pronounced and
these fell from 94% at day 0 to 9% at day 3. However, even more rapid
was the reduction in the number of transferrin receptors, which fell from
1.8×10^5 molecules bound per cell at day 0 to zero levels at day 3 (Figure
1a). The apparent half-life of these receptors was about 15 h (Noble et al.,
1989).

The opportunity was taken to measure the changes in metallothionein-
I concentrations in these cells during their maturation (Figure 1). The concentration at the start of the incubation, 34 ng/10^8 cells compared well with
that found in the lightest cells separated by density gradient centrifugation
of blood from normal rats, viz. 4 ng/10^8 cells (Morrison et al., 1988b). As
the reticulocyte count in these cells was 25%, this is equivalent to 16 ng
metallothionein-I/10^8 reticulocytes, confirming that the cells derived from
the induced reticulocytosis did not have an abnormal composition. The concentration of metallothionein decreased dramatically and was close to the

limit of detection by 48 h. The half-life of the protein was only 6.4 h, indicating that it is degraded very rapidly in the reticulocytes. However, it cannot be excluded that the metallothionein is extruded from the cell, or is converted into a form that is not immunoreactive.

The stability of the protein was considerably greater in reticulocytes isolated from rats injected with cadmium (0.5 and 1.0 mg/kg body weight) on days 6 and 8, respectively after the initial implantation of thiamphenicol (Figure 2). The half-life of the metallothionein was now 54 hours. Previous studies on the turnover of metallothionein in rat liver have shown that the cadmium-containing protein is considerably more stable than the zinc- and copper-containing forms (Bremner, 1987). The increased half-life of the cadmium-induced metallothionein in the reticulocytes helps explain the report of Tanaka et al. (1986) that metallothionein persists in erythrocytes for their entire lifespan.

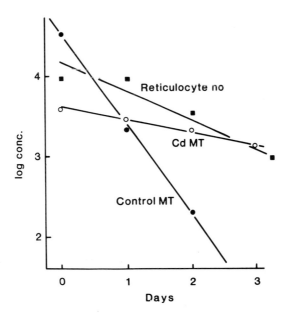

Figure 2. Decrease in metallothionein-I concentrations in reticulocytes maintained in culture after isolation from normal (●) and cadmium-dosed (○) rats. The decrease in the number of cells staining as reticulocytes is also shown (■). Details of the isolation and culture of the cells are given in Noble et al. (1989).

RELATIONSHIP BETWEEN ERYTHROPOIETIC ACTIVITY AND METALLOTHIONEIN LEVELS

As metallothionein is normally so unstable within reticulocytes and is present only in small amounts in older erythrocytes, its overall concentration in blood cells could depend on reticulocyte counts as well as on metal status. This was confirmed in studies where rats were made anemic either by inducing haemolysis with phenylhydrazine (Morrison et al., 1988b) or by feeding them on an iron-deficient diet (Robertson et al., 1989). In both cases, concentrations of metallothionein in the blood cells increased dramatically. Concentrations also increased in the liver and plasma of the rats with haemolytic anaemia but this was almost certainly part of a stress response. No such increase occurred in the iron-deficient rats and indeed kidney metallothionein levels were generally lower than those in the control rats fed *ad libitum*. Anaemia and the associated increase in erythropoietic activity do not therefore cause a general stimulation in metallothionein synthesis. The increase in its concentration in blood cells merely reflects an increase in the number of reticulocytes which have a high endogenous level of metallothionein.

This increase in blood cell metallothionein concentrations is evident even in rats that are only mildly iron-deficient (Table I). For example, blood cell metallothionein-I concentrations in rats given a diet with 15 mg iron/kg for 3 weeks were increased to 5.8 ng/mg hemoglobin. Values in the control rats, given 50 mg iron/kg diet, were only 1.8 ng/mg hemoglobin at this time. Blood hemoglobin concentrations and hematocrits in the iron-deficient rats were 102 g/l and 28%, respectively whereas those in the control rats were 142 g/l and 40%. Growth rates and food intakes were not affected by the reduced dietary iron intakes.

The increase in metallothionein-I concentrations in the cells was not maintained when the iron-deficient rats were repleted with iron (Table I). Thus, 1 week after repletion with the iron adequate diet, concentrations were reduced to 3.4 ng/mg hemoglobin, whereas those in the iron-deficient and iron-adequate rats at this time were 6.6 and 1.0 ng/mg hemoglobin, respectively. Plasma and liver metallothionein concentrations were unaffected by changes in iron intake.

An unexpected finding in the earlier studies on iron-deficient rats was that metallothionein concentrations also changed in the pair-fed control rats, whose food intake was reduced to match that of the iron-deficient animals (Robertson et al., 1989). Concentrations increased in the liver, consistent with the previously reported "stress-response" in metallothionein synthesis (Bremner, 1987), but those in the blood cells, and also in the kidneys, decreased. However, starvation reduces erythropoietic activity in rats (Fried et al., 1957) and it is likely that the reduced levels of metallothionein in

TABLE I.
Effects of Iron Depletion and Repletion on Blood and
Tissue Metallothionein-I Concentrations in Rats

	Dietary iron content (mg/kg)				
	50	15	50	15	15/50*
Weeks on diet	3	3	4	4	3/1
Blood hemoglobin (g/l)	142±8	102±5	139±5	98±10	141±9
Blood cell MT-I (ng/mg hemoglobin)	1.80±0.13	5.79±0.45	1.02±0.04	6.61±1.08	3.37±0.22
Plasma MT-I (ng/ml)	4.2±0.9	1.8±0.3	1.9±0.3	2.2±0.5	2.9±0.4
Liver MT-I (μg/g)	1.1±0.2	2.0±0.4	1.0±0.2	1.4±0.1	2.0±0.3

Means±S.E.M. (n=6) are presented.
*The rats in this group were given the Fe-deficient diet for 3 weeks followed by the Fe-adequate diet for 1 week.

TABLE II.
Effects of Protein Deficiency on Blood and Tissue Metallothionein-I Concentrations in Rats

	Dietary protein content (g/kg)		
	50	120	200
Weight (g)	118 ± 4	197 ± 5	256 ± 5
Haematocrit (%)	38.7 ± 0.7	41.8 ± 0.6	42.5 ± 0.3
Blood cells (ng MT-I/ml)	22 ± 1	53 ± 5	43 ± 2
Plasma (ng MT-I/ml)	8 ± 1	4 ± 1	4 ± 1
Liver (μg MT-I/g)	25 ± 3	8 ± 1	2 ± 1
Kidneys (μg MT-I/g)	23 ± 2	75 ± 9	56 ± 3

Rats were maintained on the diets for 19 d. Means $\pm$ S.E.M. (n = 5) are presented. Concentrations of metallothionein-I were determined by radioimmunoassay (J.N. Morrison, A.M. Wood, and I. Bremner, unpublished results).

the blood cells reflects the reduction in the numbers of reticulocytes or other immature cells. The decrease in renal concentrations cannot be explained but we have often noted a close correlation between renal and blood cell metallothionein concentrations. This has been found in rats subjected to other types of stress (Morrison et al., 1988a) and also in protein-deficient animals (see below). It is possible that renal concentrations of metallothionein are regulated by erythropoietin. Alternatively, the levels of both proteins may be controlled by some common factor.

Since protein deficiency inhibits erythropoietin production and reticulocytosis (Ito et al., 1964), the effects of different degrees of protein deficiency on metallothionein concentrations in blood and tissues of the rat were also studied. Growing rats were maintained for up to 3 weeks on a semi-synthetic diet containing 200, 120 or 50 g egg albumen/kg (Table II). Food intakes were significantly reduced in the severely protein-deficient rats (50 g protein/kg) compared with those of intermediate (120 g/kg) or normal (200 g/kg) protein status. The weights of both groups of protein-deficient rats were decreased and there was also a slight reduction in their hematocrit values. Hepatic concentrations of metallothionein-I increased in proportion to the severity of the protein deficiency and plasma concentrations also increased in the rats given 50 g protein/kg diet. However, the response in the blood cells and kidneys was more complex, insofar as the metallothionein-I concentrations increased in the rats of intermediate protein status but decreased in those that were severely protein-deficient. This pattern of response, which was observed in three separate experiments, was related to the erythropoietic activity in the rats, since the reticulocyte counts were 11, 15, and 1% in rats given diets with 200, 120, and 50 g protein/kg, respectively. However, in other studies where rats were given chow diets with

200, 120, 50, or 0 g protein/kg and then subjected to hypoxia, plasma erythropoietin levels decreased in line with the severity of the protein deficiency, with no increase at intermediate protein intakes (Anagnostou et al., 1978).

The effects of protein deficiency were rapidly reversed and blood cell and renal metallothionein concentrations returned to normal, or above normal, levels within one week of protein-deficient rats being given a protein-adequate diet (Table III). This is consistent with the rapid increase in erythropoietin production in protein-repleted rats (Anagnostou et al., 1978).

Substantial decreases in blood cell metallothionein-I levels also occur in rats made diabetic by treatment with streptozotocin (Bremner et al., 1988) (Figure 3). As this is accompanied by an increase in the plasma levels, the response in these rats is similar in some ways to that in severely protein-deficient animals. However, metallothionein concentrations increase in both the liver and kidneys of diabetic rats (Failla and Kiser, 1983), whereas renal concentrations decrease in the protein deficient animals.

CONCLUSIONS

Many analogies can be drawn between the involvement of ferritin in iron metabolism and of metallothionein in the metabolism of certain trace elements. Just as assay of circulating ferritin levels provides information on iron status, assay of metallothionein should therefore provide information on trace element status. However, interpretation of the results of metallothionein assays is inevitably more complex, since production of this protein is affected not by single element but by a range of metals and also by infection, disease, and related "stress factors." Nevertheless, assay of metallothionein could prove to be a useful confirmatory test for conditions such as cadmium or copper toxicosis and zinc deficiency. It could also be of value in the monitoring of the efficacy of nutritional support in malnourished individuals. However, it may be necessary to analyze blood cells, plasma and also urine, since the concentration of metallothionein in these samples varies in a characteristic manner in different physiological and nutritional states (Table IV).

Thus, only in zinc deficiency are metallothionein concentrations reduced in blood cells, plasma and also in urine. Blood cell metallothionein levels are not greatly affected by physical or inflammatory stress or by cytokines but they are affected by conditions that influence erythropoietic activity. However, the latter effects merely reflect changes in blood cell populations and specifically in reticulocyte counts; if results can be expressed relative to some other reticulocyte marker the apparent effects of iron and protein deficiency may disappear. Nevertheless the rapid change in blood cell me-

TABLE III.
Effects of Protein Depletion and Repletion on Blood and Tissue Metallothionein-I Concentrations in Rats

	Dietary protein content (g/kg)				
	200	50	200	50/200[a]	200/200
Weeks on diet	0	2	2	2/1	2/1
Weight		149 ± 1	270 ± 3	230 ± 5	329 ± 4
Blood cells (ng MT-I/ml)	37 ± 10	10 ± 1	24 ± 2	32 ± 3	19 ± 2
Plasma (ng MT-I/ml)	4 ± 1	3 ± 1	2 ± 1	2 ± 1	1 ± 1
Liver (μg MT-I/g)	2.8 ± 0.1	22.7 ± 2.5	1.7 ± 0.4	0.9 ± 0.3	0.2 ± 0.1
Kidneys (μg MT-I/g)	60 ± 8	35 ± 2	100 ± 7	100 ± 10	70 ± 4

Means ± S.E.M. (n = 5) are presented.

[a]The dietary protein content of this group was changed after 2 weeks from 50 to 200 g/kg and the rats were killed 1 week thereafter (J.N. Morrison, A.M. Wood, and I. Bremner, unpublished results).

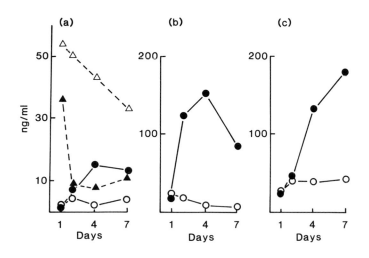

Figure 3. Effects of streptozotocin on metallothionein-I concentrations in (a) blood cells (▲) and plasma (●), (b) liver (●) and (c) kidneys (●) of rats. Concentrations in control animals are shown by the open symbols (△,○). Rats were injected with streptozotocin (100 mg/kg body weight) in 10 m*M* citrate, pH 4.5.

TABLE IV.
Factors Influencing Blood Cell, Plasma, and
Urinary Metallothionein-I Concentrations in Rats

	Blood Plasma	Blood Cells	Urine
Zinc deficiency	↓	↓	↓
Cadmium exposure	↑	↑	↑
Copper toxicity	↑	↑	↑
Stress	↑	—[a]	↑
Iron deficiency	—	↑	↓
Starvation	— or ↑	↓	↓
Protein deficiency	↑	↑ or ↓	N.d.[b]

[a]—Indicates no major effect.
[b]N.d. indicates not determined.

tallothionein levels in response to improvements in nutritional status suggests that assay of these cells could provide a sensitive index of the efficacy of nutritional therapy.

Finally, it should be remembered that these studies have been carried out in rats and that the results may not be directly applicable to humans. For example reticulocyte counts are usually lower in humans than in rats. Moreover, it cannot be assumed that little of the human blood cell metallothionein is present in leukocytes as is the case in rats. Indeed in preliminary studies with human subjects where an ELISA procedure was used for analysis of metallothionein, the concentration of the protein in leukocytes was 1-2 orders of magnitude greater than that in erythrocytes (Branca, 1989). About 20% of the total blood cell metallothionein was present in the monocytes and lymphocytes. Before metallothionein assays can be applied to human samples it may therefore be necessary to carry out prior fractionation of the blood cells.

REFERENCES

Alexander J, Forre O, Aaseth J, Dobloug J, and Ovrebo S (1982): Induction of a metallothionein-like protein in human lymphocytes. *Scand. J. Immunol.* 15: 217.

Anagnostou A, Schade S, Ashkinaz M, Barone J, and Fried W (1978): Effect of protein deprivation on erythropoiesis. *Blood* 50: 1093.

Branca F (1989): An ELISA technique for the measurement of metallothionein in man: an approach to the assessment of zinc status. *M.Sc. thesis: University of Aberdeen.*

Bremner I, Mehra RK, Morrison JN, and Wood AM (1986): Effects of dietary copper supplementation of rats on the occurrence of metallothionein-I in liver and its secretion into blood, bile and urine. *Biochem. J.* 235: 735.

Bremner I (1987): Nutritional and physiological significance of metallothionein. In *Metallothionein II.* Kägi JHR and Kojima Y, Eds., Birkhäuser-Verlag, Basel, p. 81.

Bremner I, Morrison JN, Wood AM and Arthur JR (1987): Effect of changes in dietary zinc, copper and selenium supply and of endotoxin administration on metallothionein I concentrations in blood cells and urine in the rat. *J. Nutr.* 117: 1595.

Bremner I, Morrison JN, and Wood AM (1988): Metallothionein concentrations in the blood and urine of streptozotocin treated rats. In, *Trace Elements in Man and Animals* 6. Hurley LS, Keen CL, Lonnerdal B, and Rucker RB Eds., Plenum Press, New York, p. 681.

Cousins RJ (1985): Absorption, transport and hepatic metabolism of copper and zinc: special reference to metallothionein and ceruloplasmin. *Physiol. Rev.* 65: 238.

Cousins RJ and Leinart AS (1988): Tissue-specific regulation of zinc metabolism and metallothionein genes by interleukin 1. *FASEB J.* 2: 2884.

Failla ML and Kiser RA (1983): Hepatic and renal metabolism of copper and zinc in the diabetic rat. *Am. J. Physiol.* 244: E115.

Falck FY, Fine LJ, Smith RG, Garvey JS, Schork A, England B, McClatchey KD, and Linton J (1983): Metallothionein and occupational exposure to cadmium. *Br. J. Ind. Med.* 40: 305.

Fried W, Plzak LF, Jacobson LO, and Goldwasser E (1957): Studies on erythropoiesis. III. Factors controlling erythropoietin production. *Proc. Soc. Exp. Biol. Med.* 94: 237.

Garvey JS, Vander Mallie RJ, and Chang CC (1982): Radioimmunoassay of metallothioneins. *Methods Enzymol.* 84: 121.

Ghaffar A, Aggett PJ, and Bremner I (1989): Development of an enzyme-linked immunosorbent assay for metallothionein. In, *Nutrient Availability: Chemical and Biological Aspects.* Southgate DAT, Johnson IT, and Fenwick, GR, Eds., Royal Society of Chemistry, Cambridge (Special Publication No. 72), p. 74.

Golden MHN and Golden BF (1981): Effects of zinc supplementation on the dietary intake, rate of weight gain, and energy cost of tissue deposition in children recovering from severe malnutrition. *Am. J. Clin. Nutr.* 34: 900.

Grider A, Kao K-J, Klein PA, and Cousins RJ (1989): Enzyme linked immunosorbent assay for human metallothionein: correlation of induction with infection. *J. Lab. Clin. Med.* 113: 221.

Harley CB, Menon CR, Rachubinski RA, and Nieboer E (1989): Metallothionein mRNA and protein induction by cadmium in peripheral-blood leukocytes. *Biochem. J.* 262: 873.

Hidalgo J, Giralt M, Garvey JS, and Armario A (1988): Physiological role of glucocorticoids on rat serum and liver metallothionein in basal and stress conditions. *Am. J. Physiol.* 254: E71.

Ito K, Schmaus JR, and Reissmann KR (1964): Protein metabolism and erythropoiesis. III. The erythroid marrow in protein-starved rats and its response to erythropoietin. *Acta Hematol.* 32: 257.

Mehra RK and Bremner I (1983): Development of a radioimmunoassay for rat liver metallothionein I and its application to the analysis of rat plasma and kidneys. *Biochem. J.* 213: 459.

Morrison JN and Bremner I (1987): Effects of maternal zinc supply on blood and tissue metallothionein I concentrations in suckling rats. *J. Nutr.* 117: 1588.

Morrison JN, Wood AM, and Bremner I (1988a): Effects of inflammatory stress on metallothionein-I concentrations in blood cells and plasma of rats. *Biochem. Soc. Trans.* 16: 820.

Morrison JN, Wood AM, and Bremner I (1988b): Concentrations and distribution of metallothionein-I in blood cells of rats injected with zinc or phenylhydrazine. *J. Trace Elements Exp. Med.* 1: 95.

Noble NA, Xu Q-P and Ward JH (1989): Reticulocytes I. Isolation and *in vitro* maturation of synchronized populations. *Blood* 74: 475.

Nordberg GF, Piscator M, and Nordberg M (1971): On the distribution of cadmium in blood. *Acta Pharmacol. Toxicol.* 30: 289.

Nordberg GF, Garvey JS, and Chang CC (1982): Metallothionein in plasma and urine of cadmium workers. *Envir. Res.* 28: 179.

Peavy DL and Fairchild EJ (1987): Induction of metallothionein synthesis in human peripheral blood leukocytes. *Environ. Res.* 42: 377.

Robertson A, Morrison JN, Wood AM, and Bremner I (1989): Effects of iron deficiency on metallothionein-I concentrations in blood and tissues in rats. *J. Nutr.* 119: 439.

Sato M, Mehra RK, and Bremner I (1984): Measurement of plasma metallothionein in the assessment of the zinc status of zinc deficient and stressed rats. *J. Nutr.* 114: 1683.

Sobocinski PZ, Canterbury WG, Mapes CA, and Dinterman RE (1978): Involvement of hepatic metallothioneins in hypozincemia associated with bacterial infection. *Am. J. Physiol.* 234: E399.

Tanaka K, Min K-S, Onosaka S, Fukuhara C, and Ueda M (1985): The origin of metallothionein in red blood cells. *Toxicol. Appl. Pharmacol.* 78: 63.

Tanaka K, Min K-S, Ohyanagi N, Onosaka S, and Fukuhara C (1986): Fate of erythrocyte Cd-metallothionein in mice. *Toxicol. Appl. Pharmacol.* 83: 197.

Thomas DG, Linton HJ, and Garvey JS (1986): Fluorometric ELISA for the detection and quantitation of metallothionein. *J. Immunol. Methods.* 89: 239.

Williams LM, Cunningham H, Ghaffar A, Riddoch GI, and Bremner I (1989): Metallothionein immunoreactivity in the liver and kidney of copper injected rats. *Toxicology* 55: 307.

Possible Role of Metallothioneins in Growth, Differentiation, and Carcinogenesis of Mouse Skin*

Mika Karasawa, Hiroki Hashiba and Toshio Kuroki
Institute of Medical Science
University of Tokyo
Tokyo, Japan

Chiharu Tohyama
National Institute of Environmental Studies
Ibaraki, Japan

Noriko Nishimura
Aichi Medical University
Aichi, Japan

INTRODUCTION

Metallothionein (MT) is a cysteine-rich protein with a molecular weight of 6,000 Da and characterized by binding with heavy metals. MT is present in almost all cells and inducible by a large variety of agents including heavy metals, steroid hormones and phorbol esters. Such a ubiquitous presence and inducibility suggest that MT plays important roles in cell physiology. Although several functions such as homeostatic regulation of essential ele-

*Supported in part by a Grant-in-Aid for Special Project Research, Cancer-Bioscience, from the Ministry of Education, Science and Culture of Japan.

ments, detoxification of heavy metals and scavenging of free radicals have been suggested, physiological functions of MT are still in search (Karin, 1985).

As a tissue model of MTs function, we used epidermal keratinocytes because we have been working for several years on growth, differentiation and carcinogenesis of these cells (Kuroki et al., 1988, 1989). During the course of these studies, we found that MT was highly expressed when cell growth was stimulated (Hashiba et al., 1989). We also found that 1,25-dihydroxyvitamin D_3 (1,25(OH)$_2$D$_3$) was a potent inducer of MT gene expression (Karasawa et al., 1987). In this article, we summarize these two studies which may afford new insight into physiological functions of MT.

INDUCTION OF MT IN MOUSE SKIN

It is well recognized that 12-*O*-tetradecanoylphorbol-13-acetate (TPA) binds to and thereby activates protein kinase C, and this signal is transmitted to nucleus, leading to expression of certain genes (Nishizuka, 1984; Angel et al., 1987; Lee et al., 1987a,b). MT is one of these TPA-inducible genes (Angel et al., 1986). We examined expression of MT mRNA in mouse skin treated with TPA and in papillomas produced by repeated treatment with TPA of the initiated skin (Hashiba et al., 1989).

TPA and other compounds were applied topically to dorsal skin of CD-1 mice and total RNA was extracted from the epidermis at the site of treatment by the guanidium thiocyanate/hot phenol method and purified by Cs/TFA gradient. RNA (40 to 50 μg) was loaded on a 1.5% agarose gel, transferred to a nylon membrane filter, hybridized with ^{32}P-labeled 0.4 kb EcoRI/HindIII fragment of m1pEH.4 derived from mouse MT-I cDNA, and autoradiographed. The major transcript of MT mRNA was about 0.5 kb but a weak band with 2 to 4 kb, probably a precursor of MT mRNA, was also observed.

We found that a single topical application of TPA induced MT mRNA in dose and time-dependent fashion (Figure 1). The increase of MT mRNA was apparent from 2 h after treatment with TPA and reached a peak at 8 h, returning to normal level by 24 h. The induction of MT mRNA at 4 h was dependent on TPA doses of 1 to 5 μg, a range of doses with tumor promoting effect.

We examined the inducibility of MT mRNA under various conditions using promoting and nonpromoting agents, and promotion-sensitive and -resistant strains of mice. As summarized in Table I, MT mRNA inducibility was found to correlate well with inducibility of hyperplasia, rather than tumor promotion. For example, 4-*O*-methyl TPA, a first-stage tumor promoter did not induce epidermal hyperplasia or MT mRNA. Benzoylperox-

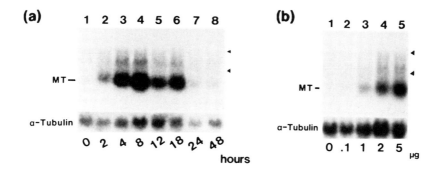

Figure 1. Time(a) and dose(b)-dependent induction of MT mRNA in mouse skin by TPA.

TABLE I.
Correlation Between Inducibility of MTmRNA and Epidermal Hyperplasia

	Promotion	MTmRNA	Hyperplasia
Compound			
TPA	+	+	+
A23187	+	+	+
Mezerein	+	+	I
Cholera toxin	−	+	+
Ethylphenylpropiolate	−	+	+
PDD	+ (weak)	+ (weak)	+ (weak)
4-*O*-Me-TPA	+	−	−
4α-PDD	−	−	−
Phorbol	−	−	−
Benzoylperoxide	+	−	−
Mouse			
Sencar	+	+	+
CD-1	+	+	+
C57BL/6	+ (weak)	+ (weak)	+ (weak)

ide, a tumor promoter did not induce hyperplasia or MT mRNA possibly because of its distinct action as a free-radical generator.

The lack of correlation between inducibility of MT mRNA and tumor promotion was further demonstrated with cholera toxin and ethylphenylpropionate, both of which showed no tumor promoting activity in two-stage carcinogenesis of mouse skin (Kuroki, 1981; Kuroki et al., 1986; Raick and Burdzy, 1973) but induced epidermal hyperplasia and MT mRNA. Localization of MT expressing cells was examined by immunochemical staining using anti-rat MT-I antibody. We found that MT positive cells are localized predominantly at the basal layer of the epidermis (Karasawa et al., in press).

Repeated applications of TPA to the initiated skin produce papillomas and at lower incidence carcinomas. We examined expression of MT mRNA in these tumors 6 months or more after termination of tumor promotion. As shown in Figure 2, high levels of MT mRNA were expressed in all papillomas examined. Immunohistochemical staining of papilloma tissues indicated that MT protein was expressed in papilloma cells, especially in those close to the basal layer, but little, if any, in stromal cells. Thus all the data obtained in this study indicate that MT is involved in cell growth through some unknown mechanisms.

REGULATION OF MT GENE EXPRESSION BY 1,25(OH)$_2$D$_3$

1,25(OH)$_2$D$_3$ has long been known as a regulatory hormone of the plasma calcium level. However, it is now accepted that the actions of this hormone are not limited to calcium homeostasis but can be extended to other biological processes including cell differentiation (Minghetti and Norman, 1988). We previously showed that 1,25(OH)$_2$D$_3$ stimulated differentiation of epidermal keratinocytes in culture by a receptor-mediated mechanism (Hosomi et al., 1983). We also found that 1,25(OH)$_2$D$_3$ was a potent inducer of MT mRNA in FRSK cells derived from fetal skin keratinocytes of rats (Karasawa et al., 1987). 1,25(OH)$_2$D$_3$ at 12 nM increased MT mRNA within

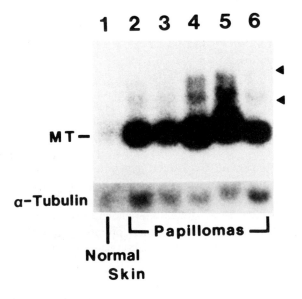

Figure 2. Constitutive expression of MT mRNA in papillomas produced by repeated treatment of TPA to the initiated skin (lane 1, normal skin; lanes 2 to 6, papillomas).

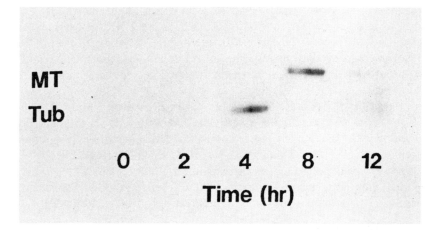

Figure 3. Nuclear run-on assay of MT gene in 1,25(OH)$_2$D$_3$-treated FRSK cells.

2 h and reached a maximum at 12 to 24 h. The induction was dependent on concentrations from 0.12 to 12 nM, the usual dose range for exerting its biological actions. The level of induction at 12 nM was almost comparable with those induced by 10 μM dexamethasone or 1 μM CdCl$_2$, indicating that 1,25(OH)$_2$D$_3$ is much more potent than those previously known.

Nuclear run-on assay was performed to clarify whether 1,25(OH)$_2$D$_3$ increases MT mRNA transcriptionally. As shown in Figure 3, elevation of transcription of MT gene was observed by the use of nuclei of FRSK cells treated with 1,25(OH)$_2$D$_3$, indicating that MT gene was transcriptionally activated by it.

Transcriptional control of genes by hormones and growth factors are now well understood thanks to recent progress of molecular biology. The receptor of 1,25(OH)$_2$D$_3$ has recently been cloned and shown to be a member of nuclear *trans*-acting receptor family that includes estrogen, thyroxine and retinoic acid receptors (Burmester et al., 1988; Baker et al., 1988). *Cis*-responsive element to which an 1,25(OH)$_2$D$_3$-receptor complex binds has also been identified in the 5′–flanking region of rat osteocalcin gene (Kerner et al., 1989).

We examined the presence of a *cis*-element that confers responsiveness to 1,25(OH)$_2$D$_3$ in MT genes. The upstream regions of human MTIITA, rat MT-I and MT-II genes, and their portions with various length were inserted into pSV0CAT and transfected to FRSK cells, MCF-7 human breast cancer cells and ROS rat osteosarcoma cells. However, we could not detect any response to 1,25(OH)$_2$D$_3$ in the regions ranging from −850 to +53 of human MT-IIA genes, from −900 to +60 of rat MT-I and MT-II gene, whereas these sequences showed responsiveness to $CdCl_2$ and dexamethasone. Co-transfection with expression vector for $1,25(OH)_2D_3$ receptor did not evoke CAT-activity in response to $1,25(OH)_2D_3$. Further experiments are needed by the use of more extreme region of upstream sequences of MT genes.

Induction of MT mRNA was also observed in liver, kidney and skin *in vivo* when mice were orally given 1-hydroxyvitamin D_3, a synthetic precursor of $1,25(OH)_2D_3$. The time course of the induction differed from those in culture. Under the condition *in vivo,* the induction of MT mRNA was not evident until 24 h and reached a maximum level at 48 to 72 h, in parallel with the increase of plasma calcium level (Figure 4). This delayed expression suggests the possibility of indirect action of $1,25(OH)_2D_3$.

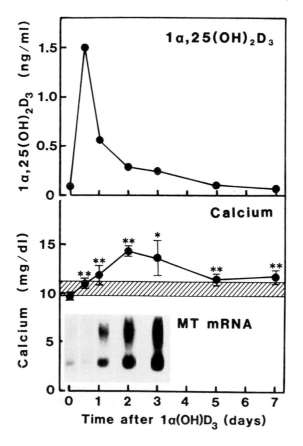

Figure 4. Induction of MT mRNA in kidney (bottom panel) in 1-hydroxyvitaminD_3-treated mice. Upper and middle panels, plasma concentrations of $1,25(OH)_2D_3$ and Ca^{2+}, respectively.

CONCLUDING REMARKS

MT is a unique molecule in its amino acid composition with an unusually high cysteine content (30%), its binding capacity to heavy metals and its inducibility by a wide range of chemicals and agents. Because of the latter characteristics, upstream sequence of MT gene is widely used as a regulator of gene expression when connected to a protein-coding region of other genes. Although structure and function of MT genes are investigated in detail, physiological functions of MT protein do not seem to draw much attention. Proposed functions for MT include detoxification of heavy metals, scavenging of free radicals and reservoir of Zn atom or cysteine molecule. However, ubiquitous presence and wide inducibility open the possibility for unforeseen biological functions of MT. Obviously, more biological experiments are needed.

REFERENCES

Angel P, Pöting A, Mallick U, Rahmsdorf HJ, Schorpp M, and Herrlich P (1986): Induction of metallothionein and other mRNA species by carcinogens and tumor promoters in primary human skin fibroblasts. *Mol. Cell. Biol.* 6: 1760.

Angel P, Imagawa M, Chiu R, Stein B, Imbra RJ, Rahmsdorf HJ, Jonat C, Herrlich P, and Karin M (1987): Phorbol ester inducible genes contain a common Cis-element recognized by a TPA-modulated trans-acting factor. *Cell* 49: 729.

Baker AR, McDonnell DP, Hughes M, Crisp TM, Mangelsdorf DJ, Haussler MR, Pike JW, Shine J, and O'Malley BW (1988): Cloning and expression of full-length cDNA encoding human vitamin D receptor. *Proc. Natl. Acad. Sci. U.S.A.* 85: 3294.

Burmester JK, Maeda N, and DeLuca HF (1988): Isolation and expression of rat 1,25-dihydroxyvitamin D_3 receptor cDNA. *Proc. Natl. Acad. Sci. U.S.A.* 85: 1005.

Hashiba H, Hosoi J, Karasawa M, Yamada S, Nose K, and Kuroki T (1989): Induction of metallothionein mRNA by tumor promoters in mouse skin and its constitutive expression in papillomas. *Mol. Carcinogenesis.* 2: 95.

Hosomi J, Hosoi J, Abe E, Suda T, and Kuroki T (1983): Regulation of terminal differentiation of cultured mouse epidermal cells by 1,25-dihydroxyvitamin D_3. *Endocrinology* 113: 1950.

Karasawa M, Hosoi J, Hashiba H, Nose K, Tohyama C, Abe E, Suda T, and Kuroki T (1987): Regulation of metallothionein gene expression by 1,25-dihydroxyvitamin D_3 in cultured cells and in mice. *Proc. Natl. Acad. Sci. U.S.A.* 84: 8810.

Karasawa M, Nishimura N, Nishimura H, Tohyama C, Hashiba H, and Kuroki T (1991): Localization of metallothionein in hair follicles of normal skin and the basal cell layer of hyperplastic epidermis: possible association with cell proliferation. *J. Invest. Dermatol.* 96: (in press).

Karin M (1985): Metallothioneins: proteins in search of function. *Cell* 41: 9.

Kerner SA, Scott RA and Pike JW (1989): Sequence elements in the human osteo-calcin gene confer basal activation and inducible response to hormonal vitamin D_3. *Proc. Natl. Acad. Sci. U.S.A.* 86: 4455.

Kuroki T (1981): Induction by cholera toxin of synchronous divisions *in vivo* in the epidermis resulting in hyperplasia. *Proc. Natl. Acad. Sci. U.S.A.* 78: 6958.

Kuroki T, Chida K, Munakata K, and Murakami Y (1986): Cholera toxin, a potent inducer of epidermal hyperplasia but with no tumor promoting activity in mouse skin carcinogenesis. *Biochem. Biophys. Res. Commun.* 137: 486.

Kuroki T, Morimoto S, and Suda T (1988): Actions of 1,25-dihydroxyvitamin D_3 on normal, psoriatic, and promoted epiderdmal keratinoocytes. *Ann. N.Y. Acad. Sci.* 548: 45.

Kuroki T, Chida K, Hosomi J, and Kondo S (1989): Use of human epidermal cells in the study of carcinogenesis. *J. Inv. Dermatol.* 92: 271S.

Lee W, Haslinger A, Karin M, and Tjian R (1987a): Activation of transcription by two factors that bind promoter and enhancer sequences of the human metallothionein gene and SV40. *Nature* 325: 368.

Lee W, Mitchell P, and Tjian R (1987b): Purified transcription factor AP-1 interacts with TPA-inducible enhancer elements. *Cell* 49: 741.

Minghetti PP and Norman AW (1988): 1,25(OH)$_2$-vitamin D_3 receptors: gene regulation and genetic circuitry. *FASEB J.* 2:3043.

Nishizuka Y (1984): The role of protein kinase C in cell surface signal transduction and tumor promotion. *Nature* 308: 693.

Raick AN and Burdzy K (1973): Ultrastructural and biochemical changes induced in mouse epidermis by a hyperplastic agent, ethylphenylpropiolate. *Cancer Res.* 33: 2221.

Chapter 28

Involvement of Metallothionein in the Prevention of Gastric Mucosal Lesions

Kazutake Tsujikawa, Takumi Imai and Tsutomu Mimura
Faculty of Pharmaceutical Sciences
Osaka University
Osaka, Japan

Noriko Otaki
National Institute of Industrial Health
Kanagawa, Japan

Masami Kimura
National Institute of Industrial Health
Kanagawa, Japan
and
Central Institute for Experimental Animals
Kawasaki, Kanagawa, Japan

SUMMARY

Zinc (Zn) administered subcutaneously to rats significantly suppressed the formation of water-immersion stress-induced gastric mucosal lesions. Metallothionein (MT) in gastric mucosal cells was slightly induced by water-immersion stress load. When rats were stressed by water-immersion stress after the administration of Zn, MT concentrations in gastric mucosal cells and serum as well as the liver significantly increased in comparison with each stress control group. Glutathione levels in gastric mucosal cells were significantly decreased by water-immersion stress load. The decrease in the intramucosal glutathione levels caused by the stress load could not be induced to return to control levels by the administration of Zn. To clarify the physiological role of MT in gastric mucosal cells, a newborn rat gastric mucosal cell culture system was utilized.

In cultured gastric mucosal cells, MT was found to be inducible by Zn. Xanthine-xanthine oxidase-induced cytotoxicity enhanced by the pretreatment with methionine sulfoximine was decreased by Zn treatment.

Intravenously administered MT-II isolated from the livers of zinc acetate treated rats suppressed the stress-induced and HCl-ethanol-induced gastric mucosal lesions.

These data indicated that (1) intra- and extracellular MTs have the anti-acute gastric mucosal lesion activity and (2) intramucosal MT functions as a physiological defensive factor, instead of glutathione, during such stress situations.

INTRODUCTION

Acute gastric mucosal lesion (AGML) is defined as a disease consisting of acute hemorrhagic erosion and/or acute gastric ulcer (Katz and Siegel, 1968). Psychological and physical stress, drug ingestion and alcohol are thought to be major causes of occurrence of AGML. The pathogenesis of AGML is not understood well, however, imbalance between aggressive and defensive factors, and weakening of the cytoprotective mechanisms are known to play important roles in the cause of the lesion (Shay and Sun, 1963). Recent studies indicate that oxygen-derived free radicals, especially the hydroxyl radical, are generated in ischemic tissue and relate to the development of stress-induced AGML (Itoh and Guth, 1985; Perry et al., 1986).

Zn compounds like zinc chloride and zinc sulfate have been shown to suppress the occurrence of AGML (Cho, 1989). Zn is known to induce MT, a low molecular weight, cysteine rich protein, in various tissues including liver. However, the biological role of MTs is not completely elucidated. Recently, it was reported that MT can scavenge hydroxyl radicals (Thornalley and Vašák, 1985).

We have hypothesized that MT might function as one of the defensive factors against the occurrence of AGML. This possibility was confirmed using a water immersion stress-induced AGML model and cultured rat gastric mucosal cells.

METHODS

Water-Immersion Stress-Induced Gastric Mucosal Lesions

Male Wistar rats weighing 200 to 250 g were used as experimental animals. Rats were subjected to stress following the method of Takagi and Okabe (1968), in which animals were immobilized in the stress cage and immersed in a water bath of $23 \pm 1°C$ to the depth of the xiphoid for 20 h.

HCl-Ethanol-Induced Gastric Mucosal Lesions

According to the method of Mizui and Doteuchi (1983), male Wistar rats weighing 200 to 250 g were deprived of food and were placed in steel wire cages for 24 h before receiving 1 ml of 150 mM HCl-60% ethanol. The rats were killed by decapitation at 1 h after administration of HCl-ethanol.

Measurement of Gastric Mucosal Lesions

The stomachs were removed, fixed in 0.5% formalin, and opened along the greater curvature. The sum of the length of all gastric mucosal lesions was measured on each rat and was used as the lesion index.

MT Assay

Rats were killed by decapitation. The trunk blood was collected and coagulated. The liver and the gastric mucosal cells were homogenized (50%, w/v) in 10 mM Tris-HCl, pH 8.6, containing 5 mM 2-mercaptoethanol, and centrifuged at $36,000 \times g$ for 1 hr at 4°C. Serum and the tissue supernatant MT were analyzed by radioimmunoassay (RIA), described by Ikei et al. (1989).

Glutathione Assay

Because glutathione (GSH) accounts for the majority of soluble-reduced sulfhydryls in cells. (Kosower and Kosower, 1978), reduced GSH concentration in gastric mucosal cells was determined by measuring total soluble-reduced sulfhydryl content without identifying the individual species of sulfhydryls by the method of Ellman (1959).

Protein Content

Protein content was determined according to the method of Lowry et al. (1951) using bovine serum albumin as a standard.

Primary Gastric Mucosal Cell Culture

Rat gastric mucosal cell culture was produced according to the procedure reported by Terano et al. (1982). The fundic area was excised from the 10- 12-day-old Wistar rats stomach and minced into 2 to 3 mm³ pieces. The minced tissues were suspended in Hank's balanced salt solution containing 0.1% collagenase and 0.05% hyaluronidase. After incubation in this medium at 37°C for 70 min, the tissues were pipetted several times and filtered through a nylon mesh. The filtrate was washed and the cells were cultured in Ham's F-12 medium supplemented with 10% FCS, 15 mM HEPES buffer and antibiotics in the collagen-coated culture dishes or plates at 37°C in a humidified 5% CO_2 incubator with the media changed daily. Three-day-old cultures, at the confluent state, were employed for this study.

³H-Thymidine Release Assay

Cytotoxicity was quantified by measuring ³H-thymidine release from prelabeled cells (Sone, 1987). Culture medium containing 1 μCi/ml ³H-thymidine was added to cultured gastric mucosal monolayers. After overnight prelabeling, the cells were washed with phosphate buffered saline (PBS) and then used for cellular injury test. After GSH depletion and/or MT induction, prelabeled monolayers were covered with 0.5 ml of Ham's F-12 medium containing 0.1 mM xanthine. After addition of test samples or vehicle controls, 50 mU/ml xanthine oxidase was added. The monolayers were incubated for up to 3 h at 37°C in a humidified 5% CO_2 incubator. After incubation for set periods in the culture condition, Ham's F-12 medium (I) was decanted and the monolayers were washed with 0.5 ml of PBS (II). (I) and (II) were combined as supernatants of cells. One ml of 0.5% Triton X-100® was added to the washed monolayers to rupture the cells. ³H-thymidine radioactivities of the cells and the supernatant were measured with a liquid scintillation counter. The percentage of ³H-thymidine released per sample was expressed as follows:

$$\text{Release (\%)} = \frac{\text{cpm of supernatant}}{\text{cpm of supernatant + cpm of cells}} = 100$$

where cpm is counts per minute, or specific release (%) due to sample or treatment action = (percent of release on treatment)—(percent of release in the intact).

Glutathione Depletion

GSH was depleted from the cultured gastric mucosal cells by pretreatment for 24 h with 0.2 mM methionine sulfoximine (MSO), an inhibitor of γ-glutamylcysteine synthetase (Owen and Meister, 1978), before cytotoxicity test.

Statistics

Student's *t*-test was employed to determine the statistical significance of the data obtained in this study.

RESULTS

Effect of Zn on Water-Immersion Stress-Induced Gastric Mucosal Lesions in Rats

Zn (as zinc acetate) was administered subcutaneously at 24-h intervals for 6 d and its effect on water immersion stress-induced AGML was examined. As shown in Table I, Zn significantly suppressed the formation of AGML by 55% and 36% at doses of 10 and 2 mg Zn/kg b. wt./d, respectively.

MT Concentrations in Rat Tissues and Serum

MT concentrations in rat gastric mucosal cells, liver and serum were determined by RIA and are shown in Table II. In the control group (44-h starvation), MT concentrations in gastric mucosal cells, liver, and serum were 15.1 ± 1.9 ng/mg protein, 1.35 ± 0.13 μg/mg protein, and 87.9 ± 16.3 ng/ml, respectively. Since slight hemolysis occurred during preparation of serum samples, MT in blood cells might have contaminated the absolute serum MT level. In water-immersion stress loaded rats, hepatic MT concentrations did not increase. However, the MT level in gastric mucosal cells and serum were 1.4- and 2.1-fold greater than the control group, respectively. When rats were loaded with water-immersion stress after the administration of Zn at a dose of 10 mg Zn/kg b. wt./d for 6 successive days, MT concentrations in gastric mucosal cells, serum and liver increased 1.9-, 2.5-, and 7.1-fold in comparison with each stress group level.

GSH Concentration in Gastric Mucosal Cells

Gastric mucosal GSH concentration in the control group was 48.5 ± 2.1 nmol/mg protein. After water-immersion stress load, the GSH level was decreased by 52% (23.1 ± 3.4 nmol/mg protein). The GSH level did not recover to control levels by the administration of Zn (Table III).

TABLE I.
Effect of Zn on Water-Immersion Stress-Induced Gastric Mucosal Lesions in Rats

Treatment	Dose (mg/kg)	No. of Rats	Lesion Index (mm)
Control	—	7	37.3 ± 3.3
Zn	2	7	$23.8 \pm 5.1*$
	10	7	$16.6 \pm 3.8**$

All values represent mean $\pm$ S.E.M. Zn was administered (as zinc acetate; s.c.) at 2 or 10 mg Zn/kg for 6 d. Significantly different from the control group: $*p < 0.05$, $**p < 0.01$.

TABLE II.
MT Concentrations in Gastric Mucosal Cells, Liver, and Serum of Rats

Treatment	No. of Rats	Gastric Mucosal Cells (ng/mg protein)	Liver (μg/mg protein)	Serum (ng/ml)
Control	8	15.1 ± 1.9	1.35 ± 0.13	87.9 ± 16.3
Stress	8	21.4 ± 3.5	1.49 ± 0.29	$183.3 \pm 8.8*$
Zn[a] + Stress	8	$41.7 \pm 3.2**$	$10.52 \pm 1.59**$	$460.7 \pm 45.6**$

All values represent mean $\pm$ S.E.M. Stress: Water-immersion stress.
[a]Zn was administered (as zinc chloride; s.c.) at 10 mg Zn/kg for 6 d.
Significantly different from the control group: $*p < 0.001$; significantly different from the stress group: $**p < 0.001$.

TABLE III.
GSH Concentration in Gastric Mucosal Cells of Rats

Treatment	No. of Rats	GSH (nmol/mg protein)
Control	10	48.5 ± 2.1
Stress	8	$23.1 \pm 3.4*$
Zn[a] + Stress	8	$26.4 \pm 3.0*$

All values represent mean $\pm$ S.E.M. Stress: Water-immersion stress.
[a]Zn was administered (as zinc chloride; s.c.) at 10 mg Zn/kg for 6 d. Significantly different from the control group: $*p < 0.001$.

TABLE IV.
Concentrations of MT and GSH in Gastric
Mucosal Cells of Rats

Treatment	No. of Rats	MT (ng/mg protein)	GSH (nmol/mg protein)
Control	9	47.8 ± 2.1	55.6 ± 5.2
Stress (7 h)[a]	10	63.1 ± 5.1*	34.7 ± 2.7**
Stress (14 h)[a]	7	63.8 ± 6.7*	39.5 ± 5.1*
Stress (20 h)[a]	9	75.5 ± 4.6***	30.6 ± 1.6***

All values represent mean ± S.E.M. Stress: Water-immersion stress.
[a]Time of stress load is in parenthesis. Significantly different from the control group: *$p < 0.05$, **$p < 0.01$, ***$p < 0.001$.

Time Courses of MT and GSH Concentrations in Gastric Mucosal Cells

Table IV shows the time courses of MT and GSH concentrations in gastric mucosal cells. The MT concentration in gastric mucosal cells increased 7 h after water-immersion stress. This concentration is significantly higher than that of the control group. The GSH concentration however significantly decreased 7 h after the stress load.

Effect of MT-II on Water-Immersion Stress-Induced Gastric Mucosal Lesions

The effect of intravenously administered MT-II on water-immersion stress-induced AGML was examined. As shown in Table V, AGML was significantly suppressed by 2.5 mg/kg b. wt. of MT-II from 24.1 ± 3.1 (control) to 7.6 ± 0.9. Even at the dose of 1.0 mg/kg b. wt., the inhibition was significant ($p < 0.01$). Cimetidine, a H_2-receptor antagonist, also suppressed the AGML at 100 mg/kg i.v. ($p < 0.001$). Since Zn is contained in MT-II, the effect of Zn on the stress-induced AGML was also tested at a dose of 0.15 mg Zn/kg b. wt., which is equivalent to the Zn in MT-II at a dose of 2.5 mg/kg b. wt. Although a slight anti-ulcerogenic activity was found in the Zn administered group, the effect was much weaker than in the MT-II administered group.

Effect of MT-II on HCl-Ethanol-Induced AGML

As shown in Table VI, in the animals treated with MT-II at doses of 2.5 mg/kg and 1.0 mg/kg b. wt. i.v., the lesion index was significantly lower (23.7 ± 3.3 and 41.2 ± 5.9, respectively) than that of the control group (66.7 ± 6.2). Zn per se (0.15 mg Zn/kg b. wt. i.v.) showed no effect. Cimetidine did not significantly suppress the AGML even at a dose of 20 mg/kg b. wt. i.v.

MT Induction in Primary Cultured Gastric Mucosal Cells

The primary cultured gastric mucosal cells reached confluence 3 days after seeding. Approximately 90% of the cells were identified as mucus-producing epithelial cells stained red with periodic acid-Schiff (PAS) reagent. Zn (100 μM as zinc chloride) could induce MT in the cultured gastric mucosal cells (Table VII).

TABLE V.
Effect of MT-II, Zn, and Cimetidine on Water-Immersion Stress-Induced Gastric Mucosal Lesions in Rats

Treatment	Dose (mg/kg)	No. of Rats	Lesion Index (mm)
1. Control	—	7	24.1 ± 3.1
MT-II	1.0	7	12.9 ± 3.8*
	2.5	7	7.6 ± 0.9**
Zn[a]	0.15	7	15.6 ± 3.1
2. Control	—	10	21.6 ± 2.0
Cimetidine	100	9	11.5 ± 2.5**

All values represent mean ± S.E.M. Each sample was administered intravenously 30 min before the stress treatment.
[a]Zn was administered (as zinc acetate; i.v.) at 0.15 mg Zn/kg. Significantly different from the control group: *p <0.01, **p <0.001.

TABLE VI.
Effect of MT-II, Zn, and Cimetidine on HCl-Ethanol-Induced Gastric Mucosal Lesions in Rats

Treatment	Dose (mg/kg)	No. of Rats	Lesion Index (mm)
Control	—	7	66.7 ± 6.2
MT-II	1.0	7	41.2 ± 5.9*
	2.5	7	23.7 ± 3.3**
Zn[a]	0.15	7	70.8 ± 6.6
Cimetidine	20.0	7	45.5 ± 8.5

All values represent mean ± S.E.M. Each sample was given intravenously 30 min before the administration of 150 mM HCl-60% EtOH (1 ml).
[a]Zn was given (as zinc acetate; i.v.) at 0.15 mg Zn/kg. Significantly different from the control group: *p <0.01, **p <0.001.

TABLE VII.
Effect of Zn on MT Concentration in Cultured Rat Gastric Mucosal Cells

Treatment	Final Concentration (μM)	MT Concentration (ng/10^6 cells)
Control	—	N.D.
Zn	50	N.D.
	100	45.2 ± 9.9

Value represents mean $\pm$ S.E.M. (n = 5). N.D.: not detectable. Cells were cultured for 24 h in Ham's F-12 medium with Zn (as zinc chloride).

TABLE VIII.
Effect of Methionine Sulfoximine (MSO) and/or Zn Pretreatment on Xanthine-Xanthine Oxidase (XO)-Induced ^{3}H-Thymidine Release from Cultured Rat Gastric Mucosal Cells

Treatment	No. of Experiments	Specific ^{3}H-Thymidine Release (%)
Control	8	28.9 ± 2.5
MSO	7	36.5 ± 2.1*
MSO + Zn (100 μM)	4	20.0 ± 2.8**
MSO + Zn (10 μM)	4	32.4 ± 3.5

All values represent mean $\pm$ S.E.M. Cells were pretreated for 24 h with 0.2 mM MSO and/or Zn (as zinc chloride) before XO treatment. Significantly different from the control group: *p <0.05. Significantly different from the MSO group: **p <0.01.

Effect of Zn and MSO on Xanthine-Xanthine Oxidase-Induced Cellular Injury

As shown in Table VIII, cultured gastric mucosal cells were injured by free radicals generated from the xanthine-xanthine oxidase reaction. The specific ^{3}H-thymidine release from the cells was 28.9 ± 2.5%. Pretreatment of cultured cells with 0.2 mM MSO increased their susceptibility to xanthine-xanthine oxidase-induced cellular injury by about 26%. Zn (100 μM as zinc chloride) inhibited MSO-enhanced xanthine-xanthine oxidase-mediated ^{3}H-thymidine release significantly.

DISCUSSION

Since MT was characterized by Kägi and Vallee in 1960, much has been studied about the physical, chemical and genetic features of this protein. Not only heavy metals but also stress stimuli have been demonstrated to induce MT in various organs. However, the function of this protein during stress has not been determined.

The stomach is highly sensitive to stress stimuli and AGML occurs quite commonly in humans due to stress. The administration of Zn, an inducer of MT, suppressed the formation of AGML. Our studies are aimed at clarifying MT function in the stomach.

The results show that MT concentrations were increased in gastric mucosal cells and serum of rats by water-immersion stress and that the mucosal MT concentration increased rapidly 7 h after water-immersion stress. Further increases of MT concentration in the mucosal cells were caused by the Zn administration to the stressed rats. From the fact that AGML markedly occurs 7 h and more after the stress load, it was suggested that intramucosal MT might function as a physiological defense factor in the stomach and regulate the occurrence of the AGML.

GSH and its redox cycle enzymes represent an important cellular antioxidant mechanism (Chance et al., 1979; Kaplowitz et al., 1985). GSH is an antioxidant available in all cells (Kosower and Kosower, 1978) and is found in particularly high concentrations in the liver and gastric mucosal cells of rats (Boyd et al., 1979) and humans (Hoppenkamps et al., 1984). Boyd et al. (1981) reported that gastric GSH depletion with diethymaleate produces AGML *in vivo*. Therefore, we determined the GSH concentration in gastric mucosal cells. Water-immersion stress load decreased GSH concentration in gastric mucosal cells. By the administration of Zn, the decrease of GSH concentration could not be rectified in spite of the increase of MT concentration in the mucosal cells.

In recent studies (Itoh and Guth, 1985; Perry et al., 1986), oxygen derived free radicals and other metabolites, which were synthesized during ischemia and reperfusion at the site of mucosal lesions, have been shown to play an important role in the pathogenesis of AGML. Moreover, the administration of agents that scavenge these active radicals such as superoxide dismutase, are reported to be effective in preventing the occurrence of AGML (Perry et al., 1986). Recently a new aspect in the biological function of MT as an efficient scavenger of hydroxyl radical has been shown (Thornalley and Vašák, 1985). Taken together, MT induced by water-immersion stress and/or the administration of Zn, should suppress the formation of AGML by scavenging hydroxyl radicals generated at the site of gastric mucosal lesions. Moreover, intravenously administered MT suppressed the formation of stress-induced and HCl-ethanol-induced AGMLs (Mimura et al., 1988). These results also suggested that MT in blood would protect the stomach by scavenging hydroxyl radicals.

Hiraishi et al. (1987) and Olson (1988) reported that gastric mucosal GSH redox mechanisms are important for protection against oxygen metabolite-mediated injury in the stomach using *in vitro* cultured gastric mucosal cells. In order to identify the protective effect of MT for superoxide radicals and relationship between GSH and MT concentrations in gastric mucosal cells, newborn rat gastric mucosal cells were cultured *in vitro*. This culture system provided valuable results for studies of cellular functions of MT in gastric mucosal cells.

In cultured gastric mucosal cells, MT was induced by 100 μM but not by 50 μM of Zn. Since the sensitivity of the RIA is several tens of ng/ml, MT induced by 50 μM Zn can not be detected. Our data showed that the oxygen metabolites induced by xanthine-xanthine oxidase caused damage to the cells. The damage was enhanced by specific depletion of GSH with MSO, γ-glutamylcysteine synthetase inhibitor. However, this damage was suppressed with Zn treatment. This result indicated that intracellular MT induced by Zn may play a role in the protection of the gastric mucosal cells instead of depleted GSH from the oxygen metabolites.

Our results indicate that intramucosal MT induced by Zn and administered MT protect the gastric mucosal cells from stress. The results support the hypothesis that mechanism of anti-AGML action of MT is scavenging of superoxide radicals.

ACKNOWLEDGMENTS

The author would like to thank Professor K. Tanaka, Kobe-Gakuin University, for technical guidance.

REFERENCES

Boyd SC, Sasame HA, and Boyd MR (1979): High concentrations of glutathione in glandular stomach. *Science Wash. D.C.* 205: 1010.

Boyd SC, Sasame HA, and Boyd MR (1981): Gastric glutathione depletion and acute ulcerogenesis by diethylmaleate given subcutaneously to rats. *Life Sci.* 28: 2987.

Chance B, Sies H, and Bovevis A (1979): Hydroperoxide metabolism in mammalian organs. *Physiol. Rev.* 59: 527.

Cho CH (1989): Current views of zinc as a gastrohepatic protective agent. *Drug Dev. Res.* 17: 185.

Ellman GL (1959): Tissue sulfhydryl groups. *Arch. Biochem. Biophys.* 82: 70.

Hiraishi H, Terano A, Ota S, Ivey KJ, and Sugimoto T (1987): Oxygen metabolite-induced cytotoxicity to cultured rat gastric mucosal cells. *Am. J. Physiol.* 253: G40.

Hoppenkamps R, Thies E, Younes M, and Siegers CP (1984): Glutathione and GSH-dependent enzymes in the human gastric mucosa. *Klin. Wochenschr.* 62: 183.

Ikei N, Kodaira T, Shimizu F, Nakajima K, Tohyama C, Saito H, Kimura M, and Otaki N (1989): New radioimmunoassay of metallothionein. *Rinsho Kensa* 33: 215.

Itoh M and Guth PH (1985): Role of oxygen-derived free radicals in hemorrhagic shock-induced gastric lesions in the rat. *Gastroenterology* 88: 1162.

Kägi JH and Vallee BL (1960): Metallothionein: a cadmium and zinc-containing protein from equine renal cortex. *J. Biol. Chem.* 235: 3460.

Kaplowitz NT, Aw TY, and Ookhtens M (1985): The regulation of hepatic glutathione. *Annu. Rev. Pharmacol. Toxicol.* 25: 715.

Katz D and Siegel HI Eds., (1968): *Progress in Gastroenterology, Vol 1*, Grune and Stratton, New York, pp. 67–96.

Kosower NS and Kosower EM (1978): The glutathione status of cells. *Int. Rev. Cytol.* 54: 109.

Lowry OH, Rosebrogh NJ, Farr AL, and Randall RJ (1951): Protein measurement with the folin phenol reagent. *J. Biol. Chem.* 193: 265.

Mimura T, Tsujikawa K, Yasuda N, Nakajima H, Haruyama M, Ohmura T, and Okabe M (1988): Suppression of gastric ulcer induced by stress and HCl-ethanol by intravenously administered metallothionein-II. *Biochem. Biophys. Res. Commun.* 151: 725.

Mizui T and Doteuchi M (1983): Effect of polyamines on acidified ethanol-induced gastric lesions in rats. *Jpn. J. Pharmacol.* 33: 939.

Olson CE (1988): Glutathione modulates toxic oxygen metabolite injury of canine chief cell monolayers in primary culture. *Am. J. Physiol.* 254: G49.

Owen WG and Meister A (1978): Differential inhibition of glutamine and γ-glutamylcysteine synthetases by α-alkyl analogs of methionine sulfoximine that induce convulsions. *J. Biol. Chem.* 253: 2333.

Perry MA, Wadhwa S, Parks A, Pickard W, and Granger DN (1986): Role of oxygen radicals in ischemia-induced lesions in the cat stomach. *Gastroenterology* 90: 362.

Shay H and Sun DCH (1963): *Gastroenterology, Vol. 1*, W.B. Saunders, Philadelphia, pp. 420–465.

Sone S (1987): *Zoku Seikagaku Jikkenkouza 8 Ketsueki*, Tokyokagakudoujin, Tokyo, pp. 781–786.

Takagi K and Okabe S (1968): The effect of drugs on the production and recovery processes of the stress ulcer. *Jpn. J. Pharmacol.* 18: 9.

Terano A, Ivey KJ, Stachura J, Sekhon S, Hosojima H, McKenzie WN, Krause WJ, and Wyche JH (1982): Cell culture of gastric fundic mucosa. *Gastroenterology* 83: 1280.

Thornalley PJ and Vašák BL (1985): Possible role for metallothionein in protection against radiation induced oxidative stress. Kinetics and mechanism of its reaction with superoxide and hydroxyl radicals. *Biochim. Biophys. Acta* 827: 36.

The Possible Role of Metallothionein in Atherogenesis

Katsuyuki Nakajima and Masakazu Adachi
Japan Immunoresearch Lab. Co., Ltd.
Takasaki, Gunma, Japan

Noriko Otaki and Masami Kimura
National Institute of Industrial Health
Kawasaki, Japan

Takeshi Tani and Takehiro Igawa
Otsuka Pharmaceutical Co., Ltd.
Tokushima, Japan

Umeko Kawaharada and Keiji Suzuki
College of Medical Care and Technology
Gunma University
Maehashi, Gunma, Japan

INTRODUCTION

The low incidence of arteriosclerosis among patients with Itai-Itai disease was first reported by Takebayashi et al. (1988) in there pathological studies of 11 subjects, registered as Cd-polluted inhabitants of Tsushima, Nagasaki in Japan. The pathogenesis of this low incidence was as yet unknown, but was discussed in relation to the high amount of heavy metal intake (Takebayashi, 1979). Since detecting the presence of metallothionein

(MT) at atheromatous lesions in the arterial intima of Japanese quail, rabbit, and man by immunohistochemical studies (Nakajima et al., 1986). We have studied the relationship between atherogenesis and the role of MT in Japanese quails (Yamamoto et al., 1989), especially MT in macrophage of atheromatous lesion. We have also found an inhibitory effect of MT for superoxide generation (Okomoto et al., 1989) and chemotaxis, using human leukocytes *in vitro* (Hunada et al., 1989). This study indicates the role of MT in leukocytes, especially at the initial stage of macrophage invasion related with superoxide generation into the arterial wall, and its subsequent preventive effect on the occurrence of atherosclerosis (Gerrity, 1981; Faggiotto et al., 1981).

MATERIALS AND METHODS

Experimental Animals

Japanese quails (15 to 20 weeks, ♂) checked by cholesterol feeding test before this study were used. The animals were divided into four groups of 8 quails each.

Group 1 was fed a normal diet. Group 2 was fed a normal diet containing Zn SO_4 (5 mg/kg/). Group 3 was fed a high cholesterol diet (0.5% cholesterol added to normal diet). Group 4 was fed a high cholesterol diet containing $ZnSO_4$ (5 mg/kg/d). The Japanese quails were kept for 8 weeks on these diets then sacrificed for the present studies.

Radioimmunoassay and Immunohistochemical Studies

Tissue and plasma MT concentrations were determined by RIA developed by N. Ikei et al. (1989). Tissues were homogenized with 10 vols. of 0.05 *M* Tris-HCl buffer (pH 8.5) and centrifuged at $18,000 \times g$ for 30 min. at 4°C. The supernatant with suitable dilution was used for MT-RIA assay. MT immunohistochemical procedure was described previously elsewhere (Umeyama et al., 1987).

Determination of Superoxide Generation and Chemotactic Activity

Granulocytes were prepared from peripheral blood taken from healthy adult volunteers. Freshly isolated granulocytes were suspended at 8×10^5 cells per ml in HBSS.

To determine the chemotactic kinetics of granulocytes, modified technique of the Boyden chamber (Boyden, 1962) system was performed, in which the number of chemotactic granulocytes on the bottom cover glass in the lower chamber were counted by using an inverted research microscope. To 8×10^5 cells of granulocytes taken from five of the volunteers, were added various amounts of MT (1.2, 6.0 μM). After preincubation with MT, they were poured into the upper chamber. FMLP with final concentration of 10^{-7} M in HBSS was used as a chemoattractant.

To estimate the ability of granulocytes to generate superoxide anion, a chemiluminescence probe with the *Cypridina* luciferin analog (CLA) (Nakano et al., 1986) was used. The light emission of CLA derived from the granulocytes mixed with MT was measured by a chemiluminescence analyzer on 5 volunteers. On the analyses, PMA and opsonized zymosan with optimal concentration were used as a stimulator.

Analysis of Lipid Contents

Plasma lipoprotein analysis was performed by the ultracentrifugation method (Havel, 1955). Cholesterol determination in the aorta was assayed by the enzymatic method (Kyowa Medix). DNA determination in the aorta was performed according to the method of Burton (Burton, 1968).

EXPERIMENTAL RESULTS

The Localization of MT in Atheromatous Lesions

MT was stained strongly in foam cells and smooth muscle cells of the atheromatous lesion of human and Japanese quails (Figures 1, 2, and 3). MT in human atheromatous aorta was found to be 12.4 μg/g wet weight (average of 11 different subjects) by RIA.

Effects of ZnSO$_4$ on the Formation of Atherosclerosis

Pathological studies indicated that Japanese quails kept for 8 weeks on a high cholesterol diet (HCD) showed severe atherosclerosis (Figure 4). Addition of ZnSO$_4$ to HCD showed markedly lower levels of atherosclerosis (Figure 5). The accumulation of total cholesterol and the cholesterol ester/DNA ratio at the aorta showed almost normal levels for the HCD + ZnSO$_4$ group when compared with the HCD group (Figures 6, 7). But the plasma T-Chol and VLDL levels of the groups fed with HCD and HCD + ZnSO$_4$ were both very high (Figures 8, 9). Immunohistochemical observation of MT at atheromatous lesions of the quails showed to be increased. MT levels of blood vessels of quails was shown highest at HCD + ZnSO$_4$ group, among the four groups.

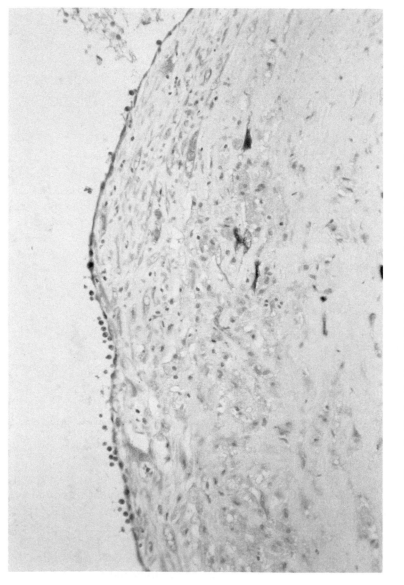

Figure 1. The localization of MT in the human arterial wall. Foam cells and smooth muscle cells are stained positively for MT (PAP method).

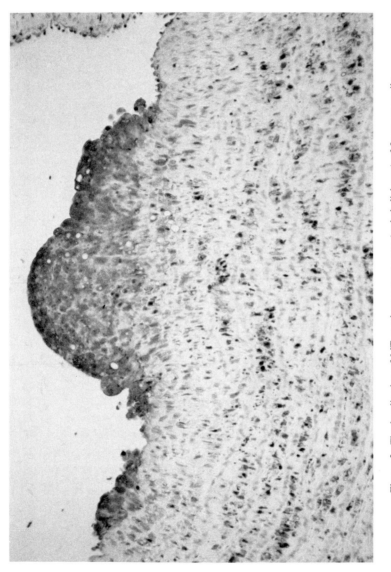

Figure 2. The localization of MT at atheromatous aorta (endothelial area) of Japanese quails. Intimal foam cells and medial smooth muscle cell positively stained for MT. In the thickened intima, foam cells in particular are strongly positive (PAP method).

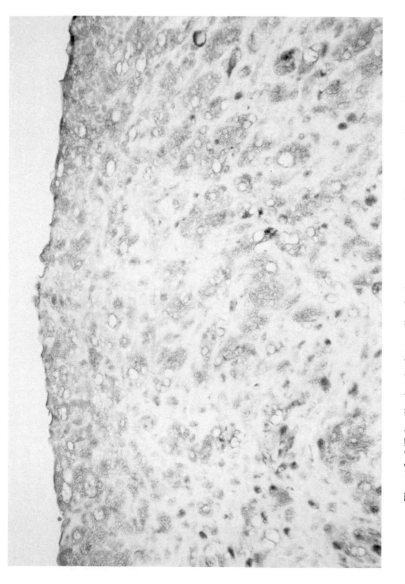

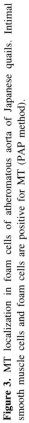

Figure 3. MT localization in foam cells of atheromatous aorta of Japanese quails. Intimal smooth muscle cells and foam cells are positive for MT (PAP method).

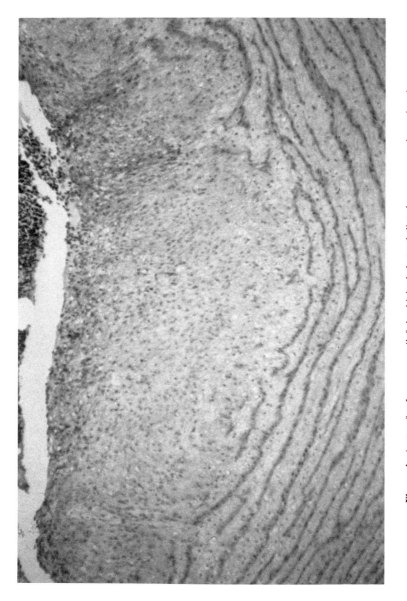

Figure 4. Aorta of a Japanese quail fed a high cholesterol diet shows severe atherosclerosis (H&E stain).

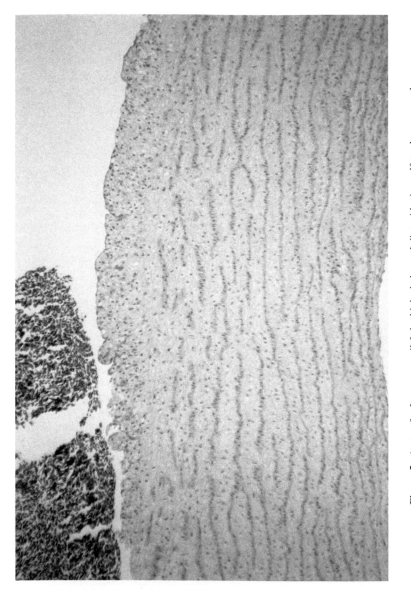

Figure 5. Aorta of a Japanese quail fed a high cholesterol diet with zinc sulfate shows normal findings (H&E stain).

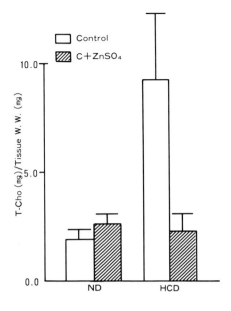

Figure 6. Effect of zinc sulfate on T-Cho (mg)/tissue w.w. (mg) ratio at arterial wall of Japanese quails when fed with normal (ND) and high cholesterol diet (HCD).

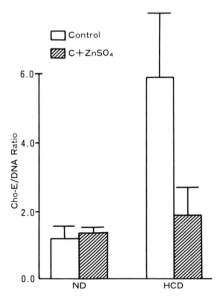

Figure 7. Effect of zinc sulfate on Cho-E/DNA ratio at arterial wall of Japanese quails when fed with normal (ND) and high cholesterol diet (HCD).

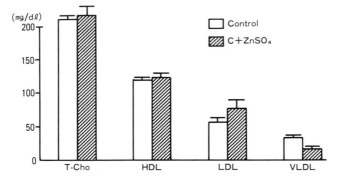

Figure 8. Effect of zinc sulfate on plasma T-Cho, HDL, LDL, and VLDL levels of Japanese quails when fed with normal diet.

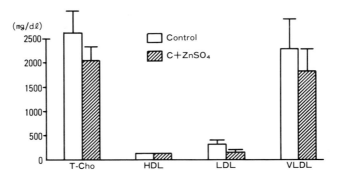

Figure 9. Effect of zinc sulfate on plasma T-Cho, HDL, LDL, and VLDL levels of Japanese quails when fed with high cholesterol diet.

Effect of MT on Superoxide Generation and Chemotactic Activity *In Vitro*

The chemotactic activity was significantly depressed in the samples containing MT with dose-dependent tendency (Table I). The activated oxygen derived from granulocytes incubated with MT was reduced with increase of MT dose (Table II). Heated MT could incompletely depress the superoxide generation.

DISCUSSION

The prevention of arteriosclerosis is presently one of mankind's most important challenges. Although the human body is well prepared for hunger,

TABLE I.
Influence of MT on Chemotaxis of Human Granulocytes
(Modified Boyden Chamber System)

	Time (min)		
	30	60	120
Added MT (μM)			
0	26.2 ± 12.3	108.6 ± 54.9	239.6 ± 124.5
1.2	20.1 ± 12.3	58.7 ± 22.0	146.1 ± 100.4
6.0	11.9 ± 5.4	50.8 ± 22.7	100.5 ± 48.6
12.0	12.0 ± 4.6	40.5 ± 20.5	75.4 ± 50.6
Heated MT (6.0 μM)	20.4 ± 8.5	59.4 ± 21.4	160.5 ± 20.5

Number of chemotactic granulocytes (mean $\pm$ S.D. per fields), MT: Metallothionein.

TABLE II.
Influence of MT on Superoxide Generation of
Human Granulocytes ($\times 10^4$ cpm)

	Added-MT (μM)		
	0	1.2	6.0
PMA-stimulated cases (n = 7)	33.9 ± 7.6	34.5 ± 12.8	22.4 ± 5.1
OZ-stimulated cases (n = 7)	25.8 ± 7.1	23.5 ± 6.8	14.8 ± 4.2

MT: Metallothionein; PMA: phorbol myristate acetate; OZ: opsonized zymosan.

it does not cope nearly as well with excess food intake, and lacks the ability for resistance against related diseases. Arteriosclerosis is a typical example of the diseases that depend on excess fat intake (Connor, 1979). Recently, several antihyperlipidemic drugs have been developed for the prevention of atherosclerosis (Barnhardt et al., 1970; Lipid Research Clinical Program, 1984).

In our study, zinc (Henzel et al., 1969; Henzel et al., 1971; Henzel et al., 1974; Pories, 1974) was markedly able to prevent the formation of atherosclerosis in quails, although plasma cholesterol and other lipid levels remained high. The addition of zinc to the high cholesterol diet of Japanese quails revealed the apparent inhibition of atherosclerosis, i.e., proliferation of smooth muscle cells and foam-cell formation in the intima, and inhibition of cholesterol deposit on the arterial wall.

Hyperlipidemia, especially high cholesterolemia, is said to be the major cause of atherosclerosis formation (Havel, 1982). Macrophages invade into the arterial wall following some initial arterial wall injury. With the presence of denatured lipoproteins (Brown and Goldstein, 1983; Steinbrecher et al., 1984) in arterial intima, this leads to atherosclerosis. This is the most commonly accepted hypothesis of the initial step of macrophage invasion and foam cell formation.

Therefore, if macrophage invasion and foam cell formation at the arterial wall can be prevented, then the progression of atherosclerosis might be controllable. Our experimental results lead us to believe that, through a still unknown mechanism, zinc may be able to prevent this macrophage invasion. Zinc did not lower the cholesterol level in plasma, however atherosclerosis of the $HCD + ZnSO_4$ group showed less severity when compared with HCD groups.

A possible explanation of this phenomenon might be that MT depressed the superoxide generation (Heinecke et al., 1986) and prevented arterial wall injuries, especially in endothelial and smooth muscle cells and also macrophage invasion into arterial wall (Heinecke et al., 1987).

As MT in leukocytes is known to be induced by Zn and Cd both *in vivo* (Shaikh and Lucis, 1972) and *in vitro* (Sone et al., 1988), it seems reasonable to assume that zinc, absorbed from the intestine into the blood, resulted in elevated MT levels in leukocytes. Induced MT might inhibit both the generation of superoxide and chemotaxis in leukocytes. As the initial stage of atherosclerosis is related to lesions of the arterial wall, leukocytes (macrophage and granulocyte), may attach to the injured region and initiate the atherosclerotic progression with superoxide generation and chemotactic function by activated macrophages. Induced MT might neutralize the condition of activated macrophage. Since MT intravenously infused to rats decreased the reperfusion damage occurring in rat hearts (Hanada et al., 1989), we can speculate that MT might neutralize free radicals (Sato et al., 1988) generated from leukocytes. If MT in leukocytes either moderates or controls this initial process with its radical scavenge function (Thornalley and Vašák, 1982; Miura et al., 1989), then the formation of atherosclerosis may be preventable in spite of having hyperlipidemia.

With Probucol® (Barnhardt et al., 1970) a known anti-atherogenic drug said to have an anti-oxidative function (Ku et al., 1989), we can estimate that the adequate amount of zinc which as a supplement, would be able to prevent atherosclerosis through the anti-oxidative effect (radical scavenger) of MT.

SUMMARY

Using experimental animals (Japanese quails), we were able to prevent severe atherosclerosis by feeding them about 10 times the normal daily intake of zinc.

At the atheromatous lesion, we found increased amounts of MT in the invased macrophage and foam cells.

The prevention of atherosclerosis seemed to be related to the anti-oxidative effect of MT in macrophage which reduced superoxide generation and attachment of macrophage to arterial wall to inhibit cholesterol deposit and proliferation of smooth muscle cells.

REFERENCES

Barnhart W, Sefranka A, and McIntosh DD, (1970): Hypocholesterol effect of 4,4'-(isopropylidenedithio)-bis-(2,6-di-*t*-butylphenol) (Probucol®). *Am. J. Clin. Nutrit.* 23: 1229.

Boyden S (1962): The chemotactic effect of mixture of antibody and antigen on polymorphonuclear leukocytes. *J. Exp. Med.* 115: 453.

Brown MS and Goldstein JL (1983): Lipoprotein metabolism in the macrophage; implications for cholesterol deposition in atherosclerosis. *Annu. Rev. Biochem.* 52: 223.

Burton K, Ed., (1968): Determination of DNA concentration with diphenylamine. *Methods in Enzymology. Vol. 12, Part B,* Academic Press, New York, pp. 163–166.

Connor WE (1979): The relationship of hyperlipoproteinemia to atherosclerosis: the decisive role of dietary cholesterol and fat. *The Chemical of Atherosclerosis.* Scanu AM, Wissler RW, and Getz GS, Eds., Marcel Dekker, New York, 1979, p. 391.

Faggiotto A, Ross R, and Harker L (1984): Studies of hypercholesterolemia in nonhuman primate I & II. *Arteriosclerosis* 4: 323.

Gerrity R (1981): Transition of blood-borne monocytes into foam cells in fatty lesions. *Am. J. Pathol.* 103: 181.

Hanada K, Ishikawa H, Imaizumi T, Hashimoto H, and Kimura H (1989): Effects of metallothionein on granulocyte chemotaxis and superoxide generation. *Dermatologica* 179(Suppl. 1): 143.

Havel RJ (1955): The distribution and chemical composition of ultracentrifugally separated lipoproteins in human serum. *J. Clin. Invest.* 34: 1345.

Havel RJ and Kane JP (1982): Therapy of hyperlipidemic state. *Annu. Rev. Med.* 33: 417.

Heinecke JW, Baker L, Rosen H, and Chait A (1986): Superoxide-mediated modification of low density lipoprotein by arterial smooth muscle cells. *J. Clin. Invest.* 77: 757.

Heinecke JW, Rosen H, Suzuki LA, and Chait A (1987): The role of sulfur-containing amino acids in superoxide production and modification of low density lipoprotein by arterial smooth muscle cells. *J. Biol. Chem.* 262: 10098.

Henzel JH, Holtman B, Keitzer FW, DeWeese MS, and Licht E (1969): Trace elements in atherosclerosis, efficacy of zinc medication as a therapeutic modality. In, *Trace Substance in Environmental Health-II.* Hemphill DD, Ed., *Proceedings of University of Missouri 2nd Annual Conference.* 1968. Columbia; Univeristy of Missouri, pp. 83–99.

Henzel JH, Keitrer FW, Lichti EL, and DeWeese MS (1971): Efficacy of zinc medication as a therapeutic modality in atherosclerosis; Follow up observations on patients medicated over prolonged periods. *Trace Substance in Environmental Health-IV.* In, Hemphill DD, Ed., *Proceedings of University of Missouri 4th Annual Conference.* 1970. Columbia; University of Missouri, pp. 336–341.

Henzel JH, Lichti EL, Shepard W, and Paone J (1974): Long-term oral zinc sulfate in the treatment of atherosclerotic peripheral vascular disease; efficacy of possible mechanisms of action. In, *Clinical Applications of Zinc Metabolism.* Pories WJ, Strain WH, Hsu JM, and Woosley RL, Eds., Charles C. Thomas, Springfield, Ill, pp. 243–259.

Ikei N, Kodaira T, Shimizu F, Nakajima K, Toyama T, Saito H, Kimura N, and Otaki N (1989): New radioimmunoassay of metallothionein (in Japanese). *Med. Technol.* 33: 215.

Ku G, Doherty NS, Wolos JA, and Jackson RJ (1988): Inhibition of Probucol® of interleukin 1 secretion and its implication in atherosclerosis. *Am. J. Cardiol.* 62: 776.

Lipid Research Clinical Program (1984): The Lipid Research Clinics coronary primary prevention trial. Results II. The relationship of reduction in incidence of coronary heart disease to cholesterol lowering. *JAMA.* 251: 365.

Miura T, Tsujikawa K, Yasuda N, Nakajima H, Haruyama M, Ohmura T, and Okada M (1989): Suppression of gastric ulcer induced by stress and HCl-ethanol by intravenously administered metallothionein-II. (Biochim. Biophys. Res. Commun. 151: 725.

Nakajima K, Adachi M, Igawa T, and Yamamoto K (1989): The localization of metallothionein in atheromatous aorta. *J. Jpn. Atheroscler. Soc.* 17: 254.

Nakano M, Sugioka K, Ushijima Y, and Goto T (1986): Chemiluminescence probe with cypridina luciferin analog, 2-methyl-6-phenyl-3,7 dihydroimidazol[1,2-a] pyrazin-3-one, for estimating the ability of human granulocytes to generate O_2^-. *Anal. Biochem.* 159: 363.

Okamoto S, Sakurai H, Ohshima S, Suzuki T, Murata K, and Nakajima K (1989): The preventive effects of Zn to the reperfusion damage of rat hearts. *J. Jpn. College Angiol.* p. 29.

Pories WJ and Strain WH (1974): Zinc sulfate therapy in surgical patients. In, *Clinical Applications of Zinc Metabolism.* Pories WJ, Strain WH, Hsu JM, and Woosley RL Eds., Charles C. Thomas, Springfield, Ill, pp. 139–157.

Sato M, Nagahama A, and Imura W (1988): Involvement of cardiac metallothionein in prevention of adriamycin-induced lipid peroxidation in the heart. *Toxicology* 53: 231.

Shaikh ZA and Lucis OJ (1972): Biological differences in cadmium and zinc turnover. *Arch. Environ. Health* 24: 410.

Sone T, Koizumi S, and Kimura M (1988): Cadmium-induced synthesis of metallothionein in human lymphocytes and monocytes. *Chem.-Biol. Interact.* 66: 61.

Steinbrecher UP, Parthasarathy S, Leake DS, Witztum JL, and Steinberg D (1984): Modification of low density lipoproteins by endothelial cells involves lipid peroxidaton and degradation of low density lipoprotein phospholipids. *Proc. Natl. Acad. Sci. U.S.A.* 81: 3883.

Takebayashi S (1979): First autopsy case, suspicion of cadmium intoxication, from the cadmium-polluted area in Tushima, Nagasaki Prefecture. I: Cadmium induced osteopathy. *Jpn. Public Health Assoc. Tokyo,* p. 124.

Takebayashi S, Harada T, Yoshimura S (1988): Clinical and pathological studies of the inhibitant who has been registrated as a cadmium-polluted subject in Tushima, Nagasaki Pref. (11th autopsy case) (in Japanese). *Environ. Health. Report.* 54: 207.

Thornalley PJ and Vašák M (1982): Possible role for metallothionein in protection against radiation-induced oxidative stress. Kinetics and mechanism of its reaction with superoxide and hydroxyl radicals. *Biochim. Biophys. Acta* 715: 116.

Umeyama Y, Saruki K, Imai K, Yamanaka K, Suzuki K, Ikei N, Kodaira T, Nakajima K, Saito H, and Kimura M (1987): Immunohistochemical demonstration of metallothionein in the rat prostate. *The Prostate* 10: 257.

Yamamoto K, Igawa T, and Tani T (1989): Ultrastructural and immunohistochemical study of experimental atherosclerosis in Japanese quail. *J. Electron Microsc.* 28: 310.

Chapter 30

Possible Application of Metallothionein in Cancer Therapy

Nobumasa Imura, Masahiko Satoh, and
Akira Naganuma
School of Pharmaceutical Sciences
Kitasato University
Tokyo, Japan

INTRODUCTION

Recent progress in studies on the physiological functions of metallothionein (MT) postulated its potencies to scavenge free radicals and to covalently bind to alkylating agents besides its well known high affinity to essential and toxic heavy metals. On the other hand, there are many anticancer drugs acting as free radical inducers or as alkylating agents as listed in Table I in addition to antimetabolites, mitotic inhibitors and heavy metal complexes like cisplatinum which may be categorized to an alkylating agent. These facts incited us to examine the effects of MT on the toxicity of various anticancer drugs of different action mechanisms.

TABLE I. Anticancer Drugs

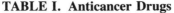

Heavy metal complex
    Cisplatin (*cis*-DDP)
Free-radical-forming antibiotics
    Adriamycin, Bleomycin
    Peplomycin (Mitomycin C)
Alkylating agents
    Cyclophosphamide
Antimetabolites
    5-Fluorouracil
Plant alkaloids
    Vinblastine

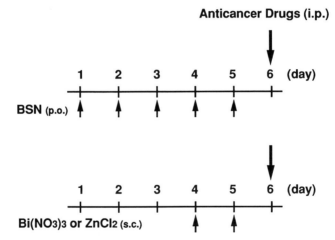

Figure 1. Administration schedule of MT-inducers and anticancer drugs.

EFFECTS OF PREADMINISTRATION OF MT INDUCERS ON TOXICITIES AND ANTITUMOR ACTIVITY OF VARIOUS ANTICANCER AGENTS

Bismuth (Bi) and Zinc (Zn) were selected as MT inducers according to the results of our preliminary experiments on their tissue specificity in MT induction. Bismuth subnitrate (BSN) was orally administered to the mice once a day for 5 days and bismuth nitrate (BN) or zinc chloride ($ZnCl_2$) was injected subcutaneously once a day for 2 days. Anticancer drugs were administered 24 h after the last administration of the MT inducers as indicated in Figure 1. According to our expectation, MT induction by Bi or

Zn compound significantly prevented the lethal effect of some anticancer drugs. Moreover, even the lethal toxicity of 5-fluorouracil (5-FU), an antimetabolite, was efficiently depressed besides those of the free radical inducers and the alkylating agents (Table II).

Further the effects of preadministration of Bi (BN was used in this series of experiments) or Zn, on the tissue specific toxicities and antitumor activity of the anticancer drugs were investigated. Meth-A fibrosarcoma cells were inoculated subcutaneously in the mice on day 0 and an MT inducer was given to the mice on day 4 and day 5, then an anticancer drug was administered on day 6. ^{203}Hg-binding assay for MT (Naganuma et al., 1987) revealed that Zn induced MT not only in the normal tissues, i.e. the bone marrow, kidneys and liver, but also in the tumor tissues in these tumor-bearing mice 24 h after the last injection. Bi induced MT in the bone marrow, kidneys and in a small amount in the liver, but not in the tumor tissues. When the MT inducers were given to the tumor bearing mice prior to cisplatinum administration, either Zn or Bi could efficiently depress the renal toxicity indicated by BUN values, and bone marrow toxicity indicated by the number of total leukocytes. Bi, which did not induce MT in the tumors, showed no effect on the antitumor activity indicated by the reduction of tumor weight. However, Zn, which induced MT in the tumor tissues, diminished the antitumor activity of this platinum complex.

Also in the case of adriamycin (ADR), both Zn and Bi could reduce its bone marrow toxicity and cardiotoxicity, the dose limiting toxicity of

TABLE II.
Effect of Pretreatment with Bismuth Subnitrate
(BSN) or ZnCl$_2$ on Lethal Toxicity of
Anticancer Drugs in Mice

Compound	Dose	Survival rate (%)[a]		
		None	BSN	ZnCl$_2$
Control	—	100	100	100
cis-DDP	35 μmol/kg	0	100	63
Adriamycin	35 μmol/kg	0	63	57
Bleomycin	800 mg/kg	14	86	100
Peplomycin	65 μmol/kg	0	43	71
Mitomycin C	60 μmol/kg	0	14	29
Cyclophosphamide	2.5 mmol/kg	0	0	86
5-Fluorouracil	4 mmol/kg	0	86	43
Vinblastine	20 μmol/kg	0	0	29

Mice were pretreated with BSN (50 mg/kg; p.o.) once a day for 5 d or ZnCl$_2$ (400 μmol/kg; s.c.) once a day for 2 d. Anticancer drugs were injected i.p. 24 h after the last administration of BSN or ZnCl$_2$.
[a]Determined 20 d after the injection of anticancer drugs.

ADR. As in the case of cisplatinum, Zn inhibited the antitumor activity of ADR, while Bi did not affect its tumor reducing activity.

Subsequent experiments with the other anticancer agents demonstrated that Zn or Bi-preadministration significantly improved the lesions in the bone marrow indicated by the decrease in the number of total leukocytes caused by bleomycin (BLM), cyclophosphamide (CPA), or 5-FU. As for the antitumor activity of these three drugs, Bi did not show any effect on their antitumor activity, but Zn diminished the antitumor activity of BLM and CPA. However, the antitumor activity of 5-FU was not affected even by Zn, regardless of its ability to induce MT in the tumor tissues. Further study is necessary to elucidate the reason why MT could depress the toxicity of 5-FU, but not its antitumor activity.

MT induction by Bi compound in the other transplantable mouse tumors than Meth-A fibrosarcoma was also examined. Bi failed to induce MT in Ehrlich tumor cells, colon adenocarcinoma 26 and 38 cells, while MT was markedly induced by Bi in the kidney of the tumor bearing mice used. In a separate experiment using colon 38 inoculated mice, we found that Bi could hardly be incorporated into the tumor tissues (Satoh et al., 1990). This may explain the inability of Bi to induce MT in the tumors.

We further examined the MT inducing ability of Bi in the human tumors. Human colon tumor and stomach tumor were inoculated subcutaneously in the nude mice, and a week later Bi was orally administered according to the protocol shown in Figure 1. MT determination at 24 h after the last administration of Bi indicated that Bi did not induce MT in human tumors, while the renal MT level was increased in the nude mice by the Bi-preadministration. These facts demonstrate that Bi is a promising MT inducer for reducing the adverse side effects of anticancer drugs without compromising their antitumor activity, in clinical cancer chemotherapy.

Actually, several groups of physicians and surgeons are interested in our method and some clinical trials using a protocol similar to ours have been carried out. A group of physicians and pharmacists in Nagoya National Hospital recently reported a clinical case in which our protocol was applied to treatment of patients having lung cancer with cisplatinum combined with 5-FU and vindesine (Takahashi et al., 1989). They examined the effect of BSN preadministration on the renal function of the patients indicated by levels of β-2-microglobulin and *N*-acetyl-β-D-glucosaminidase (NAG) excreted into the urine collected during 15 d after injection of anticancer drugs. They reported that the values of both β-2-microglobulin and NAG obtained from the patients pretreated with BSN were significantly lower than those without BSN pretreatment. They concluded that BSN preadministration was effective for reduction of renal toxicity of cisplatinum actually used in the clinical treatment.

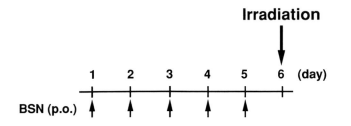

Figure 2. Experimental schedule for protection against irradiation damage by bismuth subnitrate (BSN).

TABLE III.
Effect of Pretreatment with BSN on
Lethal Effect of γ-ray (^{60}Co)
Irradiation in Mice

Pretreatment with BSN (mg/kg/d)	^{60}Co Irradiation (Gy per mouse)	Survival[a] Rate (%)
0	0	100
0	9	0
25	9	0
50	9	43
100	9	57
150	9	86
200	9	100

Mice were pretreated p.o. with BSN once a day for 5 d and irradiated with γ-ray (^{60}Co) 24 h after the last administration of BSN.
[a]Determined 30 d after γ-ray irradiation.

PROTECTIVE EFFECTS OF MT INDUCTION ON THE LESIONS CAUSED BY IRRADIATION

Considering the fact that MT may act as a free radical scavenger, we can expect its protective effect against the lesions caused by irradiation, because the damage by irradiation is known to be caused through intracellular radical formation. A few papers so far published suggested a possible protective ability of MT against irradiation (Bakka et al., 1982; Matsubara et al., 1988; Renan and Dowman, 1989).

We, then, examined the effect of Bi pretreatment on the lesions caused by gamma-irradiation using mice with the schedule of treatment shown in Figure 2 (Satoh et al., 1989). The mice were irradiated with ^{60}Co 24 h after the last administration of Bi. The survival rate of mice determined at 30 d after the irradiation (6 or 9 Gy per mouse of gamma-rays) was markedly improved by the preadministration of Bi dose-dependently (Table III).

As shown in Figure 3, the preadministration of relatively high dose of Bi significantly improved the decrease in the number of total leukocytes as an indicator of bone marrow lesions caused by gamma-irradiation. At the same time, the extent of lipid peroxidation induced in the bone marrow cells by irradiation was markedly reduced by the pretreatment with Bi. In a separate experiment, a significant increase in metallothionein level at the time point of the gamma-irradiation was observed in the bone marrow of the mice pretreated with Bi. Thus, Bi preadministration induced MT in mouse bone marrow. This induced MT might scavenge the free radicals formed by irradiation, resulting in the protection of bone marrow cells from peroxidation. It is noteworthy that, in the radiotherapy using solid tumor bearing mice, the Bi treatment did not affect the tumor reducing effect of the irradiation at all.

ANTICANCER DRUG ITSELF INDUCES MT IN TUMORS

Quite recently we examined the potency of anticancer drugs to induce MT in mouse tissues especially in the tumors. Mice were inoculated with colon adenocarcinoma 38 or Meth-A fibrosarcoma cells. A week after the inoculation various anticancer drugs were injected into the tumor bearing mice. Surprisingly, most of these drugs significantly increased the MT level in the tumor tissues.

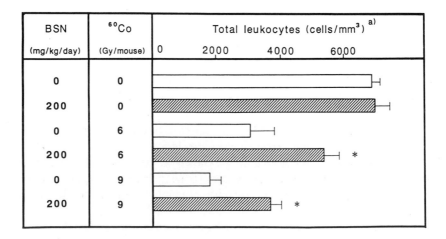

Figure 3. Effect of pretreatment with bismuth subnitrate (BSN) on number of total leukocytes in mice irradiated by gamma-ray (^{60}Co). [a]Determined 10 d after irradiation. *Significantly different from BSN-untreated mice ($p < 0.001$).

CONCLUSIONS

1. MT inducers can be used as useful tools in cancer chemotherapy and radiotherapy to protect patients from adverse side effects of drugs and gamma-ray. Bi, in particular, is a promising inducer of MT for cancer therapy, because it induces MT in the target tissues of the toxicity of anticancer drugs and irradiation without increasing MT level in tumor tissues so far examined.
2. Considering the experimental results described above together with the recent findings by ourselves (Imura et al., 1989) and by Kelley's group (Kelley et al., 1988) that cultured cells containing unusually high level of MT are resistant against various anticancer drugs, MT, once induced in the tumor tissues, may act as a multidrug resistance factor in cancer chemotherapy.
3. Therefore, the experimental result that anticancer drug itself does induce MT in the tumors may have to be taken into consideration in making protocol for cancer chemotherapy.
4. If we can reduce MT level in tumors during cancer therapy, the antitumor effects of the drugs and irradiation would be amplified.
5. If we can keep a substantial level of MT specifically in normal tissues during cancer therapy, the patients may be protected from carcinogenesis caused by secondary effects of anticancer agents or irradiation. The experiment to examine this possibility is now going on in our laboratory.

REFERENCES

Bakka A, Johnsen AS, Endresen L, and Rugstad HE (1982): Radioresistance in cells with high content of metallothionein. *Experientia* 38: 381–383.

Imura N, Naganuma A, and Satoh M (1989): Metallothionein as a resistance factor for antitumor drugs. *Jpn J. Cancer Chemother.* 16: 599–604.

Kelley S, Basu A, Teicher BA, Hacker MP, Hamer DH, and Lazo JS (1988): Overexpression of metallothionein confers resistance to antitumor drugs. *Science* 241: 1813–1816.

Matsubara J, Tajima Y, Ikeda A, Kinoshita T, and Shimoyama T (1988): A new perspective of radiation protection by metallothionein induction. *Pharmac. Ther.* 39: 331–333.

Naganuma A, Satoh M, and Imura N (1987): Prevention of lethal and renal toxicity of *cis*-diamminedichloroplatinum(II) by induction of metallothionein synthesis without compromising its antitumor activity in mice. *Cancer Res.* 47: 983–987.

Renan MJ and Dowman PI (1989): Increased radioresistance of tumor cells exposed to metallothionein-inducing agents. *Radiat. Res.* 120: 442–455.

Satoh M, Miura N, Naganuma A, Matsuzaki N, Kawamura E, and Imura N (1989): Prevention of adverse effects of γ-ray irradiation after metallothionein induction by bismuth subnitrate in mice. *Eur. J. Cancer Clin. Oncol.* 25: 1727–1731.

Satoh M, Naganuma A, and Imura N (1990): Protection against adriamycin toxicity by inducing metallothionein in appropriate tissues. *Toxicologist* 10: 81.

Takahashi A, Takagi M, Hisida H, Sakamoto Y, Takagi N, Amano H, and Ogura Y (1989): The pharmacokinetics of cisplatin and its influence on renal function according to different infusion methods (report II). Alleviation of renal impairment by bismuth subnitrate combined with Ginseng and Tang-Keui Ten. *Jpn. J. Cancer Chemother.* 16: 2405–2410.

Chapter 31

Chronic Cadmium Exposure and Metallothionein

Zahir A. Shaikh
Department of Pharmacology and Toxicology
University of Rhode Island
Kingston, Rhode Island

INTRODUCTION

Toxic exposure to many environmental and occupational hazards is monitored by analysis of the compound or its metabolites in blood or urine. This is also true for toxic metals and metal levels in body fluids are routinely used for monitoring exposure. However, in the case of cadmium there is no agreement on the value of blood cadmium measurements for monitoring the exposure. The reason is that cadmium is rapidly cleared from the blood by liver, kidney and other tissues. There it is sequestered by metallothionein (MT) and, in humans, retained with a half-life of 30 or more years. Thus, blood cadmium, which is apparently not in equilibrium with the tissue cadmium, is considered more a reflection of recent exposure rather than cumulative exposure. Urine cadmium, on the other hand, is generally agreed upon as a better indicator of body burden. An important drawback, however, is that both blood and urine are prone to external contamination during collection.

In clinical practice, ferritin, which is an intracellular protein, is quantitated in serum as a measure of iron status. Like ferritin, MT is also an intracellular protein. Because of this analogy, we wanted to test the hypothesis that, MT concentration in serum, or plasma, may be related to the body burden of cadmium. We were able to demonstrate that in both plasma and urine of rats, given multiple injections of $CdCl_2$, cadmium was associated with MT (Shaikh and Hirayama, 1979). However, determination of MT concentration was not possible because a specific immunological method to quantitate nanogram quantities of MT was not yet available (Tohyama and Shaikh, 1978). In subsequent years, a radioimmunoassay was developed (Tohyama and Shaikh, 1981) and used to measure MT in plasma and urine of cadmium-exposed rats (Tohyama and Shaikh, 1981). We soon realized that MT is better determined in urine because, due to its low molecular weight, its residence time in plasma is rather short, keeping its concentration in this compartment very low. As a result, the studies that followed concentrated on the determination of MT in urine of experimental animals and exposed human populations. This paper is a review of some of the recent findings from this laboratory.

STUDIES IN RATS

Earlier subchronic studies in rats, injected with cadmium on a daily basis for several weeks, showed that MT levels in urine of animals who had not yet developed severe renal dysfunction were reflective of the body burden, i.e., liver and kidney cadmium levels (Tohyama et al., 1981b; Lee et al., 1983). However, since most human exposure to cadmium occurs on a chronic basis, a collaborative study with Huang and Perlin was performed in which rats were put on drinking water-containing $CdCl_2$ from the time of weaning to about two years of age. Cadmium concentration in the drinking water was maintained at 0, 5, or 50 mg/l. Results of urinary MT determinations, which are described in detail elsewhere (Shaikh et al., 1989), are summarized in Figure 1. The mean control MT values ranged between 41 and 180 μg/l and did not change significantly with age. The overall group mean for the control animals was 87 μg/l. In cadmium exposed animals, the excretion of MT correlated significantly with the duration of exposure in both the 5 and 50 mg/l groups. Because of taste aversion due to cadmium, the animals in the high dose group drank significantly less water than the low dose and the control groups. As a consequence, the average weekly cadmium intake in the high dose group was approximately 8-, rather than 10-times the low dose group. The urinary MT levels were proportional to the relative cadmium intake and hence presumably also the body burden.

STUDIES IN JAPANESE POPULATIONS

For a number of years we have collaborated with Nogawa et al. on studies in environmentally exposed populations in Japan, including the Itai-

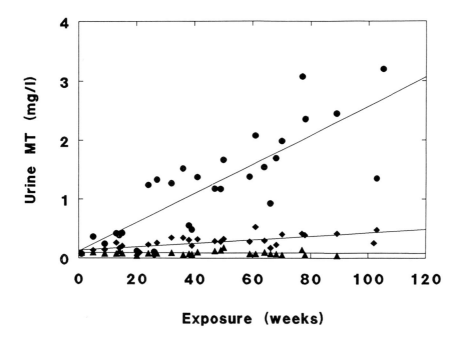

Exposure (weeks)

Figure 1. Urinary MT levels of control rats and rats maintained on drinking water containing CdCl$_2$. Urine specimens were frozen at $-20°C$ until analyzed for MT by radioimmunoassay. MT concentration was plotted against the duration of exposure and linear regression analysis was performed. Group means at each sampling time are plotted for rats maintained on distilled water (▲), 5 mgCd/l (◆), and 50 mgCd/l (●). Group mean ± S.D. for the controls was 87 ± 3 μg/l and the slope was not significantly different from zero. Regression equations for the exposed groups are: 5 mgCd/l group, Y = 2.93X + 113, r = 0.68 (*p* <0.001); 50 mgCd/l group, Y = 24.6X + 117, r = 0.82 (*p* <0.001). (Redrawn from Shaikh et al., 1989).

Itai disease patients (Tohyama et al., 1981a, 1982; Shaikh and Tohyama, 1984; Shaikh et al., 1990b; Kido et al., 1991a, b). The purpose of these studies was to evaluate the relationship of MT excretion in urine as a measure of chronic environmental cadmium exposure. Results of a recent study (Shaikh et al., 1990b), shown in Figure 2, depict the relationship of urinary MT with urinary cadmium in women living in the Kakehashi River basin—a cadmium-polluted area. As mentioned earlier, urinary cadmium level is considered an indicator of body burden. A significant correlation between cadmium and MT suggests that under chronic environmental exposure urinary MT levels must also be reflective of the cadmium body burden.

For the purpose of further evaluation, the study population was divided into control and cadmium-exposed groups based on the history of consumption of cadmium-contaminated rice. The 97.5% upper limit for the control population was determined to be 693 μg MT/g creatinine. Using this as the cut-off level, the MT data for the exposed population was evaluated for the prevalence of metallothioneinuria. These results are shown in Figure 3. It is evident that women who lived in the polluted area and also consumed cadmium-contaminated rice for about 40 years had an increased incidence of metallothioneinuria. The prevalence rates compare well to those of β_2-microglobulinuria in this population (Ishizaki et al., 1989). β_2-microglobulin is a commonly used indicator of renal tubular dysfunction. However, MT is more specific for cadmium exposure and, unlike β_2-microglobulin, its level in urine is not influenced by age of the individual. Thus, from this study, we can deduce that MT in urine is not only a measure of cumulative cadmium exposure, but perhaps also of renal tubular dysfunction due to prolonged exposure.

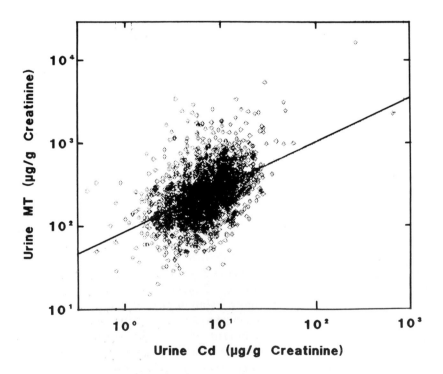

Figure 2. The relationship of urinary MT and cadmium in Japanese women living in the Kakehashi river basin. A total of 1880 individuals, 50 to 90 years of age, participated in this study and provided a sample of morning urine. Linear regression on log-transformed data was performed. The regression equation is: log $Y = 0.53$ log $X + 1.96$, r = 0.46 (p <0.001). (Replotted from Shaikh et al., 1990b).

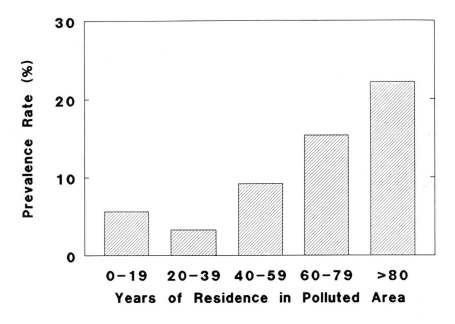

Figure 3. The prevalence of metallothioneinuria in Japanese women environmentally exposed to cadmium. The group consisted of 523 women from the Kakehashi river basin who consumed cadmium-contaminated rice on a chronic basis. Years of residence in this case implies years of exposure. The subjects were divided into five subgroups, based upon the duration of residence in the polluted area. (Adapted from Shaikh et al., 1990b).

STUDIES IN SMELTER WORKERS

We have conducted a total of three studies on workers at a cadmium smelter in the U.S. (Tohyama et al., 1981b; Shaikh et al., 1987, 1990a). As in the Japanese studies, we found that the excretion of MT in urine in this population was also directly proportional to the duration of exposure, i.e., employment at the smelter (Shaikh et al., 1987).

Two of the above-mentioned studies (Tohyama et al., 1981b; Shaikh et al., 1990a) were the result of collaboration with Ellis et al. They determined liver and left kidney cadmium levels by *in vivo* neutron activation (Ellis et al., 1980, 1981, 1984). We analyzed urinary MT concentration and compared the results with the tissue cadmium levels. As shown in Figure 4, the log of renal cadmium content correlated significantly with the log of MT concentration in urine. A similar logarithmic association was noted between hepatic cadmium and urinary MT (Figure 5). Whereas, a strong positive correlation ($p < 0.001$) exists between urinary cadmium and MT in the Japanese population, in the occupationally exposed group the correlation was not as strong ($p = 0.03$). The reason appears to be external contami-

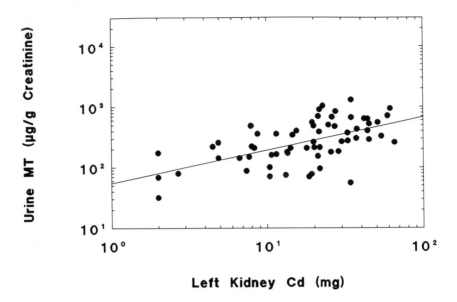

Figure 4. The relationship between urinary MT and renal cadmium in smelter workers. Spot urine samples from 68 active and retired workers were analyzed for MT. Cadmium content in left kidney was determined by *in vivo* neutron activation. Four individuals with severe renal dysfunction (data not shown) were excluded from correlation analysis. Linear regression was performed on log-transformed data. Regression equation is: $\log Y = 0.55 \log X + 1.74$; $r = 0.58$ ($p < 0.001$). (Adapted from Shaikh et al., 1990a).

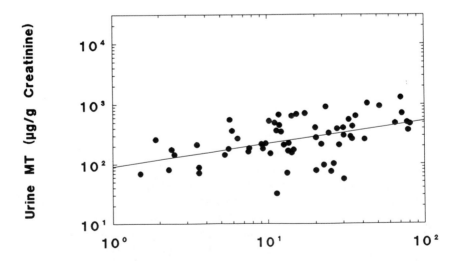

Figure 5. The relationship between urinary MT and hepatic cadmium in smelter workers. See Figure 4 for details. Regression equation is: $\log Y = 0.39 \log X + 1.96$; $r = 0.47$ ($p < 0.001$). (Adapted from Shaikh et al., 1990a).

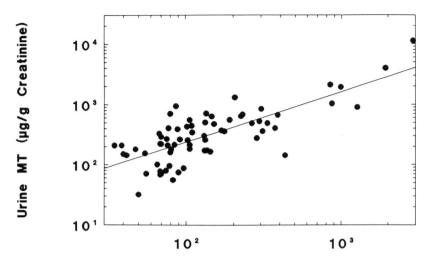

Urine Protein (mg/g Creatinine)

Figure 6. The relationship between urinary MT and protein in smelter workers. All 68 workers are included in correlation analysis. Linear regression was performed on log-transformed data. Regression equation is: $\log Y = 0.83 \log X + 0.70$; $r = 0.76$ ($p < 0.001$). (Adapted from Shaikh et al., 1990a).

nation during sample collection. Thus, in the occupational setting, due to the threat of external contamination, urinary cadmium is less reliable an indicator of individual exposure. Nevertheless, it is of value on a group basis.

Protein excretion in urine is regarded as one of the measures of renal function. It was of interest to see if urinary MT was merely an indicator of tissue cadmium levels or was also related to urinary protein excretion in exposed workers. Correlation analysis showed that indeed, not only in individuals with normal renal function (i.e., urinary protein concentration of less than 250 μg/g creatinine and β_2-microglobulin concentration of less than 500 μg/g creatinine) but also in individuals with renal dysfunction, MT was related significantly to the total protein (Figure 6). Due to its low molecular weight, MT is efficiently filtered by the kidney. While most of it is reabsorbed, a certain fraction is excreted. In the case of renal tubular dysfunction less MT, and also total filtered protein, is reabsorbed. Furthermore, there is release of MT from the proximal renal tubules due to necrosis of the epithelial cells by cadmium. There is an attractive possibility that MT can be used as a more specific indicator of cadmium-induced renal dysfunction. This conclusion is in agreement with the observations in the Japanese population where the incidence of metallothioneinuria increased with the duration of exposure (Figure 3) and the occurrence of Itai-Itai disease (Tohyama et al., 1981a).

CONCLUSIONS

Based on our data from experimental animals, an environmentally exposed Japanese population and occupationally exposed workers, summarized here, we conclude that the assay of MT in urine can be a useful addition to the battery of tests that are performed to monitor cadmium exposure and its resultant effects on the kidney. Further work is needed to determine the MT concentration associated with the onset of renal dysfunction.

ACKNOWLEDGMENTS

Studies discussed in this paper were carried out in my laboratory with the help of C. Tohyama, H. Kito, T. Kido, C. Nolan, and K. Harnett. These studies were made possible with the collaboration of K. Nogawa, K. Ellis, and P.C. Huang. This work was supported in part by U.S. Public Health Service Grant No. ESO3187.

REFERENCES

Ellis KJ, Morgan WD, Zanzi I, Yasumura S, Vartsky D, and Cohn S (1980): *In vivo* measurement of critical levels of kidney cadmium: dose-effect studies in cadmium smelter workers. *Am. J. Ind. Med.* 1: 339.

Ellis KJ, Morgan WD, Zanzi I, Yasumura S, Vartsky D, and Cohn S (1981): Critical concentrations of cadmium in human renal cortex: dose-effect studies in cadmium smelter workers. *J. Toxicol. Environ. Health* 7: 691.

Ellis KJ, Yuen K, Yasumura S, and Cohn SH (1984): Dose-response analysis of cadmium in man: body burden vs. kidney dysfunction. *Environ. Res.* 33: 216.

Ishizaki M, Kido T, Honda R, Tsuritani I, Yamada Y, Nakagawa H, and Nogawa K (1989): Dose-response relationship between urinary cadmium and β_2-microglobulin in a Japanese environmentally cadmium exposed population. *Toxicology* 58: 121.

Kido T, Shaikh ZA, Kito H, Honda R, and Nogawa K (1991a): Dose-response relationship between urinary cadmium and metallothionein in a Japanese population environmentally exposed to cadmium. *Toxicology* 65:325.

Kido T, Shaikh ZA, Kito H, Honda R, and Nogawa K (1991b): Dose-response relationship between dietary cadmium intake and metallothioneinuria in a population from a cadmium-polluted area of Japan. *Toxicology* 66:271.

Lee YH, Shaikh ZA, and Tohyama C (1983): Urinary metallothionein and tissue metal levels of rats injected with cadmium, mercury, lead, copper, or zinc. *Toxicology* 27: 337.

Shaikh ZA and Hirayama K (1979): Metallothionein in the extracellular fluids as an index of cadmium toxicity. *Environ. Health Perspect.* 28: 267.

Shaikh ZA and Tohyama C (1984): Urinary metallothionein as an indicator of cadmium body burden and of cadmium-induced nephrotoxicity. *Environ. Health Perspect.* 54: 171.

Shaikh ZA, Tohyama C, and Nolan CV (1987): Occupational exposure to cadmium: effect on metallothionein and other biological indices of exposure and renal function. *Arch. Toxicol.* 59: 360.

Shaikh ZA, Harnett KM, Perlin SA, and Huang PC (1989): Chronic cadmium intake results in dose-related excretion of metallothionein in urine. *Experientia* 45: 146.

Shaikh ZA, Ellis KJ, Subramanian KS, and Greenberg A (1990a): Biological monitoring for occupational exposure: the urinary metallothionein. *Toxicology* 63:53.

Shaikh ZA, Kido T, Kito H, Honda R, and Nogawa K (1990b): Prevalence of metallothioneinuria among the population living in the Kakehashi River basin Japan—an epidemiological study. *Toxicology* 64:59.

Tohyama C and Shaikh ZA (1978): Cross-reactivity of metallothioneins from different origins with rabbit anti-rat hepatic metallothionein antibody. *Biochem. Biophys. Res. Commun.* 84: 907.

Tohyama C and Shaikh ZA (1981): Metallothionein in plamsa and urine of cadmium-exposed rats determined by a single antibody radioimmunoassay. *Fund. Appl. Toxicol.* 1: 1.

Tohyama C, Shaikh ZA, Nogawa K, Kobayashi E, and Honda R (1981a): Elevated urinary excretion of metallothionein due to environmental cadmium exposure. *Toxicology* 20: 289.

Tohyama C, Shaikh ZA, Ellis KJ, and Cohn SH (1981b): Metallothionein excretion in urine upon cadmium exposure: its relationship with liver and kidney cadmium. *Toxicology* 22: 181.

Tohyama C, Shaikh ZA, Nogawa K, Kobayashi E, and Honda R (1982): Urinary metallothionein as a new index of renal dysfunction in "Itai-Itai" disease patients and other Japanese women environmentally exposed to cadmium. *Arch. Toxicol.* 50: 159.

Chapter

32

Meeting Synopsis and Future Directions for Metallothionein Research

Michael Webb*
10 Lagham Park, South Godstone
Surrey, England

The title of this Chapter *Meeting Synopsis and Future Directions for MT Research* is not my choice but, very kindly, has been given to me by the organizers of this meeting, Drs. Klaassen and Suzuki. Although there is a subtle difference between "future directions for research" and "directions for future research," I know and you know that dedicated scientists do not "take kindly" to anyone who has the temerity either to tell them what to do, or how to do it. Also the production of a synopsis is an unenviable occupation, practically guaranteed to gain the disfavor of one or more of the participants. Clearly, therefore, my task demands extreme diplomacy. My approach to it has been, first, to use the Proceedings of the last MT meeting in Zurich as the "most comprehensive statement of the art" at that time and to determine from them what were the outstanding questions in 1985, particularly with regard to the biological functions of these metalloproteins. Secondly, to learn from the contributions to this meeting how many of these questions have been answered during the last four years and, also, what additional questions have been raised. In this way topics for research were identified which, at least would appeal to me if I still had a laboratory and enough hands to do the work. Some of these topics, together with

Previous address: Medical Research Council Laboratories, Woodmansterne Road, Carshalton
Surrey, England

assessments of the evidence that led to them, form the major part of this Chapter. With this plan of campaign it was not possible to give a separate summary that covered all of the communications to this meeting, as this involved too much repetition. Instead, I have separated the contributions, with one exception, into appropriate groups, made mini-synopses of each group, and incorporated these into the relevant sections of my discussion. I have not obeyed in full, therefore, the dictates of the bosses. As, however, the proceedings of the meeting are to be published in full, the absence of an undoubtedly biased rehash of the papers probably does not matter greatly.

The one paper, the exception mentioned above, that does not fit into this scheme was the most impressive presentation by N. Imura et al.* which, on its merits alone, seems to deserve specific mention. Based on the observations that (1) Bi is a potent inducer of MT in the kidneys and bone marrow of experimental animals, but not in tumor tissue (Piotrowski et al., 1979; Imura et al., 1987) and (2) the nephrotoxic metabolite of *cis*-diamminedichloroplatinum, which is a dose-limiting factor in the use of the drug in the treatment of various human tumors (Bakka et al., 1981; Imura et al., 1987), N. Imura et al. have established by clinical trials that pretreatment with Bi reduces the side effects of the anticancer drug in man. Additional studies, as yet limited to mice, show that Bi pretreatment also protects against the lethal effect and bone marrow injury caused by gamma-irradiation. At present, little seems to be known about the fate of MT-bound-Pt in the kidneys of either human-beings or laboratory animals. Clearly, this needs to be investigated since, if Pt is retained, it is possible that, as in animals chronically exposed to Cd, renal damage may yet occur if the metal concentration rises above a critical level.

To plagiarize and modify, with apologies, remarks that I believe can be attributed to Enrico Fermi, "before I came to this meeting my thoughts on the functions of MT were confused. After listening to your presentations, my thoughts are still confused, but on a higher plane." Indeed, even now I am uncertain whether too much attention has been given to the metals in MT. Maybe thionein is the functional molecule. If this is so and the *metallo*thioneins are the end-products, the marked lack of discrimination in metal-binding properties of MTs, which has always been difficult to reconcile with any metal-specific function, is easier to understand. In 1985, MTs were known to be induced in response to stress and treatment with certain hormones, in addition to such metals as Zn, Cd, Cu, Hg, and Bi. Possible functions of the inducible metalloprotein were considered to include the control of the absorption, transport, storage, transfer, excretion, and detoxification of specific metals, as well as protection against various xenobiotics,

---

*Reference to papers that were presented at this meeting are given in this form since, at the time of preparation of this manuscript, the proceedings had not been paginated.

irradiation, and free radicals (see e.g., Bremner, 1987). Clearly, ideas on either induction, or function have not changed greatly over the last 4 years. Thus, of the 31 research papers presented at this meeting, 12 have dealt with either the induction of MT by emotional, sensory, and physiological stresses (C. Tohyama et al.; Y. Kojima and T. Niioka; K. Arizono et al.), (2) inflammatory agents, which include the metals Cr(III) and Fe(III) when administered i.p. (C.C. McCormick and J.C. Fleet), (3) other metallic ions, which do (K.T. Suzuki et al.), or do not (e.g Ca(II) and Sr(II); T. Maitani et al.) bind to MT, (4) organic compounds (solvents, hepatotoxins, endotoxin, indomethacin etc. (S. Onosaka and K. Tanaka; T. Maitani et al.), or the function of the Zn-metalloprotein in (a) protection against tissue damage by free radicals (A. Naganuma et al., M. Sato), (b) atherogenesis (K. Nakajima et al.) and (c) gastric mucosal lesions (K. Tsujikawa et al.). At least some of these so-called functions, either proposed, or implied in these and earlier studies, however, may well be coincidental, or secondary to alterations in metal distribution, which also may result from stress and/or hormonal changes (see also Cousins and Coppen, 1987; Koropatnick et al., 1989). Thus, as described by M. Sato, the induction of ZnMT in the livers of paraquat-dosed rats is accompanied by, but is not correlated with lipid peroxidation. At the cellular level, ionic Zn, chelated Zn and ZnMT have similar activities in the reduction of free radical formation (Cousins and Coppen, 1987). Also by analogy with dihydrolipoic acid, the oxidation of which is promoted by chelation with Cu (or Co), but prevented by chelation with Zn or Cd (Webb, 1962), CuMT and the apoprotein, thionein, might be expected to give better protection against oxidative free radicals than the ubiquitous ZnMT.

In 1985, it seemed established that MT does function in the transfer of Cd (and probably Zn) from the liver to the kidney. Thus (1) cultures of hepatocytes from the livers of normal and Cd-dosed rats secrete ZnMT and CdMT, respectively, into the medium (Thomas et al., 1987; Lloyd, 1989). (2) With the development of radioimmunoassay methods, MT has been detected at low concentrations in the plasma of normal animals and, at higher concentrations, in the plasma of animals with elevated tissue levels of MT (Bremner et al., 1987). (3) Binding sites with appreciable specificity for MT are present in the brush border membranes of rabbit kidney proximal tubules (Selenke and Foulkes, 1981). At the present meeting, further evidence for the involvement of MT in this process and in the induction of calcuria associated with the renal damage, caused by the kidney uptake of excess CdMT was presented by E.C. Foulkes and by B.A. Fowler et al. In addition the discussions that followed these and other papers, in which MT concentrations in blood and urine were measured by radioimmunological methods (I. Bremner; J.S. Garvey; Z. Shaikh) several speakers questioned whether MT in extracellular fluids and, in particular, plasma was the same at the endogenous MT of the liver. Such thoughts raise the question whether immunoprecipitation, or immunoadsorbent methods could be devised to determine if MT in plasma is glycosylated. Indeed, as at least one antibody, reactive with MT-1 and MT-2 from various sources, recognizes the epitope located within the amino-terminal heptapeptide (Kikuchi et al., 1988), such methods might be useful in studies on the kinetics of thionein synthesis, the stabilization of the nascent protein and the structurally specific binding of the metallic ions.

With the development and, as illustrated by J.S. Garvey's paper, refinement of immunohistochemical methods for the detection of minute amounts of MT in tissue sections, histopathological studies on human diseases of disordered Cu and Zn metabolism have become very popular (see e.g., Elmes, 1987; Elmes et al., 1989; Nartey et al., 1987; Janssens et al., 1982). There seems to be no sound evidence, however, that the accumulation of either CuMT, or ZnMT in these pathological states is anything more than a response to excessive tissue concentrations of these metallic ions. The elegant studies of Leone and Hamer (1987) on the abnormal Cu metabolism and regulation of gene expression in cultures of fibroblasts from the skin of Menkes' patients, for example, indicates that the mutation is likely to affect a factor, functional at an early stage in the normal regulatory pathway of Cu metabolism. The absence of this factor, which is considered to function in the synthesis of Cu-enzymes, increases the intracellular concentration of reactive Cu. Because of this, induction of MT in the cultured fibroblasts occurs at external Cu concentrations much lower than normal.

As antibodies to MT identify the protein, but not the bound metals, the method, developed and described by K.H. Summer et al., for the quantitative determination of CuMTs, which is applicable to biopsy samples of even extra-hepatic tissues, provides a new and extremely valuable analytical technique. Already it has been shown by this method that, unexpectedly, the Cu saturation levels in the hepatic MTs of patients with Wilson's disease and Indian childhood cirrhosis differ by a factor of two.

Immunohistochemical methods were used in studies by M. Karasawa et al. on the role of MT in growth, differentiation and carcinogenesis in mouse skin and by C. Tohyama and colleagues on the localization of MT in the reproductive organs of the rat. The latter authors presented extremely interesting and significant new data, which reopen the question of the involvement of ZnMT in cell proliferation and differentiation. Their results establish the presence of the metalloprotein in the glandular epithelium of the uterus, in the ovum, and in certain cells of the corpus leuteum of the female and in the spermatogenic cells, sperm and Sertoli cells of the testis, as well as in cells of the prostate, coagulating glands, seminal vesicles, and ejaculatory duct in the male. Whilst the question "What is the function of all this MT?" remains unanswered at present, the implications of the finding that seminiferous tubules with mature sperm show weak staining for MT, whereas tubules without sperm stain intensely, are obvious. With regard to the apparent involvement of MT in reproduction, it is interesting that De et al. (1989) believe that the metalloprotein functions in the establishment and maintenance of normal pregnancy in the mouse since, from the time of implantation, the embryo is surrounded by cells, which are located between the maternal and embryonic environments and actively express the MT genes.

No doubt the ability to synthesize MT is a good thing for the living organism but, clearly, it is not essential for either cellular growth, or development. Thymoma and CHO cells, in which the MT genes are transcriptionally inactive, for example, are extremely susceptible to Cd toxicity, but thrive and multiply in the normal culture media (Compere and Palmiter, 1981; Hildebrand et al., 1979). Also Hamer and colleagues (Thiele et al., 1987) have shown that, in *Saccharomyces cerevisiae,* CuMT is unessential for growth in media with adequate trace levels of Cu, but its synthesis is essential to prevent Cu-toxicity. M. Karin, in his paper, also mentioned that yeast mutants, which fail to express the CuMT gene, are very susceptible to the toxic effects of Cu. Moreover, the molecular biologists have shown conclusively that Cd-resistance which, usually, is associated with MT gene-amplification, also can be conferred by transfer of MT genes on a self-replicating plasmid (see e.g., Palmiter, 1987; Grady ct al., 1987; Durnam and Palmiter, 1987). Nevertheless, it seems unwise to assume that MT is the only factor responsible for either resistance to, or detoxification of Cd. The studies by Huang et al. (1987), Grady et al. (1987), Enger et al. (1983), Petering et al. (1987) and Suzuki and Cherian (1989) all indicate that Cd-tolerance in either the whole animal, or in cultured mammalian cells, may involve more than the detoxification capacity of MT. Also, as shown by the paper by M.P. Waalkes and colleagues, the induced resistance to Cd-carcinogenicity in the mouse testis is unlikely to be due to MT.

With regard to the proposed function of MT in essential metal homeostasis, the demonstration by Thiele et al. (1987) that MT protects against the adverse effects of too much Cu in yeast, seems to provide good evidence that the protein, thionein, acts in the detoxification of ''hyper-physiological'' concentrations of this essential, but potentially toxic cation. It seems to be accepted that, as discussed by D. Hamer et al. at the present meeting, the induction of MT gene transcription in *S. cerevisiae* provides a simple, genetically accessible model system. Nevertheless, it should not be forgotten that, in contrast with mammalian cells and organs, the induction of MT in *S. cerevisiae* (M. Karin et al.), as in *Candida glabrata* (R.K. Mehra and D.R. Winge), is transcriptionally regulated only by Cu(I) and Ag(I). Also if MT has a function in the control of Cu metabolism in mammalian cells, does it function also to detoxify excess Zn? At the Zurich meeting Vallee (1987) stated ''Zn is one of the least toxic of all the 1st transitional and

Group IIB elements and, because of this, the detoxification hypothesis is quite implausible, at least for Zn.'' Maybe though, Zn only appears to have little toxicity because all toxicity studies have been done on living systems, which have the common ability to synthesize MT. It might be worthwhile, therefore, to determine whether Zn is much more toxic to those cells in which the MT genes are non-functional, particularly as a Cd-resistant mouse hepatoma cell line, in which the MT gene has been amplified some 30-fold, is known to exhibit increased resistance to Zn (Durnam and Palmiter, 1987).

Possibly because the subject of the meeting focused attention on ''what MT does,'' rather than ''how it does it,'' little was said in either the communications, or the discussions about the structure of the metalloprotein in relation to its functions. It is well known, for example, that most mammalian MTs are mixtures of at least two isometallothioneins of different charge which, themselves, may be microheterogeneous and resolvable into further sub-forms that differ marginally in amino acid composition (Kissling and Kagi, 1979; Hunziker and Kagi, 1987). The production of multiple isoforms can be explained by the presence of multiple genes in the genome (Karin et al., 1987), but the question whether there is a biological need for them has never been answered. From the paper by C.D. Klaassen et al., it is apparent that different inducers differentially induce MT-1 and MT-2, but the patterns of induction are different in rats and mice. If, however, the functions of the isoforms are the same, the species difference in response may be interesting, but not significant. From the paper by G.K. Andrews, for example, it is apparent that, in various species of birds (turkeys, chickens, quail, and pheasants) which have only one MT-gene, all functions of MT must be accompanied by a single (metallo)-protein.

The more recent chemical studies on the structure of the MT molecule are fascinating but, in relation to the understanding of the biological functions of the metalloprotein, only add further problems. Why, for example, does Nature require the molecule to be a dumb-bell-shaped structure with a central hinge, the metal-thiolate complexes being organized into two clusters (A and B), which differ in binding affinities for specific metallic ions, in the carboxy-terminal (α) and amino-terminal (β) domains, respectively? The intriguing and comprehensive studies with genetically engineered mutant MTs, which were reported by P.C. Huang, indicate that both the composition and configuration of native MT are the most favorable for metal binding, stability and functionality. Kagi and Kojima's (1987) view that ''the presence of the two-fold pseudosymmetry and the hinged dumb-bell shaped structure suggest the participation of MT in some so far unsuspected regulatory function'' may be correct, but it is not particularly helpful in the understanding of molecular functions. It seems unlikely that, in the micro environment of the cell, MT delivers Cu from one domain and Zn from the other to separate functional sites as required, just as in the macro world a waiter with a bottle in either hand serves the appropriate wine in response to the answer to his question "would you prefer red, or white sir?". The dual metal-donor function would be aesthetically more acceptable if MT was a precursor molecule which, after cleavage at the proteinase-sensitive hinge, yielded the α and β domains as separate functional entities. Unfortunately, however, we all know that this idea is nonsense and without any supportive experimental evidence whatsoever. J.H.R. Kagi, in his paper on the solution structure of mammalian metallothioneins, showed that the cluster organizations in rat, rabbit and human MTs are identical, the common structure being determined by the conserved arrangement of the 20 cysteine residues in the peptide chains. In each domain the appropriate portion of this chain is wrapped helically around a metal-thiolate cluster. This arrangement, which is illustrated dramatically by molecular models, is difficult to reconcile with biochemical evidence on the rates of turnover of the metal and protein moieties. Thus, in Ehrlich cells with a restricted supply of exogenous Zn, the rate of loss of Zn from the endogenous MT is about three times greater than the rate of biodegradation of the protein (Petering et al., 1987). Also, whilst Gallant and Cherian (1987) find the rate of degradation of hepatic ZnMT to be more rapid in Zn-deficient than in Zn-replete newborn rats, the interesting and impressive study, reported by M. Dunn, establishes that Zn in hepatic MT (i) exchanges with other ligands in the liver and (ii) turns over rapidly, the $t_{1/2}$ being about 14 min. Clearly, more information is needed about the mechanisms of removal of the bound metals from MT and the kinetics of the biodegradation of the (metallo)protein. Such information could be relevant to (1) the work of C.D. Klaassen et al. on the biological half-times of MT-1 and MT-2 in normal, newborn Zn-dosed and Cd-dosed rats, (2) the possibility, suggested by M.G. Cherian that MT has a cysteine-storage function in newborn rats and (3) the accumulation of excessive amounts of CuMT, particularly in the liver, in certain human and animal diseases. In patients with Wilson's disease, for example, as in Bedlington terriers with an inherited defect, Cu accumulates largely as CuMT in the livers. This MT is taken up by lysosomes, uptake either being accompanied, or preceded by the polymerization of the metalloprotein. Both the monomeric CuMT and the polymer, which is considered to be identical with mitochondrocuprein and the Cu-associated protein of the histologists (see Elmes et al., 1989), seem to be extremely resistant to degradation. This resistance contrasts with the short biological half-time of the CuMT that is induced in the normal animal by the appropriate dose of Cu (Bremner et al., 1978). Whilst the reason for this difference has not been established, it may be significant that both MT-1 and MT-2 from livers of patients with Wilson's disease contain 11 to 12 g atoms Cu and 2 to 3 g atoms Zn/mole, whereas the more usually encountered (Cu-Zn)MTs seem to contain appreciably lower Cu/Zn ratios (Bremner, 1979).

It is known that the addition of Cu(I) to hepatic ZnMT *in vitro* results in the formation of $Cu_{12}MT$ (Winge, 1987), or three distinct species with stoichiometries of Cu_6MT, $Cu_{12}MT$ and $Cu_{20}MT$ (Stillman et al., 1987). It might be an interesting exercise to see what happens to these CuMTs when administered parenterally to experimental animals. If, under such conditions, the Cu-proteins are taken up by the kidneys in the same way as CdMT, maybe more information would be forthcoming about the effect of Cu content on lysosomal degradation.

In conclusion I have two further comments. Firstly, it is obvious that Vallee's statement at the Zurich meeting "MT was invented solely for Jerry Kagi to hold meetings in Switzerland, so that all of us could come to enjoy them, him, alps and all," was erroneous. Whilst we have Jerry Kagi, but not the alps with us on this occasion, it is clear that MT was not invented solely for him. Maybe Vallee's statement should be updated to read "MT was invented for Kagi, Klaassen, and Suzuki to hold meetings in Switzerland, Hawaii and, hopefully, other delightful places that are conducive to speculation. . . ." Secondly, as this is the last formal paper, may I thank firstly Drs. Klaassen and Suzuki, on behalf of all of us, for their efforts in organizing this enjoyable and productive meeting and, secondly, all of those people who, behind the scenes, have contributed so much to its success.

REFERENCES

Bakka A, Edresen L, Johnsen ABS, Edminson PD, and Rugstad HE (1981): Resistance against *cis*-dichlorodiammineplatinum in cultured cells with a high content of metallothionein. *Toxicol. Appl. Pharmacol.* 61: 215.

Bremner I (1979): Factors influencing the concentration of copper-thionein in tissues. In, *Metallothionein*. Kagi JHR and Nordberg M, Eds., Birkhäuser-Verlag, Basel, pp. 273–280.

Bremner I (1987): Nutritional and physiological significance of metallothionein. In, *Experientia Suppl. 52 (Metallothionein II)* Kagi JHR and Norberg, M, Eds., Birkhäuser-Verlag, Basel, pp. 81–107.

Bremner I, Mehra RK, and Sato M (1987): Metallothionein in blood, bile and urine. In, *Experientia Suppl. 52 (Metallothionein II)* Kagi JHR and Nordberg M, Eds., Birkhäuser-Verlag, Basel, pp. 507–517.

Compere SJ and Palmiter RD (1981): DNA methylation controls inducibility of the mouse metallothionein-I gene in lymphoid cells. *Cell* 25: 233.

Cousins RJ and Coppen DE (1987): Regulation of liver zinc metabolism and metallothionein by cAMP, glucagon and glucocorticoids and suppression of free radical formation by zinc. In, *Experientia Suppl. 52 (Metallothionein-II)* Kagi JHR and Nordberg M, Eds., Birkhäuser-Verlag, Basel, pp. 545–553.

De SK, McMaster MT, Dey SK, and Andrews GK (1989): Cell-specific metallothionein gene expression in mouse decidua and placentae. *Development* 107: 611.

Elmes ME, Clarkson JP, and Jasani B (1987): Histological demonstration of immunoreactive metallothionein in rat and human tissues. In, *Experientia Suppl. 52 Metallothionein-II)* Kagi JHR and Nordberg M, Eds., Birkhäuser-Verlag, Basel, pp. 533–537.

Elmes ME, Clarkson JP, Mahy NJ, and Jasani B (1989): Metallothionein and copper in liver disease with copper retention—histopathological study. *J. Pathol.* 158: 131.

Enger MD, Hildebrand CE, and Stewart CC (1983): Cd^{2+} responses of cultured human blood cells. *Toxicol. Appl. Pharmacol.* 64: 219.

Gallant KR and Cherian MG (1987): Changes in dietary zinc result in specific alterations of metallothionein concentrations in newborn rat liver. *J. Nutr.* 117: 709.

Grady DL, Moyzis RK, and Hilderbrand CE (1987): Molecular and cellular mechanisms of cadmium resistance in cultured cells. In, *Experientia Suppl. 52 Metallothionein-II)* Kagi JHR and Nordberg M, Eds., Birkhäuser-Verlag, Basel, pp. 447–456.

Hildebrand CE, Tobey RA, Campbell EW, and Enger MD (1979): A cadmium resistant variant of the Chinese hamster (CHO) cell with increased metallothionein induction capacity. *Exptl. Cell Res.* 124: 237.

Hunziker PE and Kagi JHR (1987): Human hepatic metallothioneins: resolution of six isoforms. In, *Experientia Suppl. 52 (Metallothionein-II)* Kagi JHR and Nordberg M, Eds., Birkhäuser-Verlag, Basel, pp. 257–264.

Imura N, Naganuma A, Satoh M, and Koyama Y (1987): Induction of renal metallothionein allows increasing dose of an extensively used anti-tumor drug *cis*-diamminedichloroplatinum. In, *Experientia Suppl. 52 (Metallothionein-II)* Kagi JHR and Nordberg M, Eds., Birkhäuser-Verlag, Basel, pp. 655–660.

Janssens AR, Van Den Hamer CJA, van Noord MJ, and Bosman F (1982): Copper and copper associated proteins in primary biliary cirrhosis. *Liver (Copenhagen)* 2: 318.

Kägi JHR and Kojima Y (1987): Chemistry and biochemistry of metallothionein. In, *Experientia Suppl. 52 (Metallothionein-II)* Kagi JHR and Nordberg M, Eds., Birkhäuser-Verlag, Basel, pp. 25–61.

Karin M, Haslinger A, Hegery A, Dietlin T, and Imbra R (1987): Transcriptional control mechanism which regulates the expression of human metallothionein genes. In, *Experientia Suppl. 52 (Metallothionein-II)* Kagi JHR and Nordberg M, Eds., Birkhäuser-Verlag, Basel, pp. 401–415.

Kikuchi Y, Wada N, Irie M, Ikebuchi H, Sawada J-I, Terao T, Nakayama S, Iguchi S, and Okada Y (1988): A murine monoclonal anti-metallothionein autoantibody recognizes a chemically synthesized amino-terminal heptapeptide common to various animal metallothioneins. *Molec. Immunol.* 25: 1033.

Kissling MM and Kägi JHR (1979): Amino acid sequences of human hepatic metallothionein. In, *Metallothionein.* Kagi JHR and Nordberg M Eds., Birkhäuser-Verlag, Basel, pp. 145–151.

Koropatnick J, Liebbrandt M, and Cherian MG (1989): Organ-specific metallothionein induction in mice by X-irradiation. *Radiat. Res.* 119: 356.

Leone A and Hamer DH (1987): Abnormal copper metabolism and regulation of gene expression in Menkes' disease. In, *Experientia Suppl. 52 (Metallothionein-II)* Kagi JHR and Nordberg M, Eds., Birkhäuser-Verlag, Basel, pp. 477–480.

Lloyd PH (1989): Role of metallothionein in the disposition of cadmium. Ph.D. thesis, University of Surrey, Guildford, England, pp. 1–459.

Nartey NO, Frei JV, and Cherian MG (1987): Hepatic copper and metallothionein distribution in Wilson's disease (hepatolenticular degeneration). *Lab. Invest.* 57: 397.

Petering DH, Krezoski S, Villalobos J, Shaw CF, and Otvos JD (1987): Cadmium-zinc interactions in the Ehrlich cell metallothionein and other sites. In, *Experientia Suppl. 52 (Metallothionein-II)* Kagi JHR and Nordberg M, Eds., Birkhäuser-Verlag, Basel, pp. 573–580.

Piotrowski JK, Szymanska JA, Mogilnicka EM, and Zelazowski AJ (1979): Renal metal binding proteins. In, *Metallothionein.* Kagi JHR and Nordberg M, Eds., Birkhäuser-Verlag, Basel, pp. 363–370.

Selenke W and Foulkes EC (1981): Binding of cadmium-metallothionein to isolated renal brush border membranes. *Proc. Soc. Exp. Biol. Med.* 167: 40.

Stillman MJ, Lau AYC, Cal W, and Zelazowski AJ (1987): Information on metal binding properties of metallothioneins from optical spectroscopy. In, *Experientia Suppl. 52 (Metallothionein-II)* Kagi JHR and Nordberg M, Eds., Birkhäuser-Verlag, Basel, pp. 203–211.

Suzuki CAM and Cherian MG (1989): Renal glutathione depletion and nephrotoxicity of cadmium-metallothionein in rats. *Toxicol. Appl. Pharmacol.* 98: 544.

Thiele DJ, Wright CF, Walling MJ, and Hamer DH (1987): Function and regulation of yeast copper-thionein. In, *Experientia Suppl. 52 (Metallothionein-II)* Kagi JHR and Nordberg M, Eds., Birkhäuser-Verlag, Basel, pp. 423–429.

Thomas DG, Dingman AD, and Garvey JS (1987): The function of metallothionein in cell metabolism. In, *Experientia Suppl. 52 (Metallothionein-II)* Kagi JHR and Nordberg M, Eds., Birkhäuser-Verlag, Basel, pp. 539–543.

Webb M (1962): Biological action of cobalt and other metals. III. Chelation of cations by dihydrolipoic acid. *Biochim. Biophys. Acta* 65: 47.

Winge DR (1987): Copper cooridnation in metallothionein. In, *Experientia Suppl. 52 (Metallothionein-II)* Kagi JHR and Nordberg M, Eds., Birkhäuser-Verlag, Basel, pp. 213–218.

INDEX

C

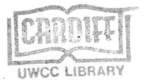